Ear Diseases of the Dog and Cat

Richard G. Harvey
BVSc, PhD, CBiol, FIBiol, DVD, DipECVD, MRCVS
Coventry, UK

Joseph Harari
DVM, MS, DipACVS
Spokane, Washington State, USA

Agnès J. Delauche
DVM, DipACVIM (Neurology), DipECVN, MRCVS
Newmarket, UK

Manson Publishing/The Veterinary Press

Second impression 2002

Copyright © 2001 Manson Publishing Ltd

ISBN 1–84076–003–6

A CIP catalogue record for this book is available from the British Library.

For full details of all Manson Publishing Ltd titles please write to:
Manson Publishing Ltd
73 Corringham Road
London NW11 7DL, UK

Tel: +44(0)20 8905 5150
Fax: +44(0)20 8201 9233

Email: manson@man-pub.demon.co.uk
Website: www.manson-publishing.co.uk

Commissioning editor:	**Jill Northcott**
Project management:	**Paul Bennett**
Text editor:	**Peter Beynon**
Layout:	**Initial Typesetting Services**
Cover design:	**Patrick Daly**
Colour reproduction:	**Tenon & Polert Colour Scanning Ltd, Hong Kong**
Printed by:	**Grafos SA, Barcelona, Spain**

Contents

Preface

Studies of disease prevalence in dogs and cats, particularly those based on hospital admission data, suggest that ear diseases are common. Estimates of the frequency of presentation range from 7.5–16.5% for dogs and 2–6.2% for cats[1–4]. However, although Grono[5] noted a presenting frequency of 4.8% for dogs, in line with other estimates, he also noted that the incidence of otitis externa detected during clinical examination of these dogs rose to between 16% and 25%. Thus, the ability of an owner to detect otitis externa does not appear to be very good. This has implications for treatment since chronic otitis results in permanent stenosis of the lumen and this is an indication for surgery.

The majority of the dogs and cats presented to veterinarians for ear disease will have otitis externa, often as a consequence of an underlying disease[6]. While early reports suggested that there was no sex predisposition for otitis externa, statistical analysis of a very large study[7] detected a significant predisposition in male dogs, although this was unexplained. Peak incidence in dogs occurs between one and four years of age [6]. Male dogs of this age group are likely to be very active and may be at increased risk as a consequence of swimming and from otic foreign bodies. The clinical signs of atopy, a major underlying cause of otitis externa, also exhibit peak incidence in this age group.

It is readily apparent that the investigation and management of ear disease, in its broadest sense, will occupy a significant proportion of a veterinary clinician's time. The concept behind this book is to provide a comprehensive source of information on the structure, function, medicine, and surgery of the ear, from *Otodectes cynotis* infection to acquired conductive deafness.

In order to assist clinicians in the diagnosis and management of ear disease, much of the book is problem oriented in approach. In addition there are clear guides to the use, and limitations, of various diagnostic aids. The practicality of the book has been enhanced by providing information on structure and function, and on the response to insult, without going into needless detail. Detailed notes on surgical techniques, coupled with clear photographic illustrations of the surgical procedures, will assist clinicians in ensuring that pitfalls are avoided. Neurologic investigations of the manifestations of vestibular disease, facial nerve paralysis, and deafness are described and the relevant differential diagnoses discussed. Extensive cross-referencing between chapters will help readers to find additional information under different headings, and the comprehensive reference lists will be of benefit to those who seek further information on this important subject.

We hope that veterinary students and clinicians will find this book a valuable source of reference and will give it the ultimate accolade – that it will become stained and tattered through frequent use.

1 Baxter M and Lawler DC (1972) The incidence and microbiology of otitis externa of dogs and cats in New Zealand. *New Zealand Veterinary Journal* **20**, 29–32.
2 Fraser G (1965) Aetiology of otitis externa in the dog. *Journal of Small Animal Practice* **6**, 445–452.
3 Baba E, Fukata T and Saito M (1981) Incidence of otitis externa in dogs and cats in Japan. *Veterinary Record* **108**, 393–395.
4 McKeever PJ and Globus H (1995) Canine otitis externa. In: *Kirk's Current Veterinary Therapy X11* (ed JD Bonagura). WB Saunders, Philadelphia, pp. 647–655.
5 Grono LR (1969) Studies of the ear mite, *Otodectes cynotis. Veterinary Record* **85**, 6–8.
6 August JR (1988) Otitis externa: a disease of multifactorial etiology. *Veterinary Clinics of North America* **18**, 731–741.
7 Hayes HM, Pickle LW and Wilson GP (1987) Effects of ear type and weather on the prevalence of canine otitis externa. *Research in Veterinary Science* **42**, 294–298.

Acknowledgements

This book could not have been written without the understanding and support of our friends and families. Colleagues who provided clinical illustrations include Jaques Penderis, Masahiko Nagata, Jane Sansom, and Janet Steiss. Simon Orr and Duncan Lascelles provided valuable criticism of the radiology and analgesia sections, respectively. We are indebted to all these colleagues.

The photomicrographs in Chapter 1 (Microscopic structure of the external ear canal) were taken using a Nikon Eclipse E600 microscope, a Nikon Model H3 automatic light meter, and a Nikon FDX 35 camera. The microscope and photographic equipment were generously loaned by Nikon UK Ltd.

The otoscopic pictures in Chapter 2 (Otoscopic appearance of the external ear canal and tympanum) were taken using a Storz 4 mm rigid endoscope, a Ricoh XR–X 3000 camera, and a Storz blitzgenerator 600. The endoscope, camera, and flash generator were generously loaned by Karl Storz Endoscopy UK Ltd.

Fujichrome Sensai II ISO 400 film was used throughout.

Richard Harvey
Joseph Harari
Agnès Delauche

Abbreviations

ATP	adenosine triphosphate
BAEP	brainstem auditory evoked potential
BAER	brainstem auditory evoked response
BAHA	bone-anchored hearing aid
CN	cranial nerve
CSF	cerebrospinal fluid
CT	computed tomography
FeLV	feline leukemia virus
FIP	feline infectious peritonitis
FIV	feline immunodeficiency virus
HCl	hydrochloride
IgE	immunoglobulin E
K^+	potassium ion
MIC	minimal inhibitory concentration
MRI	magnetic resonance imaging
Na^+	sodium ion
p/o	per os (by mouth, orally)
q6h	quaque 6 hora (every 6 hours, four times daily)
q8h	quaque 8 hora (every 8 hours, three times daily)
q12h	quaque 12 hora (every 12 hours, twice daily)
q24h	quaque 24 hora (once daily)
RTA	road traffic accident
SLE	systemic lupus erythematosus
SPL	sound pressure level
T4	thyroxine
TSH	thyroid stimulating hormone

Chapter One

The Normal Ear

GROSS AND MICROSCOPIC ANATOMY OF THE EAR: STRUCTURE AND FUNCTION

KEY POINTS

- The external ear comprises the pinna and the external acoustic meatus. It serves to collect and locate the origin of sound waves.
- The middle ear comprises the tympanic membrane, the ossicles, the auditory tube, and the tympanic cavity. It serves to transduce incoming airborne sound waves into waves in a liquid medium.
- The inner ear comprises the cochlea, the vestibule, and the semicircular canals. It interprets sound and serves to relate the head to gravity, allowing the visual system to compensate for movement and to perceive both linear and rotational acceleration.

INTRODUCTION

The ear of the dog and cat is composed of three parts: the external ear, the middle ear, and the inner ear[1-3]. Together these components allow the animal to locate a sound and the direction from which it emanates, to orientate the head in relation to gravity, and to measure acceleration and rotation of the head. Selective breeding, of dogs in particular, has resulted in a wide variation in relative size and shape of the components of the external ear. Compare, for example, the French Bulldog, the Cocker Spaniel, the German Shepherd Dog, the St. Bernard, and the Persian cat. The pinnal shape and carriage, the diameter of the external ear canal, the degree of hair and amount of soft tissue within the external ear canal, and the shape of the skull within which the middle and inner ear lie vary from one breed to another. Despite this anatomic variation the essential relationship between the various components of the external, middle, and inner ear is preserved (**1**).

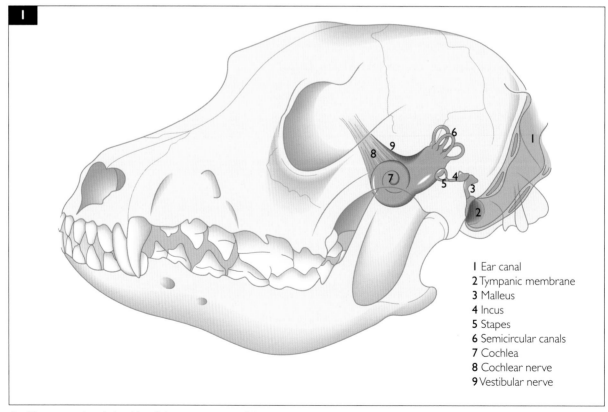

1 Ear canal
2 Tympanic membrane
3 Malleus
4 Incus
5 Stapes
6 Semicircular canals
7 Cochlea
8 Cochlear nerve
9 Vestibular nerve

1   The anatomic relationship of the components of the external, middle, and inner ear remains constant in relation to each other and the skull.

PINNA

The evolutionary role of the pinna has been as an aid to sound collection and point-of-origin location (**2, 3**). However, selective breeding of dogs has resulted in pinnae which often appear to have been designed more as lids to prevent access by foreign bodies (**4, 5**) or as vehicles to carry ornate displays

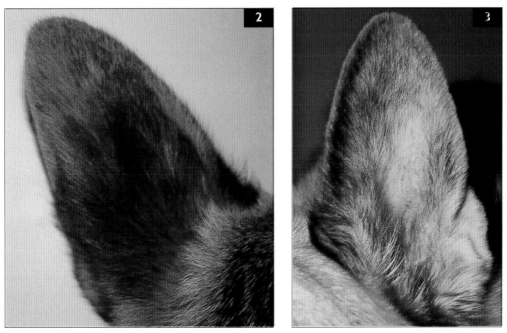

2, 3   Archetypal pinna, in this case a German Shepherd Dog. Note the even distribution of short hairs on the convex aspect (**2**). There is a variable amount of glabrous, sparsely-haired skin on the concave aspect (**3**) which is confluent with the epithelial lining of the external ear canal.

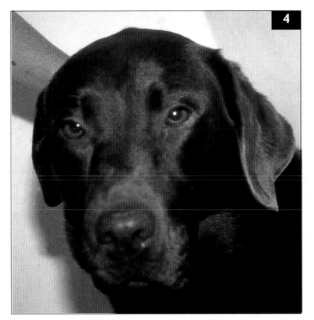
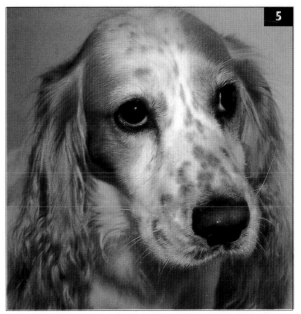

4, 5   Examples of the various pinnae which have resulted from selective breeding. Labrador Retriever (**4**), Cocker Spaniel (**5**).

of exuberant growths of hair (**6, 7**). Despite these changes the functionality of the ear appears to have been maintained. In most breeds of cats the pinna is held erect, with the exception of the Scottish Fold Cat where the distal portion of the scapha is folded rostroventrally[4].

The pinna is composed of a sheet of cartilage covered on both sides by skin (**2, 3**), which is more firmly adherent on the concave aspect than on the convex aspect[2, 3, 5]. The cartilage sheet which supports the pinna is a flared extension of the auricular cartilage. Proximally this becomes rolled to form the vertical ear canal and part of the horizontal ear canal. The major part of the external auditory meatus is contained within the auricular cartilage.

The portion of the flared auricular cartilage which forms the body of the pinna is called the scapha, although the free edges of the pinna are termed the rostral border of the helix and the caudal border of the helix, respectively[1, 3]. The anthelix is the medial ridge with the prominent tubercle that is situated on the medial aspect of the entrance to the vertical ear canal (**8**). Opposite the anthelix (**9**) is an irregularly shaped, dense plate of cartilage, called the tragus[1, 3]. This is extended caudally and medially to the antitragus and thus creates the caudal boundary of the opening into the external acoustic meatus. The rostral border of the opening is demarcated by the medial and lateral crus of the helix[1]. The tragus is an essential surgical landmark in aural surgery, because its rostral and caudal incisures mark the incision points for lateral wall resection.

The auricular cartilage becomes rolled proximal to the scapha and is termed the concha[3]. The scutiform cartilage is rostromedial to the horizontal canal, closely associated with muscular tissue[3], and it forms no part of the external ear, although the associated pad of fat, the corpus adiposum auricula, may help to provide support to the horizontal portions of the external ear canal[1].

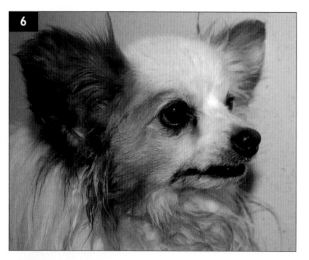

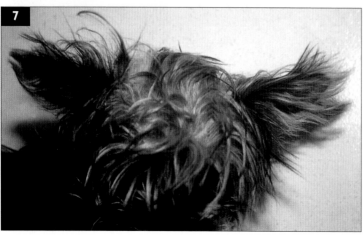

6, 7   Examples of the various pinnae which have resulted from selective breeding. Papillon (**6**), Yorkshire Terrier (**7**).

Generally the pinna is haired on the convex surface and in some breeds, such as the Cocker Spaniel and Papillon, for example, markedly so. The concave aspect may be lightly haired on the free edges and towards the tip, but towards the base it becomes essentially glabrous and is tightly adherent to the underlying cartilage. A few fine hairs are usually present around the entrance to the external auditory meatus. In breeds with hirsute ear canals, such as Cocker Spaniels, there may be profuse hair growth along the whole length of the ear canal.

The blood supply to the pinna arises from the great auricular artery, a branch of the maxillary artery[6]. The great auricular artery ascends dorsally towards the pinna just deep to the caudomedial aspect of the vertical ear canal[6]. Avascular necrosis of the pinna may follow damage to this blood vessel during resection of the vertical ear canal. The great auricular artery divides at the base of the convex aspect of the pinna. Its branches ascend the convex aspect of the pinna (**10**), wrapping around the helicine margins and penetrating the plate of the scapha to supply the concave surface[5]. The majority of the foramina through which the vessels pass to the concave aspect of the pinna are located about one third of the way along the longitudinal aspect of the scapha[1]. The auricular veins drain via the internal maxillary vein into the jugular vein.

The sensory and motor innervation of the pinna is extremely complex and is discussed in detail later (Chapter 2: Neurologic examination of the ear).

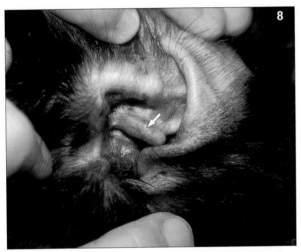

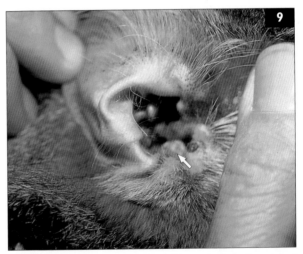

8 The prominent tubercle of the anthelix (arrow) is clearly visible on the medial aspect of the entrance to the external ear canal of this dog.

9 The tragus (arrow) is clearly visible on the lateral aspect of the entrance to the external ear canal of this cat.

10 The convex surface of the pinna of an elderly dog with an endocrinopathy. Note the prominent blood vessels following the long axis of the pinna.

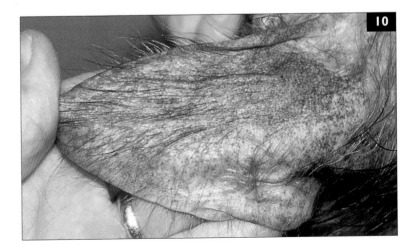

EXTERNAL AUDITORY MEATUS

The external auditory meatus serves to conduct sound waves to the tympanum. It is contained within the vertical and horizontal portions of the external ear canal.

Proximally the external auditory meatus abuts the tympanum and distally it is defined within, and bounded by, the medial faces of the various cartilaginous components at the base of the pinna. The vertical ear canal and the distal part of the horizontal canal are contained within the rolled plate (the concha) of the auricular cartilage. The free edges of the rolled auricular cartilage overlap on the medial aspect of the vertical canal and the lumen contained within becomes progressively narrower proximally. The size of the vertical canal (length and volume) correlates with body weight[7, 8]. The average length of the external ear canal within the auricular cartilage is 4.1 cm (1.6 in) (2.2–5.7 cm [0.8–2.2 in]) and its average diameter, at the level of the tragus, is 5.8 cm (2.3 in) (2.1–7.9 cm [0.8–3.1 in])[7].

The vertical canal deviates medially, just dorsal to the level of the tympanum, towards the external acoustic process. The annular cartilage is interposed between the proximal end of the auricular cartilage and the distal end of the external acoustic meatus[1]. The average length of canal within the annular cartilage is 1.2 cm (0.5 in) (0.8–1.9 cm [0.3–0.7 in])[7]. The ligamentous unions between these cartilaginous and bony tubes allow great freedom of motion to the pinna.

The epithelium and dermal tissues which line the bony and cartilaginous components of the external ear canal result in a smooth inner surface to the canal (**11**). The epithelium is sparsely haired in most, but not all, breeds and it is rich in adnexal glands (see Microscopic structure of the external ear canal).

Medial to the vertical portion of the external ear canal are branches of the auricular and superficial temporal arteries. The parotid salivary gland overlies the lateral and proximal portions of the vertical ear canal[6]. Deep to the parotid gland are the facial nerve, the internal maxillary vein, and branches of the external carotid artery[6]. The facial nerve emerges from the skull (via the stylomastoid foramen) and passes beneath the rostroventral aspect of the horizontal canal (**12**). Branches of the facial nerve and the auriculotemporal branch of the mandibular portion of the trigeminal nerve pass rostral to the vertical ear canal[6].

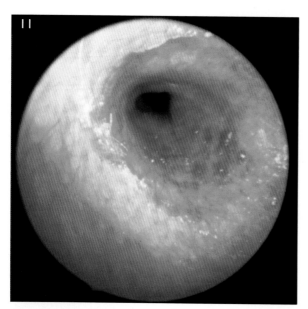

11   Otoscopic picture of a normal canine external ear canal demonstrating the smooth mural lining. Note the occasional accumulations of cerumen.

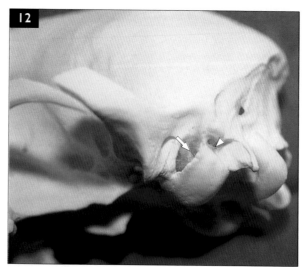

12   The caudolateral aspect of a canine skull. The external acoustic meatus (arrow) and stylomastoid foramen (arrow head) are adjacent.

MIDDLE EAR

The middle ear and auditory (eustachian) tube comprise a functional physiologic unit with protective, drainage, and ventilatory capabilities[9, 10]. The middle ear is composed of the tympanum, the ossicles, the auditory tube, and the tympanic cavities (**13**)[1, 3]. The middle ear cavities are lined with secretory epithelium (**14**). Epithelia such as this not only secrete liquid, they also absorb gas[9]. This tends to result in a slight negative pressure within the normal middle ear cavity [9]. The composition of the gas in the normal middle ear cavity of both dogs and cats has been described[11]. It appears to correlate closely to the composition of the capillary blood, rather than reflecting gaseous exchange along the auditory tube.

The three ossicles transmit sound waves impacting upon the tympanic membrane to the oval window. At this point the mechanical energy of the ossicles is transduced to pressure waves within the inner ear, to be interpreted subsequently as sound. Pressure and internal homeostasis within the inner ear is equilibrated across the round window membrane.

Tympanum

The gross appearance of the canine and feline tympanic membrane is similar[3, 4, 12]. The canine tympanum is a thin, semitransparent membrane with a rounded, elliptical outline; its mean size is 15 × 10 mm (0.6 × 0.4 in). The shorter dimension is nearly vertical, the long axis is directed ventral, medial, and cranial, and it has an area of approximately 63.3 sq mm (0.1 sq in)[1, 2, 13]. The feline tympanum is more circular in shape (8.7 × 6 mm [0.3 × 0.2 in]) and has an area of approximately 41 sq mm (0.6 sq in)[4, 12, 14]. The majority of the external aspect of the tympanum is thin, tough, and glistening (the pars tensa) with the outline of the manubrium of the malleus being clearly visible (**15**). The manubrium inserts under the epithelium on the medial aspect of the tympanum and exerts tension onto it, resulting in a concave shape to the intact membrane, rather similar to the speaker cone in a loudspeaker[3, 15]. The pars flaccida is more opaque, pink, or white in color. It is confined to the upper quadrant of the tympanic membrane and bound ventrally by the lateral process of the malleus [3, 13].

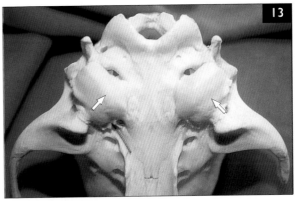

13 The caudoventral aspect of a canine skull. The paired bullae are clearly visible (arrows).

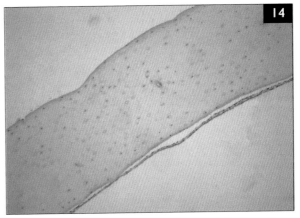

14 Photomicrograph of a section of normal bulla. Note the thin bone and the secretory epithelial lining. (Sample prepared by Finn Pathology, Diss, Norfolk, UK.)

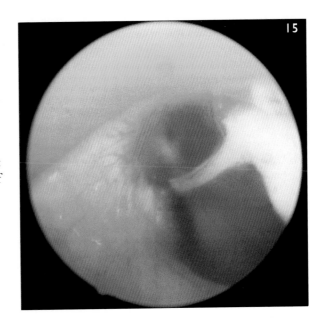

15 Otoscopic picture of a normal tympanic membrane. The manubrium of the malleus is clearly visible.

Tympanic cavities

The tympanic cavity proper, at least in anatomic terms, is one of three intercommunicating, air-filled cavities which lie directly behind the tympanum. The smallest cavity, the epitympanic cavity, lies dorsal to the tympanum and is almost entirely occupied by the head of the malleus and its articulation with the incus[1, 3]. The tympanic cavity proper is bounded laterally by the tympanic membrane (**16**). Its greatest dimension is less than 1 cm (0.4 in). Opposite the tympanum is a bony protuberance, the promontory, within which lies the cochlea. The mean volume of the canine middle ear cavity is about 2.5 cubic cm (0.15 cubic in) and this increases with body weight[8]. The volume of the feline middle ear cavity is about 0.9 cubic cm (0.05 cubic in)[16].

The largest of the three tympanic cavities is the ventral (or fundic) cavity[1]. Getty *et al*[1] compared the canine tympanic bulla to the shell of an egg, the long axis of which is some 15 mm (0.6 in) in length, set at an angle of 45% to a sagittal plane. The width and depth of the chamber are 8–10 mm (0.3–0.4 in)[3]. There is an elliptical opening in the dorsal wall which communicates with the tympanic cavity proper[1].

There are four ports of communication into the middle ear, all of which enter the tympanic cavity proper (**17**). Three of the ports, the tympanum, the round window, and the vestibular window into which the stapes connects, have membranes across their lumen. The auditory tube does not have such a membrane. The tympanum, as outlined above, is located on the lateral aspect of the tympanic cavity. The vestibular window is on the dorsolateral aspect of the promontory, on the caudomedial wall of the tympanic cavity. The round window, across whose membrane the cochlea communicates with the middle ear[17], is located in the caudal portion of the tympanic cavity proper. The ostium of the auditory tube is at the rostral extremity of the tympanic cavity[1, 18].

The ventral chamber of the feline tympanic cavity (**18**) is characterized by an incomplete bony septum[4, 19, 20, 21]. It is this septum which is visible upon opening the ventral wall of the tympanic bulla, and it divides the ventral cavity into two. The larger, ventromedial chamber is entered via a bulla osteotomy surgical approach and the smaller, dorsolateral chamber, in effect the tympanic cavity proper, lies beyond the septum. The two chambers communicate via the space between the septum and the caudomedial wall of the tympanic cavity[4, 19, 20, 21]. The round window of the cochlea, the promontory, and the postganglionic fibers of the cervical sympathetic trunk (to the eye and orbit) are in this region of the dorsomedial wall and are thus vulnerable to damage, particularly if the septum is removed during surgery[4].

Damage to these nerves leads to ipsilateral pupillary dilation and retraction of the third eyelid[4]. Sectioning of the nerves results in Horner's syndrome[4].

Ossicles

The ossicular chain comprises three bones: the malleus, the incus, and the stapes[1, 3]. The manubrium of the malleus is embedded in the central fibrous portion of the tympanum and is visible via otoscopy as a pale line across the tympanic membrane. In the dog it is about 1 cm (0.4 in) in length[1]. The malleus articulates with the incus, about 4 mm (0.2 in) in length, in the epitympanic cavity dorsal to the tympanum[3]. The incus subsequently articulates with the head of the stapes, the shortest bone in the body at about 2 mm (0.1 in) in length[1, 3]. The ossicular chain does not cross the epitympanic and tympanic cavities unsupported; ligaments attach to the bony walls of the cavities. In addition to the various ligaments there are two muscles attaching to the ossicles: the tensor tympani and the stapedius. Contraction of these muscles moves the relevant ossicle in relation to the membrane with which it is associated, significantly reducing the efficiency of sound transmission. These actions may serve a protective function, particularly from the harmful effect of low frequency sound vibrations[1].

The ratio of the length of the manubrium of the malleus to the length of the long process of the incus is known as the malleus:incus ratio. In the dog it is 2.7 ± 0.75:1 and in the cat it is 3.1 ± 0.6:1[4, 22]. These ratios are almost two to three times that of humans (ratio of 1:3) and probably explains why dogs and cats are able to hear very faint sounds which are inaudible to humans[22]. Furthermore, the ratio of the weight of the stapes to the sum of the weights of the malleus and incus is constant, as is the ratio of the cross-sectional areas of the malleus and incus to the area of the tympanum[22].

Auditory tube

The auditory tube arises in the dorsolateral wall of the nasopharynx and passes dorsocaudolaterally to enter the rostral aspect of the tympanic cavity proper (**19**)[1, 3]. In both the dog and cat it is in the order of 1.5–2 cm (0.6–0.8 in) long[3, 4, 18]. The entrance to the auditory tubes is obscured behind the soft palate, roughly midline, midway between the posterior nares and the caudal border of the soft palate[18, 23]. The distal end of the auditory tube is patent at all times[9, 10, 18], whereas the proximal, pharyngeal entrance is normally closed. It is opened by contraction of two muscles: the levator muscle and the tensor palatini muscle[9, 10, 18]. The epithelial lining of the auditory tube is continuous with that of the pharynx and it is mucociliary in nature[4, 24].

The patency of the auditory tube is ensured by the presence of a phospholipid-based surfactant, which helps to prevent closely-apposed, protein-rich mucus layers from 'sticking together'[25].

Otitis media may reflect abnormal function of the auditory tube[10, 12]. For example, reflux or aspiration of pharyngeal organisms may result in middle ear infection. Malfunction of the normal homeostatic controls will also follow edematous swelling of the epithelial lining of the auditory tube[10]. Auditory tube dysfunction is currently not considered a major etiological factor in the development of otitis media in dogs, in contrast to the situation in man[10, 12].

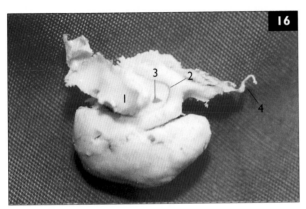

16 Silicone rubber cast of the tympanic cavities of a normal dog. This is viewed from the lateral aspect. The opening of the external acoustic meatus (1) is visible, as is the tympanic cavity (2), the promontory (3), the distal part of the auditory tube (4), and the ventral cavity, which is situated within the bulla.

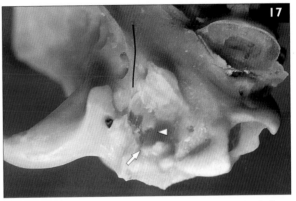

17 The caudoventral aspect of a canine skull with the bulla removed. Three of the four ports of communication are visible: the external acoustic meatus (arrow), the round window on the promontory (arrow head), and the auditory tube (delineated with a piece of nylon).

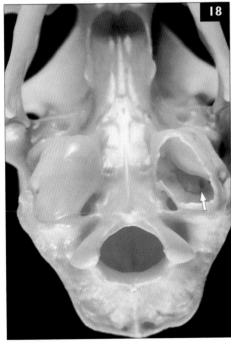

18 The caudoventral aspect of a feline skull. The left bulla has been opened and the septum is clearly visible. The promontory can be seen medial and deep to the septum (arrow).

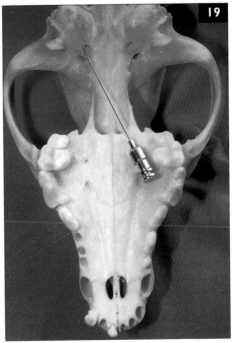

19 The ventral aspect of a canine skull. The stilette of the spinal needle enters the right bulla via the entrance taken by the auditory tube.

INNER EAR

The various tubular and spiral cavities within the petrous temporal bone that contain the components of the inner ear are called the labyrinth[1, 3, 4]. The three organs contained within the bony labyrinth are the cochlea, the semicircular canals, and the vestibule (**20**). Each labyrinthine tube and dilation contains a membranous sleeve supported and anchored by connective tissue trabeculae. The space between bone and membrane contains perilymph, whereas the membranous sleeve contains endolymph and the specialized sensory cells[1]. The membranous sleeves of the cochlea and the semicircular canals simulate the shape of their bony counterparts, whereas that of the vestibule is composed of the sac-like utricle and saccule which communicate with each other, the cochlea, and the semicircular canals[1, 4].

Vestibule

The vestibule is an irregularly shaped cavity, roughly 3 mm (0.1 in) in diameter in dogs[1, 3]. Rostrally it communicates with the scala vestibuli, caudally with the semicircular canals[3]. The medial wall contains two depressions: the elliptical recess of the utricle caudo-dorsally and the spherical recess of the saccule rostroventrally. The lateral wall contains two fenestrations: the oval window closed by the base of the stapes dorsally and the membrane-covered round window ventrally. The semicircular canals open into the vestibule caudally. The smallest foramen on the vestibular wall is that of the minute vestibular aqueduct which transports endolymph to the endolymphatic sac adjacent to the dura.

Cochlea

The spiral of the canine cochlea takes 3.25 turns around a central bony core[1]; that of the feline cochlea takes 2.75 turns[4]. The basal turn is about 4 mm (0.2 in) in diameter and the height of the bony spiral in the dog is about 7 mm (0.3 in)[1]. The whole is contained within the petrous temporal bone, although it bulges laterally into the tympanic cavity, the promontory. The cochlea contains the cochlear duct between two perilymph-filled chambers: the scala vestibuli dorsally and the scala tympani ventrally. These two chambers communicate at the apex of the cochlear duct[25]. The scala vestibuli communicates proximally with the vestibule, whereas the scala tympani terminates proximally at the level of the cochlear (round) window, which is covered by a membrane separating it from the middle ear.

The cochlear duct is triangular in shape with its base, the stria vascularis, situated at the outer lateral wall of the cochlea. A thin layer of tissue, the vestibular membrane, forms the dorsal border of the cochlear duct and this borders the scala vestibuli. The basilar membrane separates the endolymph of this duct from the perilymph of the scala tympani. Within the cochlear duct lies the organ of Corti (spiral organ), which is a sensory epithelium, composed of several types of supporting cells and hair cells, resting on a basement membrane, the basilar membrane (**21**). The hair cells have modified microvilli on their luminal surface. The tips of these hairs are embedded in a proteinaceous membrane, the tectorial membrane, which covers the hair cells and is attached medially along the cochlear duct. These structures are involved in the transduction and transmission of sound impulses, via the cochlear portion of the eighth cranial nerve, to the brain[3].

Sound waves are transmitted from the air medium of the external ear to the solid medium of the tympanum and, via a chain of three ear ossicles which extend to the vestibular window, to the fluid medium of the perilymph in the scala vestibuli. Wave flow through the perilymph in the scala vestibuli is reflected through the basilar membrane by way of the movement triggered in the endolymph of the cochlear duct. Movement of the highly organized basilar membrane causes the hair cells of the overlying organ of Corti to move and their stereocilia, which are embedded in the tectorial membrane, to bend. This action causes an impulse to be generated in the cochlear neurons which synapse with the base of the hair cells. Low frequencies cause maximal vibration of the basilar membrane at the apex of the cochlear duct, whereas high frequencies affect the proximal portion of the basilar membrane maximally[2].

Peripheral vestibular system

The vestibular system is the primary sensory system that maintains an animal's balance or normal orientation relative to the gravitational field of the Earth. It comprises the peripheral vestibular system, located in the inner ear, and the central vestibular system, located in the brainstem. Details of the central vestibular system are beyond the scope of this book. The vestibular system is responsible for maintaining the position of the eyes, trunk, and limbs in reference to the position or movement of the head at any time. This orientation is maintained in the face of linear or rotatory acceleration and tilting of the animal. This receptor for a special type of proprioception develops in conjunction with the receptor for the auditory system, the membranous labyrinth[2].

The bony labyrinth in the petrosal part of the

temporal bone consists of three communicating, perilymph-filled portions: the large vestibule, the three semicircular canals, and the cochlea. There are two openings in the bony labyrinth, the vestibular and cochlear (round) windows, which are named according to the component of the bony labyrinth in which they are located. Each is covered by a membrane and the stapes ossicle is inserted in the membrane covering the vestibular window[2].

The membranous labyrinth consists of four compartments: the saccule and utriculus within the bony vestibule; three semicircular ducts within the bony semicircular canals; and a cochlear duct within the bony cochlea (**22, 23**). The three semicircular ducts are the anterior (vertical) duct, the posterior (vertical) duct, and the lateral (horizontal) duct. Each

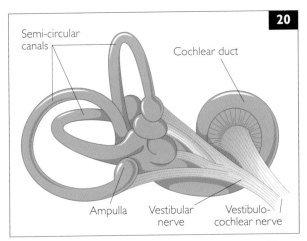

20   Schematic representation of the anatomic relationships between the various components of the middle and inner ear.

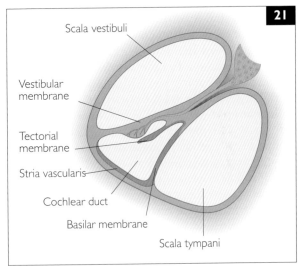

21   Sectional view of one turn of the cochlear duct. (Adapted from Morell RJ, Kim HJ, Hood LJ *et al.* (1998) Mutations in the connexin 26 gene (GJB2) among Ashkenazi Jews with nonsyndromic recessive deafness. *New England Journal of Medicine* **339**, 1500–1505, with permission.)

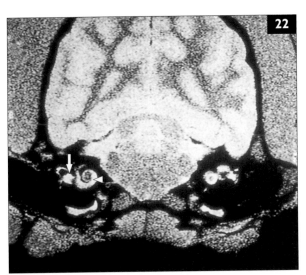

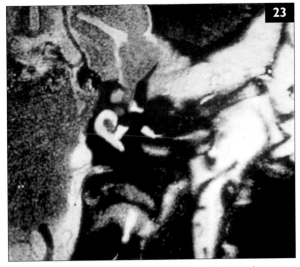

22, 23   Magnetic resonance images depicting the components of the membranous labyrinth (arrow = semicircular canal; arrow head = cochlea). (Courtesy B Dayrell-Hart.)

semicircular duct is oriented at right angles to the others; thus rotation of the head around any plane causes endolymph to flow within one or more of the ducts. Each of the semicircular ducts connects at both ends with the utriculus, which in turn connects to the saccule by way of the intervening endolymphatic duct and sac. The saccule communicates with the cochlear duct by the small ductus reuniens[2].

Each 0.5 mm (0.02 in) diameter semicircular canal describes approximately two thirds of a circle and is between 3.5 mm (0.1 in) and 6 mm (0.2 in) across, roughly at 90 degrees to each other. They lie caudal and slightly dorsal to the vestibule[1, 3, 4]. At one end of each membranous semicircular duct is a dilatation called the ampulla. On one side of the membranous ampulla a proliferation of connective tissue forms a transverse ridge called the crista ampullaris. This is lined on its medial surface by columnar epithelial cells, the neuroepithelium. On the surface of the crest is a gelatinous structure composed of a protein-saccharide material called the cupula, which extends across the lumen of the ampulla. The neuroepithelium is composed of two basic cell types: supporting cells and hair cells. The latter are in synaptic relationship to the dendritic zone of the vestibular portion of the vestibulocochlear nerve. The hair cells have 40–80 stereocilia and a single kinocilium on their luminar surface. These project into the overlying cupula. Movement of fluid in the semicircular duct causes deflection of the cupula which is oriented transversely to the direction of flow of endolymph. This bends the stereocilia and is the source of stimulus by way of the hair cell to the dendritic zone of the vestibular neuron. Each semicircular duct on one side can be paired to a semicircular duct on the opposite side by their common position in a parallel plane. Deviation of the stereocilia towards the kinocilium increases vestibular neuronal activity. These receptors function in dynamic equilibrium. They are not affected by a constant velocity of movement but respond to acceleration or deceleration, especially when there is rotation of the head[25].

Receptors (maculae) are present in the utriculus and saccule. They comprise thickened connective tissue on the surface of the membranous labyrinth, which is covered by a neuroepithelium composed of hair cells and supporting cells. The neuroepithelium is covered by the otolithic membrane, a gelatinous material on the surface of which are found calcareous crystalline bodies known as statoconia (otoliths). The hair cells are similar to those found in the crista ampullaris and their stereocilia and kinocilia project into the otolithic membrane. Movement of the otoliths away from these cell processes initiates an impulse in the vestibular neuron. The macula sacculi is oriented in a vertical direction (sagittal plane), while the macula utriculi is oriented in a horizontal direction (dorsal plane). Thus, gravitational forces continually affect the position of the otoliths in relationship to the hair cells. These are responsible for the sensation of the static position of the head and linear acceleration or deceleration. They function in static equilibrium. The macula utriculi might be more important as a receptor for sensing changes in posture of the head whilst the macula sacculi might be more sensitive to vibrations and loud sounds[2].

MICROSCOPIC STRUCTURE OF THE EXTERNAL EAR CANAL

KEY POINTS
- The normal ear canal contains a stratified squamous epidermis, hair follicles, and associated sebaceous and ceruminous (apocrine) glands.
- Breeds of dog predisposed to otitis externa, such as Cocker Spaniels, have increased amounts of glandular tissue compared to normal dogs.
- Otitis externa results in increased production of cerumen with a lower lipid content than normal, associated with increased ceruminous gland activity.
- Chronic otitis externa results in permanent changes.

NORMAL EXTERNAL EAR CANAL
The epidermis lining the external ear canal is similar in structure to that of the interfollicular epidermis of the skin, i.e. a statified cornifying epithelium with adnexal organs such as hair follicles and their associated sebaceous and ceruminous (apocrine) glands (**24, 25**)[1–4]. The underlying dermis is heavily invested with elastic and collagenous fibers (**26, 27**). Beneath the dermis and subcutis lie the rolled cartilaginous sheets of the auricular and annular cartilages which contain and support the external ear canal. The syndesmoses between these cartilage tubes, and between the annular cartilage and the osseous external acoustic process, allow great freedom of movement for the pinna[2]. The elastic and collagen fibers of the dermis allow a degree of freedom of movement for the external ear canal as well, and this can be exploited during otoscopic examination.

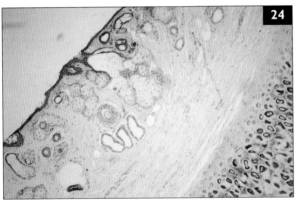

24 Photomicrograph of a section of normal canine external ear canal. Note the thin epidermis, the sparse hair follicles, sebaceous glands and ceruminous glands, and the underlying auricular cartilage.

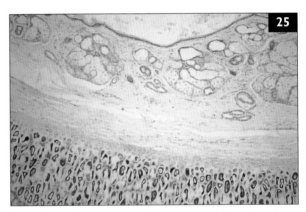

25 Photomicrograph of a section of normal feline external ear canal. Note the thin epidermis, the sparse hair follicles, sebaceous glands and ceruminous glands, and the underlying auricular cartilage.

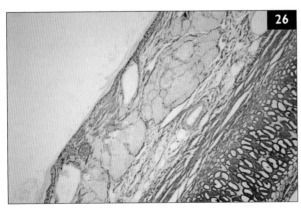

26 Photomicrograph of a section of normal canine external ear canal stained with Gomorri's stain to highlight collagen and fibrous tissue in the dermis.

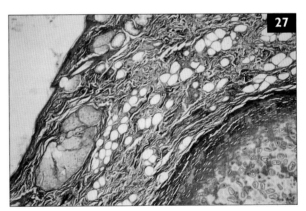

27 Photomicrograph of a section of normal canine external ear canal stained with Masson's stain to highlight collagen and fibrous tissue in the dermis.

Epidermis

The epidermis is stratified and rather thin[3–5], being only a few layers thick (**28**). The superficial topography is smooth and, on a microscopic level, composed of layers of flattened squames closely apposed and overlapping at the edges (**29**). Although no laboratory data are available, there is no reason to believe that the epidermis of the external ear canal turns over or reacts to insult any differently to the epidermis of the skin. The epidermis is punctuated by the hair follicles. In man, and presumably also in the dog and cat, the superficial epidermis and keratinized stratum corneum migrate, *en masse*, laterally from the tympanum[6]. This process is an extension of the epidermal migration on the surface of the tympanic membrane and serves to keep the proximal ear canal and tympanum free from cerumen and debris.

Hair follicles

All breeds of dog have hair follicles throughout the length of the external ear canal, although in most breeds these follicles are simple and sparsely distributed (**30**)[3]. It has been suggested[1, 2] that the density of hair follicles decreases as one progresses toward the external acoustic meatus, but recent studies[3, 4] did not describe such a distribution. The mean proportion of integument occupied by hair follicles was found to be 1.5–3.6%, with no significant spatial distribution along the canal. There was a large interdog variation[4]. However, some breeds which are predisposed to otitis externa differ from the basic pattern[3]. Thus, Cocker Spaniels exhibit a much higher concentration of hair follicles than other breeds and, furthermore, the follicles are typically compound in pattern (**31**)[3]. There is no correlation between the percentage of hair follicles within the otic integument and predisposition to otitis externa[4].

Hair is sparse or absent in the feline external ear canal[7].

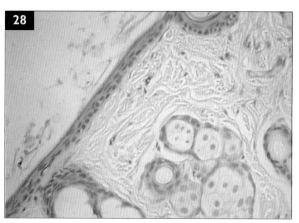

28   Photomicrograph of a section of normal canine external ear canal illustrating the thin epidermis, which is only a few cells thick.

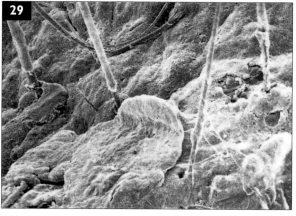

29   Scanning electron micrograph of the epithelial surface of the external ear canal. (Illustration produced by the Department of Anatomy, Royal Veterinary College, London.)

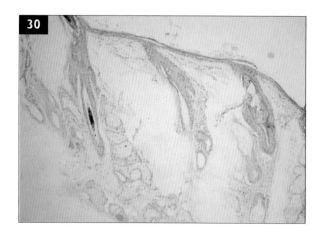

30   Photomicrograph of a section of normal canine external ear canal showing simple hair follicles.

Adnexal glands

Sebaceous glands are present in the upper dermis[1–5, 7]. They are numerous and prominent (**32**) and have a similar structure to the sebaceous glands of the skin. The mean proportion of integument occupied by sebaceous glands is 4.1–10.5%, gradually increasing from proximal to distal and peaking at the level of the anthelix[4]. There is a large interdog variation[4]. The sebaceous glands secrete principally neutral lipids[4]. In the normal dog this lipid accounts for the majority of the cerumen, along with sloughed epidermal debris[8]. This high lipid content of normal cerumen helps maintain normal keratinization of the epidermis, aids in the capture and excretion of debris which is produced within, and enters the external ear canal and results in a relatively low humidity within the lumen of the ear canal. In the cat the sebaceous glands become more prevalent and crowded proximally[5].

Ceruminous (apocrine) glands are located in the deeper dermis (**33**)[1–5]. They are characterized by a simple tubular pattern and a lumen lined by a simple cuboidal-pattern epithelium. In the normal dog and cat the ducts of the apocrine glands are virtually non-apparent. The mean proportion of integument

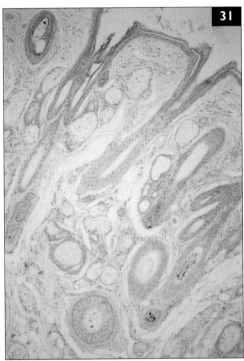

31 Photomicrograph of a section of normal canine external ear canal from a Cocker Spaniel. Note the density of the hair follicles compared to **30**, and that they are compound.

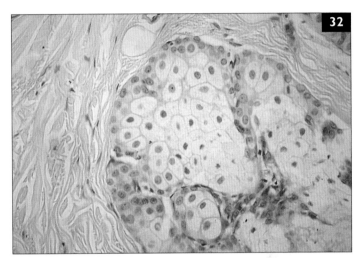

32 Photomicrograph of a section of normal canine external ear canal showing a higher power view of a sebaceous gland.

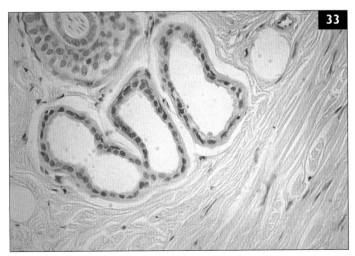

33 Photomicrograph of a section of normal canine external ear canal showing a higher power view of an apocrine gland.

occupied by apocrine glands is 1.4–4.5%, gradually decreasing from proximal to distal and peaking at the level of the tympanic membrane[4]. There is a large interdog variation[4]. The apocrine glands contain acid mucopolysaccharides and phospholipids[5].

Overall, these data[4] suggest that the ratio of apocrine to sebaceous gland decreases from proximal to distal, tending to produce a more aqueous cerumen in the deeper ear canal, possibly more conducive to epidermal migration. The more lipid nature of cerumen at the distal end may facilitate water repulsion.

Breed variations

Fernando[5] observed that the external ear canals of longhaired breeds of dogs and those with fine hair contained more sebaceous and apocrine glandular tissue, which was also better developed, than dogs with short hair.

Breeds predisposed to otitis externa also have abnormal morphometric ratios compared to normal dogs[3]. Specifically, they exhibit an increase in the overall amount of soft tissue within the confines of the auricular cartilage, an increase in the area occupied by the apocrine glands, and an increase in the apocrine gland area compared to that of the sebaceous glands (**34**). Overall, the breeds of dog predisposed to otitis externa have increased apocrine tissue. If this increased volume of apocrine tissue is actively secreting, the concentration of lipid within the cerumen will fall[4], humidity within the ear canal will rise, and maceration, followed by infection and otitis externa, will follow. Increased moisture and surface maceration creates an environment particularly favorable to gram-negative bacteria. Theoretically, the increased apocrine secretions in the ear canals of these dogs should result in a cerumen with a lower pH than normal and an environment not conducive to gram-negative colonization. It may be that the acidifying effect of increased ceruminous gland secretion is not sufficient to overcome the effects of humidity, inflammation, and surface maceration.

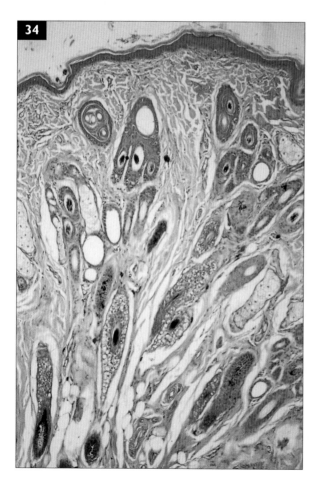

34

34 Photomicrograph of a section of normal canine external ear canal from a Cocker Spaniel. Note the much more closely packed dermis than that in **30**. There is more hair follicle and more glandular tissue.

Response to insult and injury

The epidermis of the external ear canal reacts to inflammation by increasing its rate of turnover and increasing in thickness; it becomes hyperplastic (**35**)[9, 10]. There may be surface erosions and ulceration, particularly with gram-negative infections. The dermis becomes infiltrated with inflammatory cells (**36**) and fibrosis will follow (**37, 38**). The mean proportion of integument occupied by connective tissue falls from 85.9–91.5% to a mean of 66.5–75.2% in cases of chronic otitis, a reflection of the relative and absolute increase in glandular tissue[4].

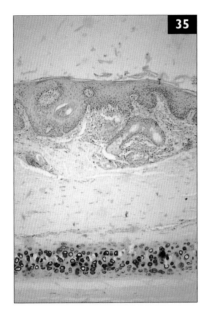

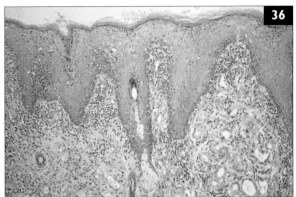

36 Photomicrograph of a section of canine external ear canal exhibiting epidermal hyperplasia, a thickened stratum corneum, and a moderate dermal inflammatory infiltrate.

35 Photomicrograph of a section of feline external ear canal demonstrating epidermal hyperplasia.

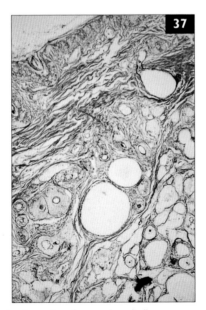

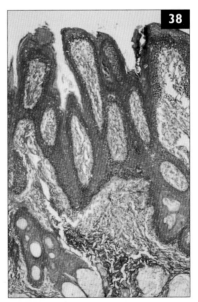

37 Photomicrograph of a section from a chronically inflamed canine external ear canal which has been stained with Gomorri's stain to highlight fibrosis. Compare the amount of fibrous tissue and the thickness of the dermis with **26**.

38 Photomicrograph of a section from a chronically inflamed canine external ear canal which has been stained with Masson's trichrome. Compare the amount of epidermal and dermal tissue with **27**.

In the early stages of otitis externa there is hyperplasia of the sebaceous glands, and their ducts may become dilated[10]. If chronic otitis persists, the apocrine glands become hyperplastic with cystic dilatation of the glands and ducts (**39, 40**). Thus, in ears from dogs with chronic otitis the proportion of integument occupied by sebaceous glands increases from a mean of 5.2% to a mean of 19.2%, significantly more than in normal ears[4]. The proportion occupied by apocrine glands increases from a mean of 10.1% to 17.1%, significantly more than in normal ears[4].

Papillary proliferation of ceruminous glands and ducts may obliterate the lumen of the external ear canal in some cases (**41–45**)[10]. In very chronic cases ossification of the tissues may take place.

> Even very early changes in the lining of the external ear canal have the potential to become permanent, and it is for this reason that the most common surgical procedure practiced upon the external ear, the Zepp resection, fails so often. Once any degree of luminal stenosis has occurred, lateral wall resection is not indicated. Vertical ablation is necessary.

Similar changes take place in the feline ear canal, although the papillary changes in the ceruminous glands may be sufficiently florid that discrete polyps occur[10].

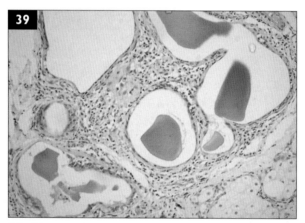

39 Photomicrograph of a section from a chronically inflamed canine external ear canal which has moderate dilation of the apocrine glands.

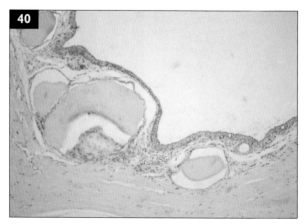

40 Photomicrograph of a section from a chronically inflamed feline external ear canal. Note the massively dilated apocrine glands which are distorting the epithelium into the lumen.

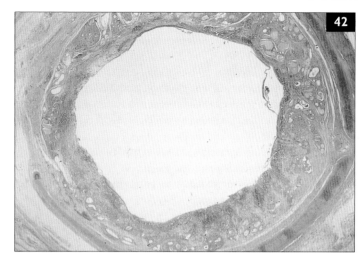

41 Cross-section of hyperplastic external ear canal demonstrating almost complete obstruction of the lumen.

42 Photomicrograph of a cross-section of an inflamed external ear canal. There is thickening of the soft tissue within the confines of the cartilage, resulting in reduced luminal cross-section.

43 Photomicrograph illustrating folds of hyperplastic epithelium reducing the lumen cross-section.

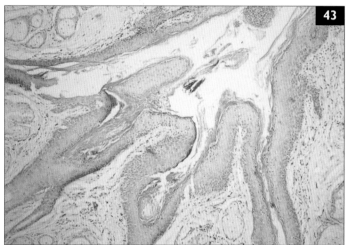

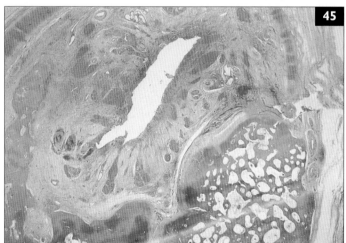

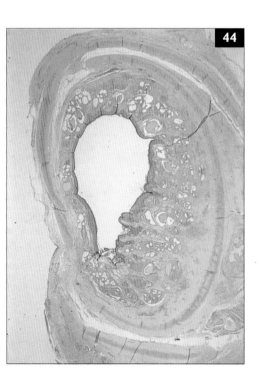

44, 45 Photomicrographs of two chronically inflamed canine external ear canals. Note the almost complete loss of lumen.

MICROSCOPIC STRUCTURE OF THE TYMPANUM AND MIDDLE EAR

KEY POINTS

- The tympanum, middle ear cavities, and auditory tube all possess epithelia which react to injury in a similar fashion to epithelial surfaces elsewhere in the body.
- Epithelial migration occurs on the tympanum as a mechanism to maintain auditory function.
- Auditory tube dysfunction may be more important than is currently recognized.

TYMPANUM

Microscopic structure

The components of the tympanic membrane are arranged in three layers (**46, 47**): an outer keratinizing epithelium, a central lamina propria, and an inner mucosa of pharyngeal origin[1, 2]. There are no hair follicles, or sebaceous or apocrine glands, on the tympanum[1].

The pars flaccida tends to be thicker than the pars tensa and it contains irregular, loosely packed collagen bundles[3, 4, 5], whereas the pars tensa is more dense and contains tightly packed collagen fibers[6, 7]. The outer collagen bundles are radial in arrangement, whereas the inner bundles are arranged in a circular pattern, helping to maintain the acoustic properties of the membrane under varying conditions[1]. Elastin fibers are found in both the pars tensa and the pars flaccida of the dog and in neither area of the cat[6]. The reason for this disparity is not known. The lamina propria of both dogs and cats contains abundant mast cells[6], although their function is unclear[1].

Epithelial migration

Superficial epithelial cells on the human tympanum migrate centripetally from the umbo, and it appears that this is a mechanism for clearing epithelial and ceruminous debris from the tympanum which, if it accumulated, would impair hearing[8]. The epithelial migration may also have a role in repair of tympanic perforation[9]. The cleavage line between stationary and migrating cells is at the level of the nucleated squames, rather than the stratum corneum, although the mechanism of the migration is not clear[10]. In some experimental animals, such as the guinea pig, the movement is not centripetal but rather follows the line of the underlying collagen fibers[1]. The mechanics of tympanic epithelial migration in the dog and cat have yet to be established.

Reaction to insult and puncture

Reaction to irritants

Experimental studies have demonstrated that the epithelium of the tympanum responds similarly to that of the external ear canal and other squamous epithelia when exposed to irritants. There is thickening of the tympanic epithelium, particularly of the stratum corneum, and an increase in epithelial turnover time, as measured by an increased rare of basal cell mitoses[11].

The tympanic epithelium also responds to chronic inflammation (**48, 49**) within the middle ear, even if there is no tympanic rupture. There is hyperplasia of the epithelium on the lateral side and loss of the mucosa on the medial side[12]. If the otitis media continues, the hyperplastic epithelium migrates through the lamina propria into the middle ear where it keratinizes, leading to cholesteatoma[12].

Puncture of the tympanum

Puncture of the tympanum most commonly arises as a result of infection or trauma[13]. The well-documented sequence of hemostasis, inflammation, fibroblastic and collagenous proliferation, and epithelialization, which characterizes healing of skin wounds[14], is not followed in the tympanum[15]. In particular, the epithelium migrates over and bridges the defect before a granulation bed is established beneath[10, 13, 15]. This adaptation presumably results in a more rapid restoration of tympanic function than might be achieved if the cutaneous pattern was followed. Thus, simple, elective myringotomy wounds heal rapidly and even excision myringectomy wounds heal within 3–8 weeks[16, 17].

46, 47 Photomicrographs of normal tympanic membrane. Note the insertion of the malleus in **47**. The three layers are clearly visible. (Sample prepared by Finn Pathology, Norfolk, UK.)

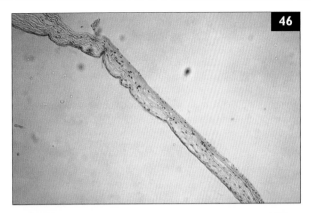

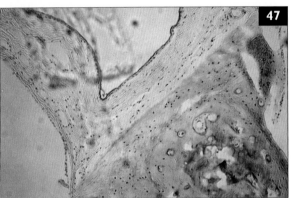

48, 49 Photomicrographs of inflamed tympanic membrane. Note the overall increase in thickness (compare with **46**), the increased cellularity of the central lamina propria, and the hyperkeratosis of the outer epithelial layer. (Sample courtesy D Heripret, Clinique Frgis, Paris, France; sample prepared by Finn Pathology, Norfolk, UK.)

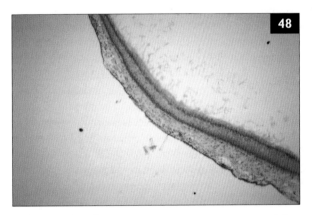

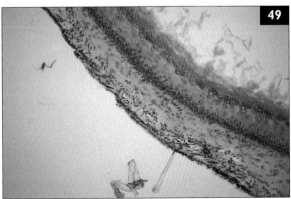

MIDDLE EAR

The epithelial lining of the normal middle ear is a modified respiratory pattern with a squamous or cuboidal appearance (**50**)[18]. A few ciliated and secretory cells are scattered among the epithelial cells. There is a thin lamina propria between the epithelium and the periosteum overlying the bone of the tympanic bulla[18].

When exposed to irritant chemicals, which may enter via a punctured tympanum for example, the epithelium responds with a range of inflammatory reactions proportional to the toxicity of the chemical and, presumably, its concentration and the period of exposure. There may be a mild and potentially reversible perivascular dermatitis with hypersecretion of mucus into the middle ear cavity[12, 18, 19]. If the irritation continues, the low cuboidal or squamous epithelium becomes columnar with a papillary appearance[18]. Secretory cells are visible between some of the columnar epithelial cells. Glandular or even cystic structures may be found within the granulation tissue; they may become so large that they fill the middle ear (**51, 52**). The lamina propria underlying the epidermis thickens and may take on the appearance of loose, edematous granulation tissue[18, 19, 20] with collagen, and even bone, being laid down as chronic changes take place. New bone deposition occurs on both the luminal and extraluminal bone of the tympanic bulla. At worst, a necrotizing inflammation may occur, with a thick, cellular neutrophil-rich exudate filling the middle ear cavity and an underlying osteomyelitis[12, 18, 19, 20].

Chronic inflammation within the middle ear cavity may lead to loss of the mucosal surface of the tympanum[15] and, ultimately, to cholesteatoma formation[12, 20]. Cholesteatomas are slowly enlarging, cystic lesions within the middle ear cavity. They are lined by stratified squamous epithelium and keratin squames are shed into them[20, 21]. Cholesteatomas are thought to arise when a pocket of the tympanic membrane comes into contact with, and adheres to, inflamed mucosa within the middle ear[12, 20, 21].

AUDITORY TUBE

The canine auditory tube is lined with pseudostratifed ciliated and non-ciliated columnar epithelium interspersed with goblet cells[22]. Cilia predominate at the proximal end of the auditory tube. This is presumably an adaptation to facilitate mucus clearance into the nasopharynx, while at the same time providing a mechanism to limit bacteria ascending from the nasopharynx[22, 23]. Goblet cells are more numerous at the distal, tympanic end. The goblet cells may be the source of the surface tension-lowering substance detected in the canine auditory tube[24, 25]. This surfactant is a complex mixture of lecithin, lipids, and polysaccharides, which helps to keep the auditory tube patent. Infection or allergic reactions, for example, may compromise epithelial function, resulting in decreased clearance of middle ear secretions and decreased patency of the auditory tube. These changes have been postulated as possible causes of otitis media in man[26]. Whether auditory tube dysfunction is a factor in the etiology of canine otitis media is not known.

ROUND WINDOW MEMBRANE

The round window membrane is located in the medial wall of the middle ear. It separates the scala tympani of the cochlea from the cavity of the middle ear and provides a means of communication between the two[27]. The structure of the round window membrane is essentially similar to that of the tympanum. There are three layers, the middle layer being composed of connective tissue[27]. However, unlike the tympanum both outer layers are thin epithelium. Morphologic evidence suggests that the round window membrane has an important role in the movement of substances between the inner and middle ear and, as such, it plays a role in both homeostasis and ototoxicity[27].

50 Photomicrograph of a section of normal canine bulla from a dog. Note the thin mucosa overlying the bone. (Sample prepared by Finn Pathology, Norfolk, UK.)

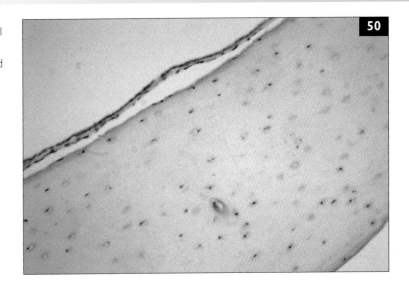

51, 52 Photomicrographs of inflammatory tissue taken from the middle ear of a dog with otitis media. Note the increase in thickness of the epithelium, associated with a chronic inflammatory reaction. Cystic changes are beginning.

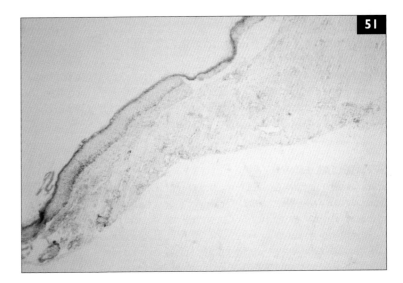

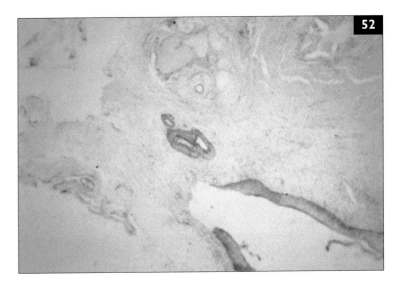

MICROCLIMATE OF THE EXTERNAL EAR CANAL

KEY POINTS

- The principal factor affecting the microflora within the external ear canal is the microenvironment.
- Temperature and relative humidity within the external ear canal are very stable.
- The mean temperature within the external ear canal is between 38.2°C (100.7°F) and 38.4°C (101.1°F), some 0.6°C (33.1°F) lower than the rectal temperature.
- The mean relative humidity in the external ear canal is 88.5%.
- The mean pH of the normal external ear canal is 6.1 in males and 6.2 in females.
- Otitis externa is associated with a rise in relative humidity and a rise in pH within the external ear canal.
- Cerumen is composed principally of lipid and sloughed epithelial cells.
- In cases of chronic otitis externa the lipid component of cerumen decreases.
- Lateral wall resection results in a fall in both temperature and relative humidity within the external ear canal.

EPITHELIAL LINING

The external ear canals are lined such that the underlying cartilaginous architecture and the intercartilaginous joints are covered by a smooth, clean epithelial surface (**53**). The epithelial surface is composed of closely apposed squames which are covered by a variable, but usually thin, layer of cerumen and adherent debris (**54, 55**). There is a constant, outward movement of cerumen[1, 2]. Squames detach (**56, 57**) and move distally in the cerumen, thus keeping the tympanum clear of debris and providing a mechanism for removing sloughed epithelial and glandular secretions from the external ear canal.

TEMPERATURE

In a series of studies the temperature within the external ear canal of dogs was 38.2–38.4°C (100.7–101.1°F)[3, 4, 5]. These studies were performed over 25 years apart with very different technologies, and for such close results to be achieved is remarkable. There was no significant difference between breeds of dog or whether there was a pendulous pinna or not[3, 4]. The temperature within the external ear canal rises significantly if otitis externa is present: mean 38.9°C (102°F)[5]. The temperature within the external ear canal is a mean of 0.6°C (33.1°F) lower than rectal temperature.

One study[3] was performed in Australia where the environmental temperature tends to be high. Nevertheless, as the day grew progressively hotter the temperature within the external ear canal only rose 0.3°C (32.5°F) compared to a rise of 6.4°C (43.5°F) in the environment. This illustrates very well how the environment within the ear canal is effectively buffered from the external environment.

RELATIVE HUMIDITY

In one study the mean relative humidity within the external ear canal of 19 dogs was 80.4%[6]. This was remarkably stable throughout the day[6], with a recorded rise within the ear of only 2.3% compared to 24% in the external environment, again illustrating the buffering effect of the tissues surrounding the external ear canal. Grono[6] suggested that the high relative humidity in the external ear canal was such that the meatal epithelium would readily become hydrated and macerated, an ideal environment for bacterial proliferation. In cases of otitis externa the relative humidity was somewhat higher (mean 89%) than normal, but not significantly so. The influence of a pendulous pinna was not reported.

pH

The range of pH in normal dogs is 4.6–7.2[6]. The mean pH is slightly lower in males than in females (6.1 compared to 6.2). The pH rises in otitis externa. Grono[7] measured the pH in cases of otitis externa and found the mean to be 5.9 (range 5.9–7.2) in acute cases and 6.8 (range 6.0–7.4) in chronic cases. Grono also measured the pH of the external ear canals of dogs and recorded the bacteria which were isolated from some of these cases. Non-parametric (Mann Whitney) analysis of Grono's data by the authors showed that in cases of otitis externa associated with *Pseudomonas* spp. the pH is significantly higher (mean 6.85, $p > 0.05$) than in cases of otitis externa in which no *Pseudomonas* spp. are isolated (mean 5.7).

53 Otoscopic view of the normal external ear canal. Note the clean, smooth epithelial surface.

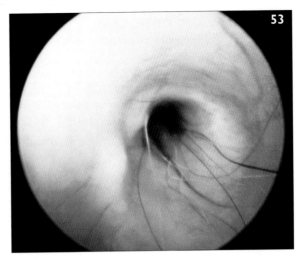

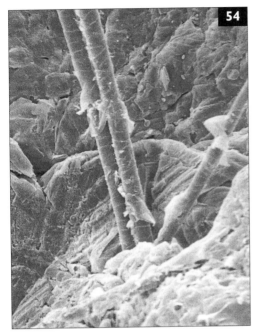

54, 55 Scanning electron micrographs of the epithelial surface of the external ear canal of a dog (**54**) and a cat (**55**). Note the cerumen coating the hair shafts and squames such that individual squame borders cannot clearly be seen. (Electron micrographs produced by the Department of Anatomy, Royal Veterinary College, London, UK.)

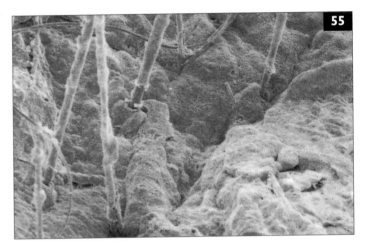

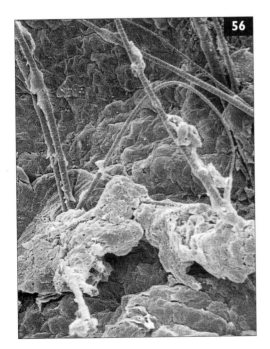

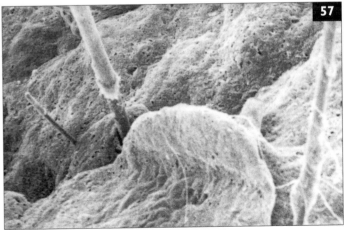

56, 57 Scanning electron micrographs illustrating squames in the process of detaching in a canine ear canal (**56**) and a feline ear canal (**57**). (Electron micrographs produced by the Department of Anatomy, Royal Veterinary College, London, UK.)

CERUMEN IN NORMAL AND OTITIC EARS

Cerumen coats the lining of the external ear canal (**58, 59**). It is composed of lipid secretions from the sebaceous glands, ceruminous gland secretion[8], and sloughed epithelial cells. The lipid component of dogs' cerumen can vary widely, as does the type of lipid within the cerumen, although margaric (17:0), stearic (18:0), oleic (18:1), and linoleic (18:2) fatty acids are the most common[9, 10]. A range of 18.2–92.6% (by weight) of lipid content was found in the external ear canals of normal dogs and in some cases there was wide disparity between the left and right ears. This variation presumably reflects individual variation in concentration and activity of ceruminous glands. In man, cerumen type ('wet' or 'dry') is a simple mendelian trait[11]. Whether there is a simple genetic control of canine or feline cerumen type is not known. Oleic and linoleic acid have antibacterial activity[12, 13], although the effects of these fatty acids, and others, against bacteria and *Malassezia pachydermatis* within the ear canal is less clear[10].

In cases of otitis externa the lipid content of the cerumen falls significantly to a mean of 24.4%, compared to a mean of 49.7% from normal ears[9]. This fall in lipid content may reflect the hypertrophy of apocrine glands which accompanies chronic otitis externa[14]. The decreased lipid component of cerumen may account for the increase in relative humidity reported in the external ear canals of dogs with otitis externa[6]. This, plus the decrease in antibacterial activity, may allow increased bacterial multiplication.

EFFECT OF SURGERY ON THE ENVIRONMENT OF THE EXTERNAL EAR CANAL

Lateral wall resection results in a fall in both temperature and humidity within the external ear canal, as might be expected. In one study of 12 dogs the temperature in the resected ears was reduced by a mean of 0.6°C (33.1°F) compared to the contralateral, normal ears[3]. Furthermore, the relative humidity in resected ear canals falls by a mean of 10%[6]. Whether this change in temperature and humidity is sufficient to explain the clinical improvement which follows lateral wall resection is debatable. Certainly it increases local drainage and this may be all that is necessary.

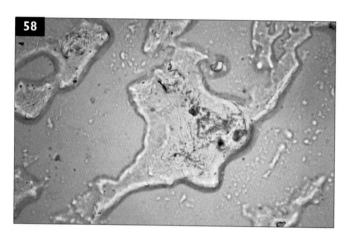

58 Photomicrograph of normal cerumen. Note the high proportion of amorphous lipid material to squame.

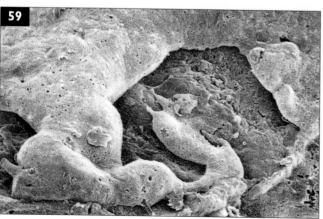

59 Scanning electron micrograph illustrating cerumen on the epithelial surface of a cat's external ear canal. (Electron micrograph produced by the Department of Anatomy, Royal Veterinary College, London, UK.)

MICROBIOLOGY OF THE CANINE EXTERNAL EAR CANAL

KEY POINTS

- The bacterial flora of the canine external ear canal is principally a gram-positive flora, similar to that of the interfollicular epidermis.
- The vertical portion of the external ear canal contains more bacteria than the horizontal portion.
- Not all external ear canals contain significant numbers of bacteria or yeast.
- Otic inflammation is accompanied initially by an increase in the number of bacteria and a shift towards coagulase-positive staphylococci.
- Chronic inflammation in dogs is accompanied by increased numbers of gram-negative bacteria.
- *Malassezia pachydermatis* is regarded as an opportunistic pathogen.
- Otitis media may be present in over 80% of cases of otitis externa.
- The bacterial flora in the inner ear may be different from that of the external ear.

NORMAL FLORA OF THE CANINE EXTERNAL EAR CANAL

Bacteria

The approach to investigating the bacterial flora of the normal ear canal has usually been to insert a sterile swab an unspecified distance into the vertical ear canal, collect a sample, and then inoculate the material onto appropriate culture plates. Collation of the various publications on this subject[1–7] is difficult because of the methods and classifications of results employed in each study. Furthermore, the failure of these studies to define otitis externa, or the limits of normality, hampers detailed comparison. However, most authors agree that a proportion of dogs appear to carry no viable bacteria within their external ear canals. When bacteria are recovered, the gram-positive flora predominate, with both coagulase-positive and coagulase-negative staphylococci being recovered from a large percentage of normal ear canals (*Table 1*).

Consideration of *Table 1* reveals a disparity in the reported recovery of bacteria between Grono and Frost[3] and the other studies. Grono and Frost reported a lower incidence of ears yielding no bacterial growth and a higher incidence of gram-negative bacteria, particularly coliforms, compared to the other studies. This might relate to the location of the institution in which the studies were performed. Grono and Frost carried out their work in a subtropical region (Queensland, Australia) whereas the other studies were performed in temperate climates. Humidity and temperature within the external ear canal increases (albeit within

Table 1: A summary of the microbial flora (% incidence) of the external ear canal of normal dogs. Note the incidence of ears from which no growth was recorded. Note also how the results from Grono and Frost[3] showed a much higher incidence of gram-negative carriage than the other studies.

Reference number	Number of ears	No growth	Mala	CPS	CNS	Strp	Crn	Psd	Prt	Col
1	156	40.0	ND	42.9	combined	0	0	0	0	<0.5
2	70	ND	ND	54.3	combined	32.9	15.7	0	0	5.7
3	124	1.6	35.9	47.6	74.2	15.3	25.8	2.4	1.6	42.7
4	279	ND	15.8	9.6	13.6	3.6	1.8	0	0	0.4
5	600	22.7	20.7	28.7	73.7	14.3	11.0	0	0	1.6
6	42	26.2	14.3	19.0	ND	ND	ND	ND	ND	ND
7	60	ND	28.3	1.6	3.2	0	5	0	0	0
Mean		**22.7**	**23.0**	**17.5**	**41.2**	**10.2**	**11.9**	**0.4**	**0.3**	**7.27**

Mala = *Malassezia pachydermatis* ; CPS = coagulase-positive *Staphylococcus* spp.; CNS = coagulase-negative *Staphylococcus* spp. and *Micrococcus* spp.; Strp = *Streptococcus* spp.; Crn = *Corynebacteria* spp.; Psd = *Pseudomonas* spp.; Prt = *Proteus* spp.; Col = coliforms; combined = coagulase-positive and coagulase-negative staphylococci counts combined; ND = not done narrow limits) as environmental temperature and humidity increases[8, 9]. Furthermore, the incidence of canine otitis externa increased with seasonal increases in rainfall and humidity [10]. It is possible that the higher humidity and higher environmental temperatures in tropical and subtropical regions result in a degree of maceration within the external ear canal and an increased carriage of gram-negative organisms.

Only one study specifically investigated the bacterial flora of the horizontal ear canal[11]. Fourteen of the 51 ears sampled yielded no growth, and when bacteria were recovered they were reported to be in very low numbers. Thus, although some of the organisms involved in otitis externa can be recovered from a normal external ear canal, they are usually very scarce or absent from the horizontal portion of the canal.

One quantitative study investigated the carriage of staphylococci within the external ear canal of ten normal dogs[12]. Both coagulase-negative and coagulase-positive staphylococci were recovered from the vertical and horizontal ear canals, although not from all the canals. The number of staphylococci was very similar to that obtained from normal interfollicular epidermis. A detailed, albeit qualitative, study of the staphylococcal flora in normal ears[13] revealed several (five) species of coagulase-negative staphylococci in the canine ear canal and four in the feline ear canal.

Consideration of the above suggests that the relationship between normal flora and disease is not straightforward. Potential pathogens such as coagulase-positive staphylococci can be recovered from ear canals in the absence of evidence of disease, just as they can be found on the normal interfollicular epidermis of the skin[12]. It seems reasonable to consider that these organisms cannot proliferate unless inflammation or maceration occurs within the ear canal, and it was for this reason that August[14] considered microorganisms as perpetuating causes rather than primary or predisposing causes of otitis externa. This theory also highlights the value of otic cytology as an adjunctive aid in assessing the relevance of bacteriologic results. Failure to detect changes consistent with otitis externa suggests that any organisms found on cultures are part of the normal flora.

The bacterial flora of the normal feline external ear canal has not been reported[15], although it may be envisaged that it is broadly similar to that of the dog.

Fungi

Malassezia pachydermatis

Malassezia pachydermatis is a yeast-like fungus commonly isolated from both normal and diseased external ear canals of dogs and cats. The number of organisms recovered varies, as does the rate of recovery of the yeast from ear canals. Thus recovery rates of between 14.3% and 37% have been reported for healthy dogs[3–7, 16]. There appears to be the same environmental effect on the carriage of *M. pachydermatis* in normal ears as there is on gram-negative bacteria, with a higher rate of recovery in tropical and subtropical regions compared to temperate areas (*Table 1*). Currently, the organism is regarded as an opportunist pathogen, capable of causing inflammatory changes in the ear canal, at least in the presence of moisture[17]. This is not to minimize its importance as a potentiator of chronic, or acute, otic inflammation, but it serves to suggest to the clinician that a search for underlying causes of the inflammation should be made.

Other yeast-like fungi

Malassezia sympodialis was reported to be present in the external ear canals of both normal cats and those with mild otic pruritus[18]. The pathogenic status of this organism is not known. A small study from Spain[19] reported that *M. pachydermatis* represented only 3% of the yeast isolates from cases of otitis externa and that *Candida* spp. and *Cryptococcus* spp. were more prevalent. It may be that the local environment (hot and dry climate) and the microbiologic methods used influenced this result.

Candida albicans has been recovered from normal ear canals of dogs and cats[2, 4]. However, the organism is only rarely implicated in otitis externa. In one incident, *C. albicans* was implicated as the prime agent in an outbreak of apparently contagious otitis externa in 76 foxhounds[20].

Other fungi

Fraser[21] reported on the fungal flora of 35 healthy dogs and 277 dogs with otitis externa. In addition to yeast he recovered six species of fungi from 11% of the normal ear canals. *Aspergillus* spp., *Penicillium* spp., and *Rhizopus* spp. accounted for 70% of the strains from normal ears and were presumably contaminants rather than members of the normal otic flora.

Given that most cases of infectious otitis externa originate in the horizontal canal[11], the clinician should ensure that both bacteriologic and cytologic samples are taken from this area and that precautions are taken to prevent contamination by microorganisms within the vertical ear canal.

MICROBIAL CHANGES ASSOCIATED WITH OTITIS EXTERNA

The overall changes in bacterial flora associated with otitis externa are qualitative and quantitative (*Table 2*); the number of bacteria increases and the proportion of various species changes (compare *Tables 1* and *2*). The incidence of recovery of staphylococci in general, and of coagulase-positive staphylococci in particular, increases[2, 5, 13]. More particularly, the incidence of recovery of *Pseudomonas* spp. and *Proteus* spp. increases[1-5, 20-30].

Early studies[2] reported that *Proteus* spp. and *Pseudomonas* spp. were commonly isolated from certain breeds of dog, particularly the Cocker Spaniel, but not recovered from others such as the Miniature Poodle. The authors postulated that Miniature Poodles presented with acute, painful ear disease with a short time course, whereas Cocker Spaniels were notorious for exhibiting chronic otitis externa, permitting contamination with gram-negative organisms. A more rational explanation is that Cocker Spaniels are anatomically prone to narrow, hirsute ear canals and to defects in keratinization. Both of these factors are likely to predispose to chronic otitis externa and gram-negative bacterial infection, particularly if the humidity within the external ear canal is elevated because of a pendulous pinna. Miniature Poodles, on the other hand, might well have hirsute canals but they are often affected by atopy. Atopy is associated with an inflamed, erythematous otitis, at least at first, which is not exudative. Such changes mimic those on the skin and might be sufficiently aberrant to favor colonization by *Staphylococcus intermedius* and *M. pachydermatis*, but not *P. aeruginosa*.

The most common bacteria recovered from otitis externa in cats' ears were coagulase-positive staphylococci (54.8%). Gram-negative bacteria such as *Pseudomonas* spp. and *Proteus* spp. were only rarely recovered from feline otitis externa[20].

The fungal flora of the ear canal also changes in otitis externa (*Tables 1* and *2*) and almost all of the increase results from an increased incidence of *M. pachydermatis*. Thus, Fraser[21] recovered *M. pachydermatis* from 36% of normal ear canals and

Table 2: A summary of the microbial flora (% incidence) from the external ear canal of dogs with otitis externa. Note the number of ears from which no growth was recorded. Note also the shift toward the carriage of gram-negative flora when compared to *Table 1*.

Reference number	Number of ears	No growth	Mala	CPS	CNS	Strp	Crn	Psd	Prt	Col
1			ND	79.3	combined	56.0	ND	3.4	3.4	3.4
2	62	ND	ND	80.6	ND	6.5	19.4	12.9	12.9	7.7
3	716	9.9	35.9	30.9	8.0	12.6	3.1	34.6	20.8	7.3
4	115	18.3	54.2	32	ND	1.0	1.0	9.0	9.0	4.0
5	69	ND	34.8	22.6	1.9	4.2	1.8	18.1	3.9	5.6
6	160	26.2	14.3	19.0	ND	ND	ND	ND	ND	ND
7	116	ND	82.8	37.9	20.7	8.6	6.0	16.4	3.4	2.5
20	60	ND	63	51.8	combined	29.6	ND	3.7	14.8	25.9
22	371	ND	51.5	66.6	combined	25.8	ND	11.3	14.8	
22	87	ND	56	32	ND	1	1	9	9	ND
24	669	22.3	19.3	16.3	combined	ND	ND	ND	ND	ND
26	389	ND	2.1	32.1	0.5	9.0	0.5	20.1	13.4	ND
27	59	ND	ND	47.5	3.4	25.4	1.7	5.1	13.6	ND
29	293	ND	35.8	33.8	combined	6.5	ND	3.8	3.1	ND
30	36	ND	50	41.6	combined	25	ND	25	19.4	13.8
Mean		**24.8**	**41.6**	**44.7**	**6.9**	**15.1**	**4.1**	**13.5**	**10.9**	**8.8**

Mala = *Malassezia pachydermatis*; CPS = coagulase-positive *Staphylococcus* spp.; CNS = coagulase-negative *Staphylococcus* spp. and *Micrococcus* spp.; Strp = *Streptococcus* spp.; Crn = *Corynebacteria* spp.; Psd = *Pseudomonas* spp.; Prt = *Proteus* spp.; Col = coliforms; Combined = coagulase-positive and coagulase-negative staphylococci counts combined; ND = not done from 44% of cases of otitis externa. However, the incidence of fungi was unchanged; indeed the number of isolations of *Aspergillus* spp., *Penicillium* spp., and *Rhizopus* spp. was reduced in otitic ear canals.

OTITIS MEDIA AND OTITIS EXTERNA

Otitis media is thought to be an important cause of recurrent otitis externa, as the presence of bacteria in the middle ear may act as a focus for reinfection. The presence of an intact tympanum does not rule out otitis media since it can repair in the presence of otitis media. There may be quantitative and qualitative differences in microbial isolates from either side of an intact tympanum[31], perhaps suggesting that topical otic medications fail to cross the tympanum, resulting in different populations of bacteria. The implication of this is that separate samples from both the middle and external ear must be taken for bacterial culture and sensitivity testing if otitis media and otitis externa are present.

EFFECTS OF TREATMENT ON THE OTIC MICROFLORA

Only a few published studies (summarized in *Table 3*) have investigated the otic microflora before and after appropriate treatment[15, 17, 18]. There were dramatic reductions in the numbers of organisms recovered after treatment, with a marked increase in the number of ears from which no growth was recorded (86% compared to a pretreatment rate of 21%) in one of the studies[17]. However, in several cases which responded well to treatment, and were pronounced cured, the original organisms could still be recovered.

Therefore, clinical cure does not always necessitate microbial elimination. It may well be that in a number of cases the other agents within polypharmaceutical preparations, such as glucocorticoids and antimycotics in particular, affect inflammation, epidermal proliferation, and bacterial adhesion to such an extent that microbial multiplication is not possible. Therefore, although viable bacteria can be recovered from ear canals post treatment, they are unable to adhere, multiply, or cause infection.

Table 3: The microbial flora (% of incidence) of canine external canals before treatment and after appropriate treatment had resulted in resolution of the condition. Note that after treatment had resulted in resolution it was still possible to recover microflora from the external ear canals.

Source	No growth	Mala	CPS	CNS	Strp	Crn	Psd	Prt	Col
Before (a)	ND	63.0	51.8	combined	29.6	ND	3.7	14.8	25.9
After (a)	ND	0	11.1	ND	11.1	ND	0	7.4	18.5
Before (b)	ND	53.3	46.7	combined	33.3	ND	6.7	13.3	43.3
After (b)	ND	0	10.0	ND	10.0	ND	0	10.0	3.3
Before (c)	50	52.3	51.5	combined	0.4	2.1	6.0	3.4	2.1
After (c)	203	8.9	4.3	combined	0	0	3.4	0.9	0.9
Before (d)	ND	45	17	15	5.2	ND	8.2	2.3	3.0
After (d)	ND	9.1	7.5	6.4	2.2	ND	3.8	2.3	0

Before (a) = before treatment with miconazole, prednisolone, and polymixin[20]

After (a) = after resolution of the otitis externa[20]

Before (b) = before treatment with diethanolamine fusidate, framycetin, nystatin, and prednisolone[24]

After (b) = after resolution of the otitis externa[24]

Before (c) = before treatment with fucidin, framycetin, nystatin, and prednisolone[20]

After (c) = after resolution of the otitis externa[20]

Before (d) = before treatment with neomycin, monosulfiram, and betamethasone[17]

After (d) = after resolution of the otitis externa[17]

Mala = *Malassezia pachydermatis*; CPS = coagulase-positive *Staphylococcus* spp.; CNS = coagulase-negative *Staphylococcus* spp. and *Micrococcus* spp.; Strp = *Streptococcus* spp.; Crn = *Corynebacteria* spp.; Psd = *Pseudomonas* spp.; Prt = *Proteus* spp.; Col = coliforms; combined = coagulase-positive and coagulase-negative staphylococci counts combined; ND = not done or not recorded

REFERENCES

GROSS AND MICROSCOPIC ANATOMY OF THE EAR: STRUCTURE AND FUNCTION

1 Getty R, Foust HL, Presley ET and Miller ME (1956) Macroscopic anatomy of the ear of the dog. *American Journal of Veterinary Research* **17**, 364–375.

2 Fraser G, Gregor WW, Mackenzie CP, Spreull JSA and Withers AR (1970) Canine ear disease. *Journal of Small Animal Practice* **10**, 725–754.

3 Evans HE (1993) *Miller's Anatomy of the Dog*. 3rd edn. (ed HE Evans) WB Saunders, Philadelphia, pp. 988–1008.

4 Hudson LC and Hamilton WP (1993) *Atlas of Feline Anatomy for Veterinarians*. WB Saunders, Philadelphia, pp. 228–239.

5 Henderson RA and Horne RD (1993) The pinna. In *Textbook of Small Animal Surgery*. 2nd edn. (ed D Slatter) WB Saunders, Philadelphia, pp. 1545–1559.

6 Smeak DD (1998) Total ear canal ablation and lateral bulla osteotomy. In *Current Techniques in Small Animal Surgery*. 4th edn. (ed MJ Bojrab) Williams and Wilkins, Baltimore, pp. 102–109.

7 Huang H-P (1993) *Studies of the Microenvironment and Microflora of the Canine External Ear Canal*. PhD Thesis, Glasgow University.

8 Forsythe WB (1985) Tympanographic volume measurements of the canine ear. *American Journal of Veterinary Research* **46**, 1351–1353.

9 Bluestone CD and Doyle WJ (1988) Anatomy and physiology of the eustachian tube and middle ear related to otitis media. *Journal of Allergy and Clinical Immunology* **81**, 997–1003.

10 Bluestone CD (1983) Eustachian tube function: physiology, pathophysiology, and role of allergy in pathogenesis of otitis media. *Journal of Allergy and Clinical Immunology* **72**, 242–251.

11 Ostfield E, Blonder J, Crispin M and Szeinberg A (1980) The middle ear gas composition in air-ventilated dogs. *Acta Otolaryngology* **89**, 105–108.

12 Chole RA and Kodama K (1989) Comparative histology of the tympanic membrane and its relationship to cholesteatoma. *Annals of Rhinology and Laryngology* **98**, 761–766.

13 Neer TM (1982) Otitis media. *Compendium on Continuing Education* **4**, 410–416.

14 Nummela S (1995) Scaling of the mammalian middle ear. *Hearing Research* **85**, 18–30.

15 Secondi U (1951) Structure and function of the lamina propria of the tympanic membrane in various mammals. *Archives of Otolaryngology* **53**, 170–181.

16 Huang GT, Rosowski JJ, Flandermeyer DT, Lynch TJ and Peak WT (1997) The middle ear of a lion: comparison of structure and function to domestic cat. *Journal of the Acoustic Society* **101**, 1532–1549.

17 Goycoolea MV and Lundman L (1997) Round window membrane. Structure, function, and permeability: a review. *Microscopy Research and Technique* **36**, 201–211.

18 Rose WR (1978) The eustachian tube. I: General considerations. *Veterinary Medicine/Small Animal Clinician* **73**, 882–887.

19 Boothe HW (1998) Ventral bulla osteotomy: dog and cat. In *Current Techniques in Small Animal Surgery*. 4th edn. (ed MJ Bojrab). Williams and Wilkins, Baltimore, pp. 109–112.

20 Seim HB III (1993) Middle ear. In *Textbook of Small Animal Surgery*. 2nd edn. (ed D Slatter) WB Saunders, Philadelphia, pp. 1568–1576.

21 Trevor PB and Martin RA (1993) Tympanic bulla osteotomy for treatment of middle-ear disease in cats: 19 cases (1984–1991). *Journal of the American Veterinary Medical Association* **202**, 123–128.

22 El-Mofty A and El-Serafy S (1967) The ossicular chain in mammals. *Annals of Otology, Rhinology and Laryngology* **76**, 903–909.

23 Hopwood PR and Bellenger CR (1980) Cannulation of the canine auditory tube. *Research in Veterinary Science* **28**, 382–383.

24 Sucheston ME and Cannon MS (1971) Eustachian tube of several mammalian species. *Archives of Otolaryngology* **93**, 58–65.

25 Hills BA (1984) Analysis of eustachian surfactant and its function as a release agent. *Archives of Otolaryngology* **110**, 3–9.

MICROSCOPIC STRUCTURE OF THE EXTERNAL EAR CANAL

1 Fraser G (1961) The histopathology of the external auditory meatus of the dog. *Journal of Comparative Pathology* **71**, 253–258.

2 Getty R, Foust HL, Presley ET and Miller ME (1956) Macroscopic anatomy of the ear of the dog. *American Journal of Veterinary Research* **17**, 364–375.

3 Stout-Graham M, Kainer RA, Whalen LR and Macy DW (1990) Morphologic measurements of the external ear canal of dogs. *American Journal of Veterinary Research* **51**, 990–994.

4 Huang H-P (1993) *Studies of the Microenvironment and Microflora of the Canine External Ear Canal*. PhD Thesis, Glasgow University.

5 Fernando SDA (1966) A histological and histochemical study of the glands of the external auditory canal of the dog. *Research in Veterinary Science* **7**, 116–119.

6 Johnson A, Hawke M and Berger G (1984) Surface wrinkles, cell ridges and desquamation in the external auditory canal. *Journal of Otolaryngology* **13**, 345–354.

7 Scott DW (1980) Feline dermatology: a monograph. *Journal of the American Animal Hospital Association* **16**, 426–433.

8 Huang HP, Fixter LM and Little CJL (1994) Lipid content of cerumen from normal dogs and otitic canine ears. *Veterinary Record* **134**, 380–381.

9 Fernando SDA (1966) Certain histopathologic features of the external auditory meatus of the cat and dog with otitis externa. *American Journal of Veterinary Research* **28**, 278–282.

10 Van der Gaag I (1986) The pathology of the external ear canal in dogs and cats. *Veterinary Quarterly* **8**, 307–317.

MICROSCOPIC STRUCTURE OF THE TYMPANUM AND MIDDLE EAR

1 Lim DJ (1995) Structure and function of the tympanic membrane: a review. *Acta Oto-rhino-laryngolica belg.* **49**, 101–115.

2 Evans HE (1993) *Miller's Anatomy of the Dog*. 3rd edn. (ed HE Evans) WB Saunders, Philadelphia, pp. 988–1008.

3 Secondi U (1951) Structure and function of the lamina propria of the tympanic membrane in various mammals. *Archives of Otolaryngology* **53**, 170–181.

4 Filogamo G (1949) Recherches sur la structure de la membrane du tympan chez les differents vertebres. *Acta Anatomica* **7**, 248–272.

5 Lim DJ (1968) Tympanic membrane. Electron microscopic observations. Part 11: Pars flaccida. *Acta Otolaryngologica* **66**, 515–532.

6 Chole RA and Kodama K (1989) Comparative histology of the

tympanic membrane and its relationship to cholesteatoma. *Annals of Rhinology and Laryngology* **98**, 761–766.

7   Lim DJ (1968) Tympanic membrane. Electron microscopic observations. Part I: Pars tensa. *Acta Otolaryngologica* **66**, 181–198.

8   Litton W (1963) Epithelial migration over the tympanum and external canal. *Archives of Otolaryngology* **77**, 254–257.

9   Reeve DR (1977) Some observations on the diurnal variation of mitosis in the stratified squamous epithelium of wounded tympanum. *Cell, Tissue Research* **9**, 253–263.

10 Broekaert D (1990) The migratory capacity of the external auditory canal epithelium: a critical mini review. *Acta Oto-rhino-laryngologica belg.* **44**, 385–392.

11 Monkhouse WS, Moran P and Freedman A (1988) The histological effect on the guinea pig external ear of several constituents of commonly used aural preparations. *Clinical Otolaryngology* **13**, 121–131.

12 Sennaroglu L, Özkul A, Gedikoglu G and Turan E (1998) Effect of intratympanic steroid application on the development of experimental cholesteatoma. *Laryngoscope* **108**, 543–547.

13 Boedts D (1995) Tympanic membrane perforations. *Acta Oto-rhino-laryngolica belg.* **49**, 149–158.

14 Dyson M (1997) Advances in wound healing physiology: the comparative perspective. *Veterinary Dermatology* **8**, 227–233.

15 Makino K, Amatsu M, Kinishi M and Mohri M (1990) Epithelial migration in the healing process of tympanic membrane perforations. *Archives of Otorhinolaryngology* **247**, 352–355.

16 Truy E, Disant F and Morgon A (1995) Chronic tympanic membrane perforation: an animal model. *American Journal of Otology* **16**, 222–225.

17 Steiss JE, Boosinger TR, Wright JC and Pillai SR (1982) Healing of experimentally perforated tympanic membranes demonstrated by electrodiagnostic testing and histopathology. *Journal of the American Animal Hospital Association* **28**, 307–310.

18 Little CJL and Lane JG (1991) Inflammatory middle ear disease of the dog: the pathology of otitis media. *Veterinary Record* **128**, 293–296.

19 Mansfield PD, Steiss JE, Boosinger TR and Marshall AE (1997) The effects of four commercial ceruminolytic agents on the middle ear. *Journal of the American Animal Hospital Association* **35**, 479–486.

20 Little CJL, Lane JG, Gibbs C and Pearson GR (1991) Inflammatory middle ear disease in the dog: the clinical and pathological features of cholesteatoma, a complication of otitis media. *Veterinary Record* **128**, 319–322.

21 Ruedi L (1959) Cholesteatoma formation in the middle ear in animal experiments. *Acta Otolaryngologica* **50**, 233–242.

22 Harada Y (1977) Scanning electron microscopic study on the distribution of epithelial cells in the eustachian tube. *Acta Otolaryngolica* **83**, 284–290.

23 Sucheston ME and Cannon MS (1971) Eustachian tube of several mammalian species. *Archives of Otolaryngology* **93**, 58–64.

24 Birken EA and Brookler KH (1972) Surface tension lowering substance of the canine eustachian tube. *Annals of Otology* **81**, 268–271.

25 Mendenhall RM, Mendenhall AL and Tucker JH (1966) A study of some biological surfactants. *Annals of the New York Academy of Sciences* **130**, 902–919.

26 Bluestone CD (1983) Eustachian tube function: physiology, pathophysiology, and role of allergy in pathogenesis of otitis media. *Journal of Allergy and Clinical Immunology* **72**, 242–245.

27 Goycoolea MV and Lundman L (1997) Round window membrane. Structure, function, and permeability: a review. *Microscopy Research and Technique* **36**, 201–211.

MICROCLIMATE OF THE EXTERNAL EAR CANAL

1   Litton W (1963) Epithelial migration over the tympanum and external canal. *Archives of Otolaryngology* **77**, 254–257.

2   Broekaert D (1990) The migratory capacity of the external auditory canal epithelium: a critical mini review. *Acta Oto-rhino-laryngologica belg.* **44**, 385–392.

3   Grono LR (1970) Studies of the microclimate of the external auditory canal in the dog. I: Aural temperature. *Research in Veterinary Science* **11**, 307–311.

4   Huang H-P, Shih H-M and Chen K-Y (1998) The application of an infrared tympanic membrane thermometer in comparing the external ear canal temperature between erect and pendulous ears in dogs. In *Advances in Veterinary Dermatology, Volume 3.* (eds KW Kwochka, T Willemse and C von Tscharner) Butterworth Heinemann, Oxford, pp. 57–63.

5   Hui-Pi Huang and Hui-Mei Shih (1998) Use of infrared thermometry and effect of otitis externa on external ear canal temperature in dogs. *Journal of the American Veterinary Medical Association* **213**, 76–79.

6   Grono LR (1970) Studies of the microclimate of the external auditory canal in the dog. III: Relative humidity within the external auditory meatus. *Research in Veterinary Science* **11**, 316–319.

7   Grono LR (1970) Studies of the microclimate of the external auditory canal in the dog. II: Hydrogen ion concentration of the external auditory meatus in the dog. *Research in Veterinary Science* **11**, 312–315.

8   Fernando SDA (1966) A histological and histochemical study of the glands of the external auditory canal of the dog. *Research in Veterinary Science* **7**, 116–119.

9   Huang HP and Little CJL (1994) Lipid content of cerumen from normal dogs and otitic canine ears. *Veterinary Record* **134**, 380–381.

10 Huang HP, Little CJL and Fixter LM (1993) Effects of fatty acids on the growth and composition of *Malassezia pachydermatis* and their relevance to canine otitis externa. *Research in Veterinary Science* **55**, 119–123.

11 Roeser RJ (1997) Physiology, pathophysiology, and anthropology/epidemiology of human ear canal secretions. *Journal of the American Academy of Audiology* **8**, 391–400.

12 Gutteridge JMC, Lamport P and Dormandy TL (1974) Autoxidation as a cause of antibacterial activity in unsaturated fatty acids. *Journal of Medical Microbiology* **7**, 387–389.

13 Knapp HR and Melly MA (1986) Bactericidal effects of polyunsaturated fatty acids. *Journal of Infectious Diseases* **154**, 84–94.

14 Stout-Graham M, Kainer RA, Whalen LR and Macy DW (1990) Morphologic measurements of the external ear horizontal canal of dogs. *American Journal of Veterinary Research* **51**, 990–994.

MICROBIOLOGY OF THE CANINE EXTERNAL EAR CANAL

1   Gustafson B (1954) Otitis externa hos hund. *Nordic Veterinærmedicin* **6**, 434–442.

2   Fraser G (1961) Factors predisposing to canine external otitis. *Veterinary Record* **73**, 55–58.

3   Grono LR and Frost AJ (1969) Otitis externa in the dog. *Australian Veterinary Journal* **45**, 420–422.

4   Sharma VD and Rhodes HE (1975) The occurrence and microbiology of otitis externa in the dog. *Journal of Small Animal Practice* **16**, 241–247.

5   McCarthy G and Kelly WR (1982) Microbial species associated with the canine ear and their antibacterial sensitivity patterns.

Irish Veterinary Journal **36**, 53–56.

6 Chengappa MM, Maddux R and Greer S (1983) A microbiologic survey of clinically normal and otitic ear canals. *Pet Practice* **78**, 343–344.

7 Marshall MJ, Harris AM and Horne JE (1974) The bacteriological and clinical assessment of a new preparation for the treatment of otitis externa in dogs and cats. *Journal of Small Animal Practice* **15**, 401–410.

8 Grono LR (1970) Studies of the microclimate of the external auditory canal of the dog. I: Aural temperature. *Research in Veterinary Science* **11**, 307–311.

9 Grono LR (1970) Studies of the microclimate of the external auditory canal of the dog. III: Relative humidity within the external auditory meatus. *Research in Veterinary Science* **11**, 316–319.

10 Hayes HM, Williams Pickle L and Wilson GP (1987) Effects of ear type and weather on the hospital prevalence of canine otitis externa. *Research in Veterinary Science* **42**, 294–298.

11 Dickson DB and Love DN (1983) Bacteriology of the horizontal ear canal of dogs. *Journal of Small Animal Practice* **24**, 413–421.

12 Harvey RG and Lloyd DH (1995) The distribution of *Staphylococcus intermedius* and coagulase-negative staphylococci on the hair, skin surface, within the hair follicles and on the mucous membranes of eleven dogs. *Veterinary Dermatology* **5**, 75–81.

13 Uchida Y, Tetsuya N and Kitazawa K (1990) Clinicomicrobiological study of the normal and otitis externa ear canals in dogs and cats. *Japanese Journal of Veterinary Science* **52**, 415–417.

14 August JR (1988) Otitis externa: a disease of multifactorial etiology. *Veterinary Clinics of North America* **18**, 731–742.

15 Scott DW (1980) Feline dermatology: a monograph. *Journal of the American Animal Hospital Association* **16**, 426–433.

16 Fraser G (1961) The fungal flora of the canine ear. *Journal of Comparative Pathology* **71**, 1–5.

17 Mansfield PD, Boosinger TR and Attleburger MH (1990) Infectivity of *Malassezia pachydermatis* in the external ear canal of dogs. *Journal of the American Animal Hospital Association* **26**, 97–100.

18 Bond R, Anthony RM, Dodd M and Lloyd DH (1996) Isolation of *Malassezia sympodialis* from feline skin. *Journal of Medical and Veterinary Mycology* **34**, 145–147.

19 Blanco JL, Guedeja-Marron J, Hontecillas R, Suarez G and Garcia M-E (1996) Microbiological diagnosis of chronic otitis externa in the dog. *Journal of Veterinary Medicine* **43**, 475–482.

20 McKellar, QA, Rycroft, A, Anderson L and Love J (1990) Otitis externa in a foxhound pack associated with *Candida albicans*. *Veterinary Record* **127**, 15–16.

21 Fraser G (1961) The fungal flora of the canine ear. *Journal of Comparative Pathology* **71**, 1–5.

22 Fraser G, Withers AR and Spreull JSA (1961) Otitis externa in the dog. *Journal of Small Animal Practice* **2**, 32–47.

23 Baxter M and Lawler DC (1972) The incidence and microbiology of otitis externa of dogs and cats in New Zealand. *New Zealand Veterinary Journal* **20**, 29–32.

24 Krogh HV, Linnel A and Knudsen PB (1975) Otitis externa in the dog: a clinical and microbiological study. *Nordic Veterinærmedicin* **27**, 285–295.

25 Baba E, Fukata T and Saito M (1981) Incidence of otitis externa in dogs and cats in Japan. *Veterinary Record* **108**, 393–395.

26 Blue JL and Wooley RE (1977) Antibacterial sensitivity patterns of bacteria isolated from dogs with otitis externa. *Journal of the American Veterinary Medical Association* **171**, 362–363.

27 Nesbitt GH and Schmitz JA (1977) Chronic bacterial dermatitis and otitis: a review of 195 cases. *Journal of the American Animal Hospital Association* **13**, 442–450.

28 Webster FL, Whyard BH, Brandt RW and Jones WG (1974) Treatment of otitis externa in the dog with Gentocin Otic. *Canadian Veterinary Journal* **15**, 176–177.

29 Rycroft AK and Saban HS (1977) A clinical study of otitis externa in the dog. *Canadian Veterinary Journal* **18**, 64–70.

30 Hallu RE, Gentilini E, Rebuelto M, Albarellos GA and Otero PE (1996) The combination of norfloxacin and ketoconazole in the treatment of canine otitis. *Canine Practice* **21**, 26–28.

31 Cole LK, Kwochka KW, Kowalski JJ and Hillier A (1998) Microbial flora and antimicrobial susceptibility patterns of isolated pathogens from the horizontal ear canal and middle ear in dogs with otitis media. *Journal of the American Veterinary Medical Association* **212**, 534–538.

Chapter Two

Diagnostic Procedures

- **Otoscopic appearance of the external ear canal and tympanum**

- **Cytologic characteristics of normal and abnormal ears**

- **Neurologic examination of the ear**

- **Radiographic features of the normal and abnormal ear**

- **Imaging the middle and inner ears**

- **Electrophysiologic procedures**

- **Other investigatory procedures**

- **References**

OTOSCOPIC APPEARANCE OF THE EXTERNAL EAR CANAL AND TYMPANUM

KEY POINTS

- Do not examine the ear in isolation. Obtain a history and examine the animal first.
- Ear canals may require cleaning before a proper examination is possible.
- Always examine both ears, even if a unilateral problem is suspected.
- Adequate restraint is essential. Use a sedative or neuroleptanalgesia if necessary.
- Cats require general anesthesia before they are subjected to otoscopic examination.
- Remember that the presence of hair in the external ear canal is normal in some dogs.
- Do not expect to visualize *Otodectes cynotis* unfailingly. Use a microscope as well as an otoscope.

SEDATION FOR OTOSCOPY AND AURAL EXAMINATION

In order properly to examine the entire length of the ear canal, adequate restraint is necessary as the external ear canal must be manipulated into as straight a line as possible. This is achieved by gently grasping the pinna and pulling it, and the attached auricular cartilage, up and away from the sagittal plane.

Otoscopic cannulae are hard, often cold, and have sharp ends; it hurts when a cannula is thrust into an inflamed ear canal. In small dogs and cats, and animals with painful or tender ear canals, this process is resented and the clinician will require chemical restraint or general anesthesia. McKeever and Richardson[1] advocated a mixture which provides approximately 20 minutes sedation, sufficient to allow thorough examination and cleaning of both ears:

- Ketamine (1.36–2.2 mg/kg)
- Midazolam (0.023 mg/kg)
- Acepromazine (0.023 mg/kg)
- All mixed in the same syringe and injected slowly intravenously.

One alternative would be xylazine injection (1–2 mg/10 kg i/v), which should provide about 20 minutes reasonable sedation. Another alternative is detomidine (20–40 mcg/kg i/v), which will produce moderate sedation and has the great advantage that it can be reversed by intramuscular injection of its antagonist atipamezole. However, there are two disadvantages with this regime: it is very expensive (mitigated by giving buprenorphine at the same time), and there is a risk of inducing a cardiac arrhythmia if potentiated sulphonamides are administered at the same time.

NORMAL APPEARANCE OF THE EXTERNAL EAR CANAL AND TYMPANUM

The normal external ear canal is smooth, pale in color, and contains minimal discharge (**60, 61**). A small amount of pale yellow or brown cerumen (**62, 63**) may be seen in some cases and this is normal[3]. Occasionally, there may be a hair shaft in the horizontal canal (**64, 65**). In some breeds, such as Cocker Spaniels, Miniature and Giant Schnauzers, Airedales, and other terriers, for example, there are hair follicles the whole length of the external ear canal[1, 3]. The diameter of the vertical portion of the external canal varies from breed to breed but at its base, where it apposes the horizontal portion, it is 5–10 mm (0.2–0.4 in) in diameter[2]. The horizontal canal is approximately 2 cm (0.8 in) in length[2].

The normal tympanum is thin, pale gray in color (described as rice paper-like), and translucent (**66**). It is visible via otoscopy in about 75% of normal ears[4]. Cerumen, debris, or hair prevents a clear view of the tympanum in the other ears[4]. The shape of the tympanum is elliptical, mean 15×10 mm (0.6×0.4 in), with the short axis nearly vertical[2]. The initial otoscopic view is restricted to the posterior quadrant of the pars tensa and the pars flaccida[5, 6]. Manipulation

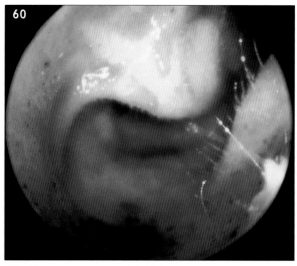

60 The upper portion of the feline external ear canal.

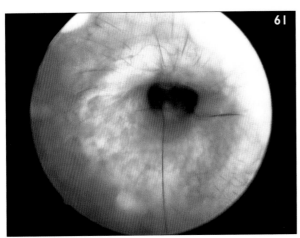

61 A normal horizontal external ear canal of a dog. There is an even, pale color with a smooth contour. A few fine hairs may be seen.

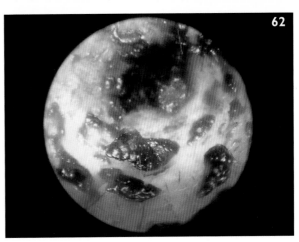

62 Patchy brown cerumen adhering to the walls of a normal external ear canal.

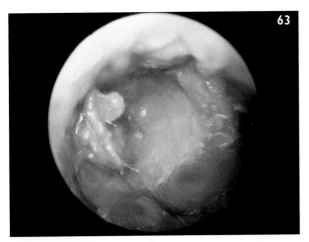

63 Yellowish cerumen near the tympanum.

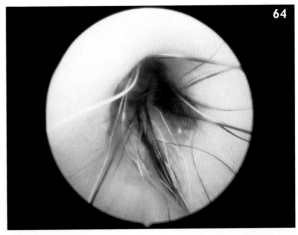

64 Tufts of hair emerging from the horizontal ear canal.

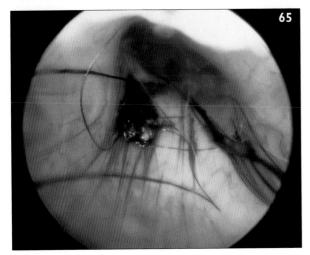

65 Hair and adhering cerumen emerging from the horizontal ear canal.

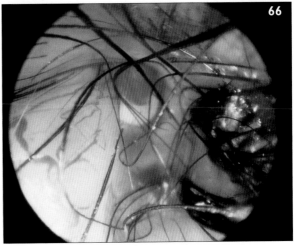

66 A normal, translucent tympanic membrane, in this instance partially hidden by hair and cerumen.

of both the external ear canal and the otoscope will usually bring the majority of the manubrium (**67**) and the larger portion of the pars tensa into view[5, 6]. The external aspect of the tympanum, as viewed with an otoscope, is divided into two unequal parts by the manubrium of the malleus. This is attached along the medial aspect of the tympanum and exerts tension onto it, resulting in a concave shape to the intact membrane.

ABNORMAL APPEARANCE OF THE EXTERNAL EAR CANAL

Inflammation results in edema, erythema, and warmth (**68**). Given that the glandular tissues of the external ear canal are contained within a cartilaginous tube, any swelling will result in a reduction in the diameter of the lumen. In many cases the concave aspect of the pinna will also be affected (**69**). In most cases the inflammation affects the entire ear canal but in some instances it will be localized to either the horizontal or, more usually, the vertical canal. Bilateral inflammation confined to the concave aspect of the pinna and the vertical canal, particularly if there is little discharge, is very suggestive of atopy (**70**). Indeed, erythema of the entire canal in the absence of significant discharge or other pathology is highly suggestive of allergy. Atopy, dietary intolerance, and neomycin sensitivity should all be considered in the differential diagnosis.

Inflammation also results in increased secretion from the glands within the epithelial lining of the canal and a shift away from a lipid to an aqueous constitution[7, 8]. Continued inflammation results in maceration of the stratum corneum, loss of barrier function, and the outward movement of transepidermal fluid. Discharge accumulates within the external ear canal (**71–73**) and microbial proliferation occurs. The color of the discharge may vary from light yellow to dark brown and it may be aqueous, thin, or pus-like in nature. Animals with severe or generalized defects in keratinization may exhibit a greasy yellow discharge that has a purulent appearance but which may be sterile and non-inflammatory in nature. Medications may result in a thin, shiny covering over the mural epithelium.

> The color and nature of the otic discharge may give some clues to the microbial population within the external ear canal, but prescribing treatment solely on the basis of the nature of this discharge is inadvisable.

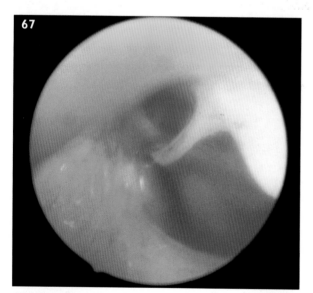

67 The tympanic membrane with the manubrium of the malleus clearly visible.

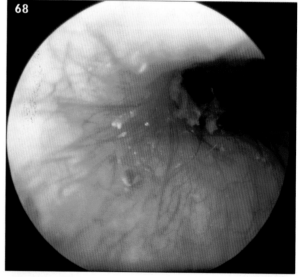

68 Erythematous otitis in a case of atopy. There is erythema and some degree of swelling, resulting in loss of luminal cross-section.

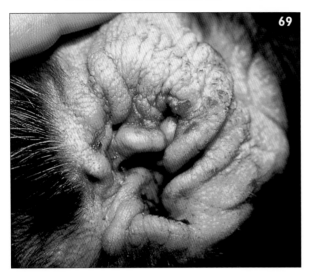

69 External ear canal of an atopic dog. There is erythema, hyperplasia, and lichenification.

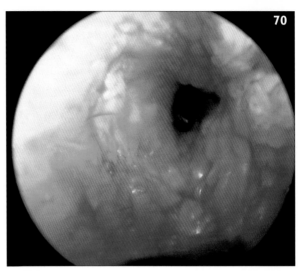

70 Erythema, hyperplasia, moderate fissure formation, and a tendency to ulcerate and bleed very easily, even after otoscopy, are commonly seen in ear canals of atopic dogs.

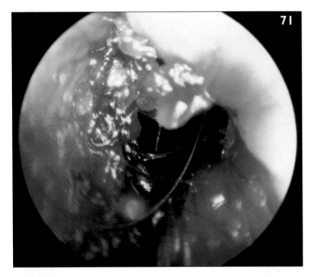

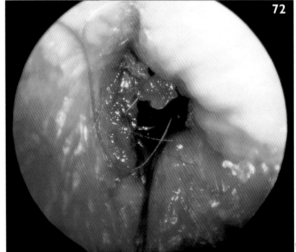

71–73 Erythema, hyperplasia, loss of luminal cross-section, and partial obstruction of the lumen by cerumen.

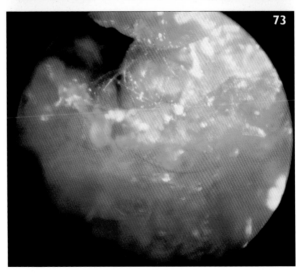

The presence of erosions and ulcers in the external ear canal should be noted (**74**). Frank ulceration is uncommon and is usually associated with gram-negative bacterial infection. Rare causes of otic ulceration are autoimmune diseases and otic neoplasms. The finding of ulcers within the external ear canal mandates samples for both cytologic evaluation and bacterial culture and sensitivity testing.

Otoscopic examination may reveal the presence of ectoparasites, such as *Otodectes cynotis* or *Otobius megnini*. Otodectic mites are often accompanied by the presence of a crumbly brown discharge (**75**). Not all infestations are inflammatory. Failure to detect otodectic mites during otoscopic examination does not preclude infestation, and microscopic examination of cytologic samples is necessary.

Epidermal hyperplasia, nodules, tumors, polyps, and foreign bodies within the external ear canal are easily visualized during otoscopy (**76**), although cleaning of the external ear canal may be necessary. This is particularly the case for cats where the whole canal may fill with purulent discharge if an otic tumor or polyp is present (**77**).

> Otoscopic examination of the tympanum in dogs with otitis externa is difficult.

The tympanum should be examined for color, texture, and integrity; it is usually dark gray or brown in cases of otitis externa[1]. In contrast to normal dogs it is only possible adequately to visualize the tympanum in 28% of ears affected with otitis externa[4]. If tears or holes in the tympanum (**78, 79**) indicate that otitis media is present (although an intact tympanum does not rule out otitis media), then failure adequately to visualize the tympanum, let alone a tear, suggests that diagnosis of otitis media, exclusively via otoscopy, is not reliable. Bulging of the tympanum may indicate an accumulation of exudate within the middle ear, whereas retraction (and a concave appearance) suggests a partially filled middle ear with obstruction of the auditory tube[5].

Tympanic defects may heal in the presence of infection in the middle ear. Thus, diagnosing otitis media on the sole basis of a ruptured tympanum is unreliable.

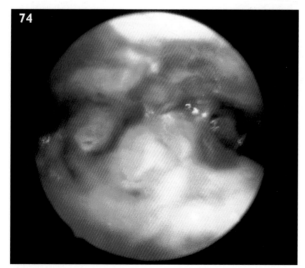

74   Hemorrhagic foci associated with focal ulceration in a case of gram-negative bacterial infection.

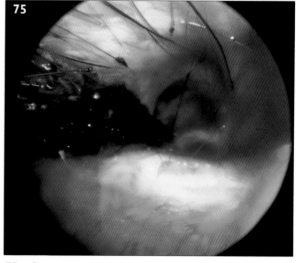

75   Crumbly, dry, blackish brown cerumen associated with *Otodectes cynotis* infestation.

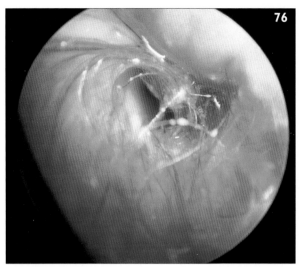

76 Grass awn, cerumen, and associated erythema in the external ear canal of a dog.

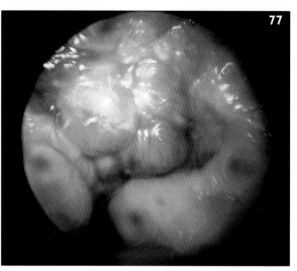

77 Polyp in the external ear canal of a cat.

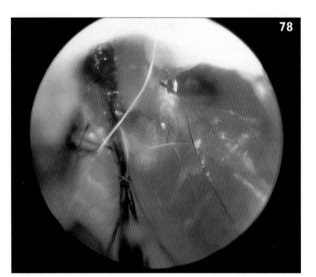

78 Acute tear in the tympanic membrane of a dog associated with grass awn penetration.

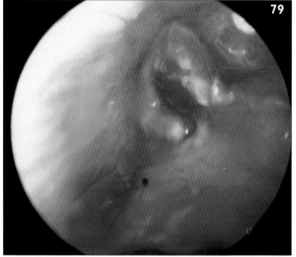

79 Chronic otitis media and otitis externa have resulted in a thickened, opaque, ruptured tympanic membrane.

CYTOLOGIC CHARACTERISTICS OF NORMAL AND ABNORMAL EARS

KEY POINTS
- Cytologic samples should be taken before ear cleaning is undertaken.
- Both external ear canals should be sampled, preferably from the horizontal canal.
- There is no reliable correlation between the physical nature of the discharge and a particular microbe.
- Examination of unstained, oil-mixed cerumen is a reliable method of determining infestation with *Otodectes cynotis*.
- Information on the organisms within the canal and the type and nature of the inflammatory response may be obtained from microscopic examination of stained smears.
- Modified Wright's stains such as Diff-Quik are ideal stains for in-house use.

INTRODUCTION
Otodectic otitis (**80**) is often associated with a crumbly, rather dryish discharge (**81**), similar to coffee grounds[1]. However, there is no clear-cut relationship between the gross characteristics of any otic discharge and the species of microorganism with which it is associated, e.g. staphylococcal, gram-negative, or malassezial[2, 3].

Cytologic examination of otic exudate is a rapid, in-house test which provides diagnostically and

> Cytologic examination of otic discharges should become part of the routine work up in all but the most obvious cases of otitis externa, such as those caused by foreign bodies.

therapeutically useful information[2–5]. In many cases, information from cytologic examination of cerumen is more accurate than that from samples submitted for microbiologic culture and sensitivity testing (*Table 4*). Furthermore, the clinician can assess the significance of any microorganisms in the light of other ceruminal characteristics, such as the presence of nucleated squames, proteinaceous debris, and inflammatory cells. This is particularly exemplified in the case illustrated (**82**) of a Cocker Spaniel with chronic, bilateral otitis associated with a thick, greasy exudate. Gross examination of the discharge (**83, 84**) might suggest that a malassezial, or even a gram-negative, infection was responsible but cytologic examination (**85**) does not support this. Although there are increased numbers of squames and microbes visible, the lack of any inflammatory cells suggests a ceruminous otitis externa, probably associated with a more generalized defect in keratinization, rather than infection.

Table 4: Sensitivity and specificity of cytologic examination versus culture and sensitivity of selected Classes of microbes recovered from the external ear canals of dogs[3].

Class of microbe	Cytology	Culture and sensitivity
Gram-positive cocci		
Sensitivity	84%	59%
Specificity	100%	100%
Gram-negative rods		
Sensitivity	100%	69%
Specificity	100%	100%
Yeast		
Sensitivity	100%	50%
Specificity	100%	100%

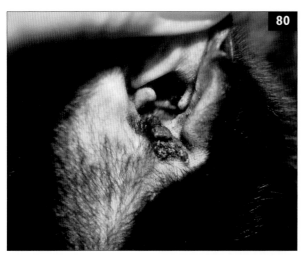

80 Typical appearance of cerumen associated with *Otodectes cynotis* – dark, dry, and crumbly. As in this case, it is not always associated with inflammation in the ear canal.

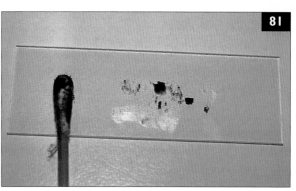

81 The dry, crumbly nature of the cerumen can be appreciated when it is rolled onto a glass slide.

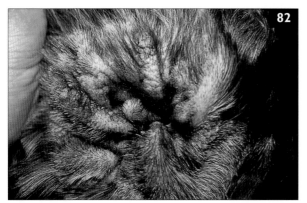

82 External ear canal of a Cocker Spaniel with chronic otitis externa.

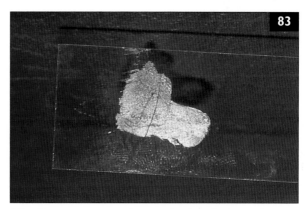

83 Gross appearance of an unstained cytologic sample – thick and white.

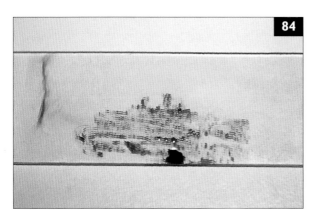

84 Gross appearance of a Diff-Quik-stained sample – thick and blue, suggestive of a high cell content.

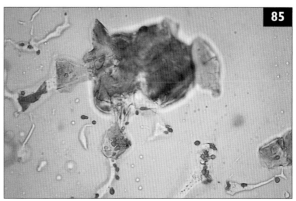

85 High-power photomicrograph from the Cocker Spaniel in **82**. Note the yeast and cocci on and around the squames, and the absence of inflammatory cells.

SAMPLES AND STAINS

The most useful sample for otic cytology is a swab taken from the ear canal which is then rolled onto a clean glass slide. If feasible, samples should be taken from the horizontal portion of the external ear canal of both ears[4, 5]. In large dogs it is usually possible to collect a shielded sample using, for example, an alcohol-sprayed otoscope cone. In small dogs and cats collecting a shielded sample is difficult and vertical canal samples will have to suffice[5]. If otitis media is suspected, a shielded sample should be taken from the middle ear in addition to that from the external ear canal.

Most clinicians advocate using modified Wright's stains such as Diff-Quik[1, 4]. Alcohol-based stains are more useful than aqueous preparations (e.g. new methylene blue) because of the lipid nature of the otic discharge[4]. Griffin[1] advocated heat fixing of obviously waxy preparations in order to prevent solvent-associated leaching of lipid. Since all cerumen contains lipid it would seem appropriate to heat fix all samples, but opinion is divided on this issue[4–6]. Subtle information may be lost if heat fixing is not performed, but generally it is not necessary unless samples are to be kept for future examination. Commercial laboratories usually perform a Gram's stain because although more time consuming, it does allow assessment of the classification of organisms by both morphology (coccus, rod, diphtheroid) and Gram's stain status. Generally, Gram staining is too cumbersome and time consuming for practitioners to consider it as a rapid, in-house stain[6].

Knowledge of morphology and Gram's stain status allows a recommendation for treatment[1, 4]. In addition

> Cytologic examination of gram-stained smears of cerumen has proved to be more sensitive in detecting microorganisms within the external canal than culture[2,3,4,7].

to allowing visualization of the microbial populations of the external ear canal, cytology also allows the physical nature of the cerumen to be assessed, in terms of keratinaceous debris and the lipid content of the cerumen[7, 8].

Stained samples should be air-dried and examined for evenness of stain and for depth of stain, which is usually deeper in intensity as the cell count increases. A coverslip should be applied prior to microscopic examination[5]. Initial low-power examination is followed by high power examination, and this is usually sufficient for accurate classification of any microorganisms and identification of any cells present[5, 6].

GROSS EXAMINATION OF CYTOLOGIC PREPARATIONS

Gross examination of fresh and stained smears reflects the lipid and cellular content of cerumen. Normal cerumen has a high lipid content and a low concentration of intact cells, usually squames. Unstained preparations are all but invisible in direct light (**86**) reflecting the low cell content of cerumen. Increasing cell content, particularly if it is inflammatory in nature, is reflected in the increased opacity of the cerumen.

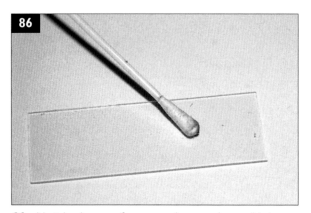

86   Unstained smears from normal ear canals are all but invisible.

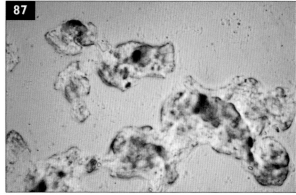

87   Photomicrograph of a cytologic sample from a normal ear. Note the low cell content in the cerumen.

NORMAL CYTOLOGIC CHARACTERISTICS

Cerumen does not take up stain because of its high lipid content (**87**), although ghost outlines of lipid droplets may be seen occasionally (**88**). Low numbers of anucleate, epithelial cells may be detected, although in normal ears they are not excessive (**89**). When there is inflammation of the epithelial lining of the external ear canal the rate of cellular turnover increases and nucleated squames may be seen in the cerumen (**90**). Low numbers of *Malassezia pachydermatis* and staphylococci may be identified adhering to shed squames (**91, 92**). Leucocytes are usually absent from normal cerumen[4].

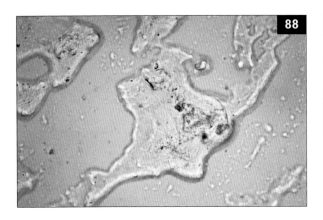

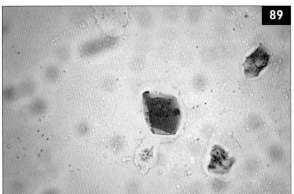

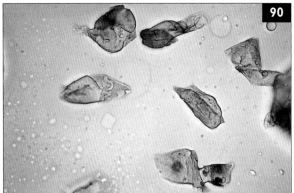

88 Outlines of lipid are visible, even after fixing and staining with Diff-Quik.

89 Photomicrograph of a cytologic sample from a normal ear, with a few squames apparent.

90 Photomicrograph demonstrating increased numbers of squames, some of which are nucleated.

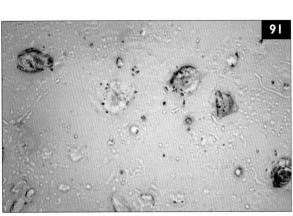

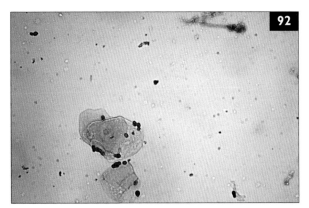

91 Photomicrograph demonstrating a few anucleate squames with a few staphylococci apparent.

92 Photomicrograph demonstrating a few anucleate squames with low numbers of yeast apparent.

ABNORMAL CYTOLOGIC CHARACTERISTICS
Cerumen
The lipid content of cerumen from inflamed external ear canals is lower and the cell count is usually higher than that in normal ear canals[8]. This is reflected in the gross appearance of the stained smear, which appears bluer in a sample from an otitic ear (**93**) than in that from a normal ear (**94**).

Keratinocytes
In acute cases of otitis externa, or cases of very short duration, there will be very little change in the epithelial shedding of squames. In chronic cases, such as those associated with defects in keratinization or atopy, the epithelial lining of the external ear canal reacts to the inflammation and the hyperplasia may result in the appearance of both anucleate and nucleated squames and debris (**95**).

Autoimmune disorders, in particular pemphigus foliaceus, may result in acantholysis. Single, nucleated, well-defined acanthocytes may be shed from erosions in the ear canal, often surrounded by adherent neutrophils (**96**), i.e. a positive Tzank test.

Inflammatory cells
In samples taken from dogs and cats with acute otitis externa there may be little change in the cellular population, but in most cases there will be neutrophils and proteinaceous debris (**97**). More chronic otitis results in the appearance of macrophages as well as neutrophils within the exudate[5]. In cases of bacterial otitis the increasing concentration of toxins may result in the appearance of toxic neutrophils (**98**) and indicate that the

> Abnormal cytologic samples from ear canals may reflect aberrations in lipid content, squame characteristics, and the inflammatory cell population, and in changes in the microflora.

external ear canal should be flushed before treatment is initiated[1].

Neoplastic cells
Intraluminal neoplasms may shed cells into the cerumen but it is unusual to find diagnostically useful material in this discharge[9]. Cells from adenocarcinomas tend to exfoliate in sheets or clusters, whereas squamous cell carcinomas shed large, densely-staining individual cells with prominent nucleoli[5].

Bacteria
The normal microbial population of the ear canal is dominated by staphylococci. In the early stages of otic inflammation the numbers of staphylococci increase, particularly the numbers of *Staphylococcus intermedius* (**99**).

Care should be taken when pronouncing that staphylococci are present in cerumen or on the squames, as cocci may be confused with:
- Debris in poorly-maintained Diff-Quik (filter the stain regularly).
- Or with pigment granules within the squames (melanin granules are usually brown in color rather than the blue-black color of staphylococci).

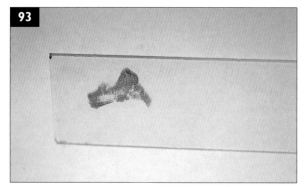

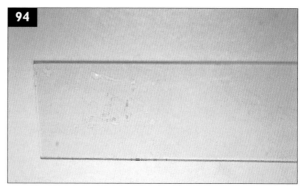

93, 94 Gross cytologic samples from an otitic and a normal ear canal. The otitic ear (**93**) contains a higher cell content and appears much bluer, when stained, than the smear from the normal ear (**94**).

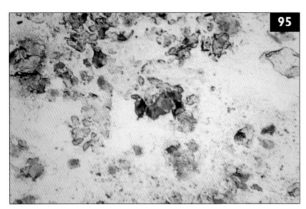

95   Photomicrograph from an acute case of otitis externa. There are anucleate and nucleated squames present.

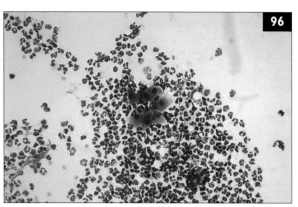

96   Photomicrograph of a stained smear from a pustule in a case of pemphigus foliaceus. Compare the 'clean' neutrophils and rounded-up, nucleated squames in this Tzank test-positive smear with the cells and neutrophils in **97** and **98**.

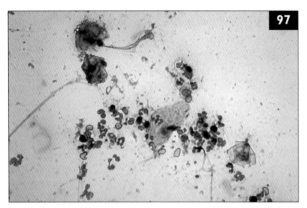

97   Photomicrograph of a small group of squames with surrounding neutrophils.

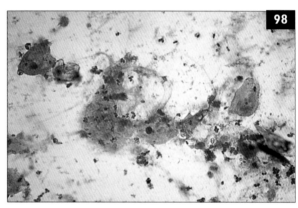

98   Photomicrograph illustrating squames, proteinaceous debris, and dark, pyknotic neutrophils.

99   Photomicrograph of a dense group of cells with large numbers of staphylococci apparent.

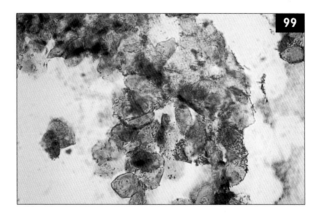

Occasionally the otic flora remains staphylococcal in nature but most commonly it becomes dominated by gram-negative bacilli, in particular *Escherichia coli*, *Proteus* spp., and *Pseudomonas* spp. These changes in bacterial shape (i.e. coccoid to rod) are easily detected by microscopic examination of cytologic samples (**100**)[5, 6]. Cocci cannot be reliably classified as either staphylococci or streptococci on the basis of clumping or chain formation, respectively, since this is not usually observed[4]. With experience, clinicians may be able to detect that staphylococci are larger than streptococci[4].

Generally, even in first opinion cases, the observation of bacilli should prompt sampling for bacterial culture and sensitivity testing[4]. This is particularly important if Gram's staining is not performed, since clinicians cannot differentiate *Pseudomonas* spp. from *Clostridium* spp. or *Bacillus* spp.[4]. Unless a recurrent case is involved it is not usually necessary to submit samples from otitis externa associated with cocci for bacterial culture and sensitivity testing. Indeed, in one study[7] testing achieved a sensitivity of 59% for gram-positive cocci and 69% for gram-negative rods, compared with 100% sensitivity with cytologic examination (*Table 4*).

Yeast

Malassezia pachydermatis is a member of the normal canine otic microflora[10], although it has the potential for opportunistic pathogenicity. At least two species of malassezial yeast can be isolated from feline ear canals, *M. pachydermatis* and *M. sympodialis*[11]. The presence of yeast (**101**) must, therefore, be interpreted with caution. Evidence of increased numbers of yeast (arbitrarily more than 5 to 10 per high-power field [**102**][1, 4, 5]) and an associated inflammatory reaction (**103**) should be sought before disease status is decided. Malassezial yeast are flask or peanut-shaped whereas candidial yeast are round in appearance, although this distinction is not easily made.

The importance of cytologic evaluation was exemplified in two studies which reported that demonstration of malassezial infection by cultural methods achieved a sensitivity of 82% and 50% respectively[1, 7]. In addition to relative insensitivity, malassezial culture is expensive and time consuming, resulting in unnecessary cost and delay in treatment compared to cytologic assessment[2].

Ectoparasites

It is often easy to visualize *Otodectes cynotis* within the external ear canal simply by using an otoscope. However, since very low numbers of mites have been associated with otitis externa[12] it is not surprising that they will be missed in some cases, particularly if there is an accumulation of debris or discharge within the canal. Therefore, microscopic examination of cytologic preparations is indicated if otodectic mange is suspected. Cerumen is deposited on a glass slide and mixed with mineral oil prior to microscopic examination[2]. Otodectic mites have a characteristic appearance (**104, 105**).

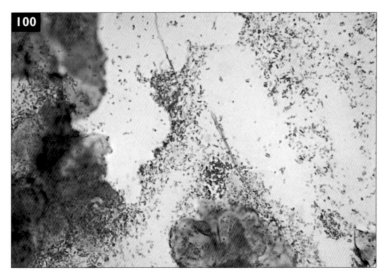

100 Photomicrograph illustrating squames and vast numbers of bacilli.

101 Photomicrograph illustrating yeast.

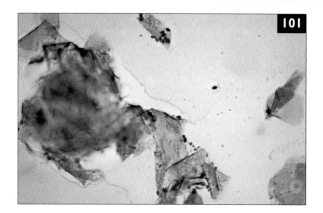

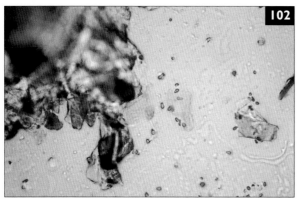

102 Photomicrograph illustrating yeast in sufficient numbers to be associated with disease.

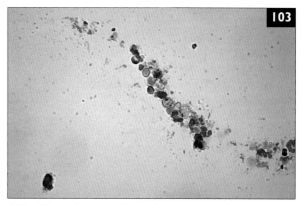

103 Photomicrograph illustrating yeast and inflammatory cells.

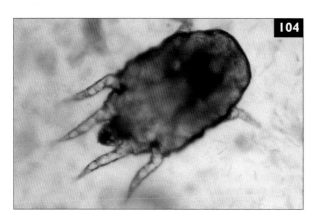

104 Photomicrograph of an adult otodectic mite.

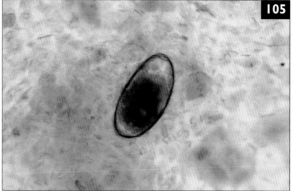

105 Photomicrograph of an ovum recovered from the cerumen of an ear infected with *Otodectes cynotis*.

NEUROLOGIC EXAMINATION OF THE EAR

KEY POINTS
- The neurologic examination of the ear is complicated by the multiplicity of sensory and motor innervation.
- Meaningful assessment of the sense of hearing is extremely difficult without the use of complex equipment.

SENSORY AND MOTOR FUNCTION OF THE PINNA AND THE EXTERNAL EAR CANAL
Sensory function
The sensory innervation of the external ear canal is extremely complex and involves multiple nerves. Evaluation of the sensory innervation of the pinna and external ear canal is dependent on a knowledge of the extensive overlap in sensory field that exists between various cutaneous nerves as well as the role these cutaneous afferents play in eliciting the pinna reflex (**106–111**).

The convex surface of the pinna is innervated by:
- Branches of the second cervical nerve (**107**):
  - The dorsal cutaneous branch of the second cervical nerve;
  - The great auricular nerve (a branch of the ventral cutaneous branch of C2).
- Branches of the trigeminal nerves (**106**)[1]:
  - The third cervical nerve;
  - The mandibular branch of the trigeminal nerve (**111**).

The concave surface of the pinna is innervated by:
- Branches of the facial nerve:
  - Middle internal auricular branch of the facial nerve (**108**);
  - Lateral internal auricular branch of the facial nerve;
  - Caudal internal auricular branch of the facial nerve (**109**).
- The second cervical nerve[1].

The horizontal canal is innervated by:
- A branch of the facial nerve (lateral internal auricular branch)[2].

The proximal part of the external acoustic meatus and the tympanum is innervated by:
- The auriculotemporal nerve (from the mandibular branch of the trigeminal nerve)[3].

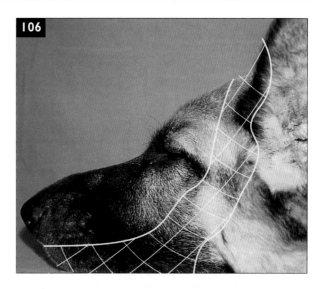

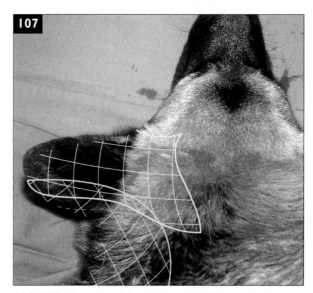

106, 107 Lateral and dorsal views of a German Shepherd Dog marked up to illustrate the principal areas of innervation of the convex aspect of the pinna. Note that the central portion is innervated by branches of the cervical nerve. Overlap zones occur at the free edges. **106** Mandibular branch of the trigeminal nerve. **107** Greater auricular nerve (caudal part of the pinna) and greater occipital nerve (both from the second cervical nerve) innervating the rostral part of the pinna.

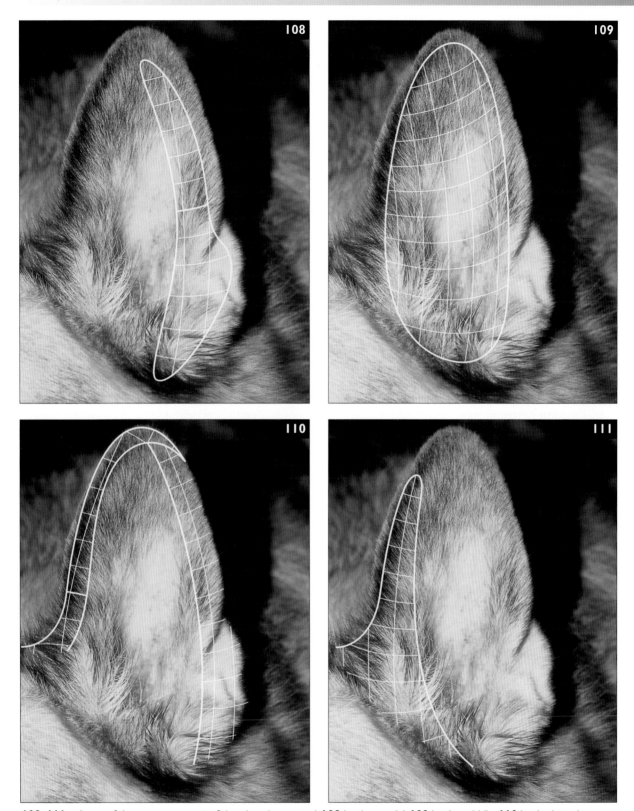

108–111 Areas of the concave aspect of the pinna innervated: **108** by the caudal, **109** by the middle, **110** by the lateral internal auricular branches of the facial nerve, **111** by the mandibular branch of the trigeminal nerve. Note that the central portion is innervated by other branches of the facial nerve. Overlap zones occur at the free edges.

Motor function

The facial nerve provides motor innervation for all of the muscles of the external ear[3] and represents the efferent limb of the pinnal reflex.

A branch of the mandibular branch of the trigeminal nerve innervates the tensor tympani muscle. It is this muscle which is responsible for maintaining the tension of the tympanic membrane as it vibrates in response to sound waves.

The stapedial branch of the facial nerve innervates the stapedius muscle, which is responsible for reducing movement of the stapes ossicle[3].

Assessing the sensory and motor innervation of the pinna and the external ear canal

The pinnal reflex

Gentle pinpoint stimulation of the convex or concave surface of the pinna with a blunt instrument (such as an artery forceps) elicits a twitch of the pinna – a test of sensory innervation. Stimulation of the central portion of the pinna on the convex surface tests the 2nd cervical nerve reflex while stimulation on the concave surface tests the facial nerve. Attempting to interpret this reflex by stimulating the cranial or the caudal margin of the pinna is inadvisable because of the overlap of different cutaneous nerves[1].

The motor function of the ear is evaluated by the pinnal reflex. It can also be evaluated by the Preyer's reflex which is manifested by a twitch of both pinnae in response to any auditory stimuli. However, care must be taken to interpret the absence of reflex due to bilateral deafness as a bilateral paralysis of the facial nerve.

NB: The pinnal scratch reflex is a pathologic sign which must not be confused with the pinnal reflex. Rubbing the tip of the pinna between finger and thumb elicits a vigorous scratch reflex in the ipsilateral hindlimb, particularly in dogs with scabies or pediculosis. This reflex is not pathognomonic but it is highly reliable.

Assessing the sense of hearing

Evaluation of the sense of hearing during a physical examination is dependent upon behavioral reactions to sound and it is therefore subject to misinterpretation. Crude assessment involves startling the animal with a loud noise such as a clap or a whistle[4]. The only objective means of evaluating the hearing ability in animals is based on electrophysiologic assessment of electric potentials triggered along the auditory pathway by an audible stimulus such as a click. The equipment used consists of a signal-averaging computer recording the response of the brainstem time, locked with the stimulus. The test is called brainstem auditory evoked responses (BAER) or potentials (BAEP). BAER not only detects auditory deficits but it may also indicate the location of the lesion[4] (see Electrophysiologic procedures).

Assessing the sense of balance

Evaluation of the vestibular division of the vestibulocochlear nerve is based on a number of tests such as examination of the posture, gait, and head position, and precise observation of the position and movements of the eyes (physiologic nystagmus) in relation to the position of the head. The animal should be left to ambulate freely in the examination room during initial discussion with the owner; then it should be walked and trotted in straight lines on a lead. The position of the head should be observed carefully at rest and in motion. Physiologic nystagmus should be elicited by gentle oscillation of the head in the horizontal plane in both directions, and the presence of positional strabismus should be evaluated during dorsal extension or ventral flexion of the head (compare with *Table 15* [Comparative neurologic signs of vestibular disease] in Chapter 7: Neurologic signs related to inner ear disease). A complete neurologic examination, including evaluation of proprioception and cranial and spinal segmental reflexes, should be performed in order to establish the presence of vestibular disease and to localize it to either side, and to differentiate peripheral versus central vestibular syndrome (compare with Chapter 7: Neurologic signs related to inner ear disease).

RADIOGRAPHIC FEATURES OF THE NORMAL AND ABNORMAL EAR

KEY POINTS
- Careful positioning is the key to radiographic interpretation of the tympanic bullae.
- The most useful views are the dorsoventral, rostrocaudal (open mouth), and lateral oblique views.
- Given the individual variation between animals, comparison of one side with the other is often the only way of making a diagnosis. Therefore, perfect positioning is essential.

INTRODUCTION
Radiographic examination is a useful tool in the investigation of ear disease in both the dog and the cat. Principally, it is utilized for the diagnosis of disease affecting the middle ear, although there are some indications for radiographic examination of the external ear canal.

The radiological anatomy of the petrous temporal bones, and the associated components of the middle ear, is complex and subject both to breed and individual variation, particularly in the dog[1-5]. Consequently, a thorough knowledge of the spatial relationships between the skull and the ear is essential if the radiographs are to be interpreted correctly[3]. However, pathologic changes to the region are unlikely to be symmetrical. Thus, provided a good quality, symmetrical radiographic image is obtained, useful information may be acquired by comparing one side with the other[2, 3]. *Table 5* summarizes the most common radiographic changes seen with external and middle ear disease.

> The key to successful radiological diagnosis of ear disease is the positioning of the animal for radiography[3].

Table 5: Summary of the radiographic changes associated with clinical pathology in the external and middle ear[4, 7, 8, 9, 11].

Condition	Increased soft tissue opacity	Sclerosis and thickening of the bulla wall*	Lysis of the bulla wall	Sclerosis, thickening, or lysis of the petrous temporal bone	Calcification of the external ear canals
Otitis externa	++	–	–	–	+
Otitis media	++	+	+/-	+	+
Otitis media associated with osteomyelitis	+	+/–	++	+	–
Neoplasia of the middle or external ear	++	+/–	+++	+	–
Inflammatory polyp	++	+	–		–

* Bilateral sclerosis and thickening of the bulla wall is normal in elderly cats

NORMAL RADIOGRAPHIC FEATURES
NB:

- Dolichocephalic (or oligocephalic) heads are long and narrow, e.g. as in the Rough Collie or Saluki.
- Mesaticephalic heads are more rounded, e.g. as in the Doberman Pinscher or Labrador Retriever.
- Brachycephalic heads are short and wide, e.g. as in the English Bulldog and the Pekingese.

Any one of several radiographic views will provide information on the middle ear but no one view can provide a complete picture. Therefore, at least two different radiograph views must be included in any radiographic investigation. The three most frequently used radiographic views are the lateral oblique, the dorsoventral, and the rostrocaudal (open mouth) views. Lateral and ventrodorsal views may occasionally be required.

Lateral oblique view (112, 113)
Advantages. Good visualization of the tympanic bulla and petrous temporal bone.

Disadvantages. General anesthesia is necessary. Only one bulla can be visualized at a time. Not easily repeatable, even in the same animal, so side-to-side comparison is difficult[6].

Positioning. The animal is placed in lateral recumbency with the head parallel to the film and the bulla of interest nearest the to film. The jaw should be closed. Either the head is rotated around this long axis until the sagittal plane lies at about 20° to the horizontal, the bulla to be radiographed remaining ventral, or the nose is elevated some 15–20% to achieve separation of the bullae on the plate[6]. The beam should be centered to the base of the ear to project the bulla clear of other structures.

Interpretation. The bullae appear as thin-walled, crisply outlined bone structures with a smooth external border (**114, 115**)[7]. Air shadow should be visible in the external ear canal[7]. Predominantly lytic changes on the rostroventral wall of the bulla are usually associated with chronic inflammation[7]. Lytic changes within the petrous temporal bone may reflect either inflammation or neoplasia[7, 8].

Rostrocaudal (open mouth) view (116, 117)
Advantages. Good visualization of both tympanic bullae. Good view for diagnosing otitis media[4, 9].

Disadvantages. General anesthesia is necessary and the endotracheal tube must be removed. Can be difficult to obtain perfect pictures without fine-tuning, especially with brachycephalic breeds.

Positioning. The animal must be in dorsal recumbency. The head is positioned with the sagittal plane and hard palate vertical to the film. The tongue must be brought as far forward as possible and tied to the mandible with tape[8]. The interpupillary line must be parallel to the film. In dolichocephalic breeds the primary beam is centered through the open mouth parallel to the hard palate[5]. In mesaticephalic breeds it may be necessary to angle the hard palate slightly away from the vertical (perhaps 10° or so[4]). In brachycephalic breeds the hard palate may need to be angled up to 20° away from the vertical in order to avoid superimposing the bullae on the wings of the atlas[5]. Alternatively, the center of the beam can be angled rostrocaudally, at up to 30° angling towards the hard palate. The beam can be centered on the base of the tongue[10].

Interpretation. The bullae appear as thin-walled, symmetrical bone opacities at the base of the skull (**118**)[7]. Overlying soft tissues may produce the appearance of middle ear pathology. This must be interpreted with care.

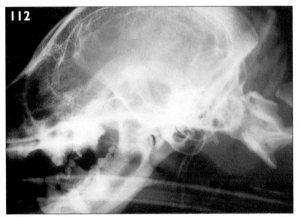
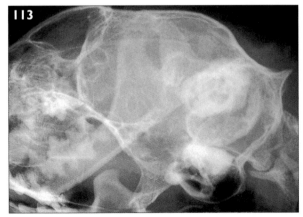

112, 113 Lateral oblique radiographs of the head of a dog (**112**) and a cat (**113**) demonstrating optimal positioning for visualizing the tympanic bullae, which are clearly visible.

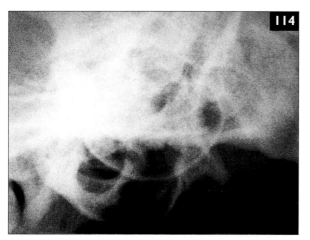

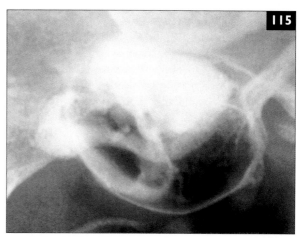

114, 115   Close ups of the normal tympanic bullae of a dog (**114**) and a cat (**115**) in the lateral oblique view.

116, 117   Rostrocaudal (open mouth) radiographs of the head of a dog (**116**) and a cat (**117**) demonstrating how the tympanic bullae are skylined.

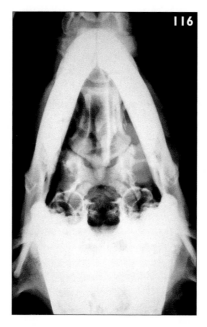

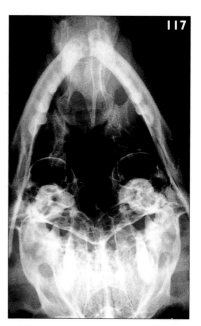

118   Close-up rostrocaudal (open mouth) view of the tympanic bullae of a cat. Near perfect positioning is important for this view as one is looking for subtle changes that may only be apparent by comparing one side with the other.

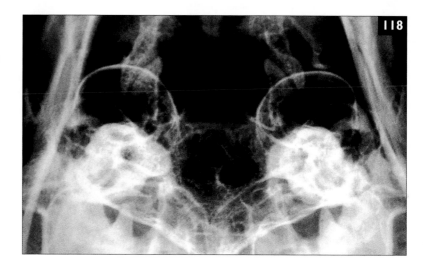

Dorsoventral view (119, 120)

Advantages. Anesthesia may not be necessary, although in most cases it will allow better positioning. In some patients sedation may suffice. It is easier to achieve good bilateral symmetry with this view than with the ventrodorsal view, as the mandibles provide stability against lateral rotation[6]. Good view for diagnosing otitis media[4].

Disadvantages. Because the calvarium is further from the plate it is magnified and this can induce some artefactual distortion[6]. However, this is more than outweighed by the advantage of having the bullae close to the plate.

Positioning. The animal is placed in ventral recumbency, under general anesthesia or heavy sedation. Care must be taken to ensure that the animal is aligned symmetrically with the interpupillary line parallel to the film[6]. The hard palate must be parallel to the table and the animal adjusted so that the base of the skull is as close to the film as possible[6]. This may require support with radiolucent blocks of foam under the rostral mandible or sandbags over the cervical spine, or both. The beam should be centered at the intersection of two imaginary lines: a sagittal line, and a lateral line, at right angles to the sagittal line, drawn through the estimated position of the tympanic membranes.

Interpretation. The bullae should exhibit bilateral symmetry and appear as fine, crisp, distinct, linear bony opacities[7]. Some distortion and masking may occur due to superimposition of the petrous temporal bones[6]. Air shadow should be visible in the external ear canals.

Lateral view (121, 122)

Advantages. Standard view; lots of reference material.

Disadvantages. General anesthesia is necessary. Not ideal for visualizing individual tympanic bullae as they are superimposed if a true lateral position is achieved.

Positioning. Place the animal in lateral recumbency and adjust the head to true lateral with the sagittal plane parallel to the film and the interpupillary line vertical[6]. This may require foam padding to achieve a true lateral. The calvarium, nasal pharynx, and larynx should be included in the view. The beam should be centered between the ear and the eye.

Interpretation. The bullae appear as thin-walled, crisply outlined bony structures with a smooth external border (**123, 124**), but in a true lateral view they will be superimposed, making for difficult interpretation[6]. Air shadow and, if present, the thickened walls of the horizontal ear canal may be visible[6].

Ventrodorsal view (125, 126)

Advantages. Standard view; lots of reference material. Good view for diagnosing otitis media[4].

Disadvantages. Requires general anesthesia. This position is not suitable for brachycephalic breeds[5]. The sagittal crest tends to make the skull fall laterally, making exact positioning difficult[6].

Positioning. The animal is placed in dorsal recumbency, under general anesthesia. Care must be taken to ensure that the animal is aligned symmetrically. The hard palate must be parallel to the table. This may require support under the rostral mandible or under the cervical spine, or both. Intraoral tape, positioned immediately caudal to the canine teeth and then tied to the table, may help in positioning the mandible. The beam should be centered at the intersection of two imaginary lines: a sagittal line, and a lateral line, at right angles to the sagittal line, drawn through the estimated position of the tympanic membranes.

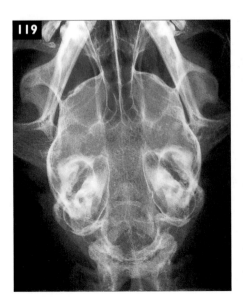
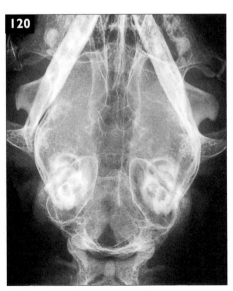

119, 120 Dorsoventral radiographs of the head of a dog (**119**) and a cat (**120**). Note the appearance of the bullae and the difficulty in visualizing them using this position compared with the lateral oblique and rostrocaudal (open mouth) views.

Interpretation. The superimposition of the petrous temporal bones makes the bullae walls appear thicker, and this can make evaluation of subtle changes more difficult. The bulla of the cat contains an additional inner bony wall which appears in this view (**126**)[6].

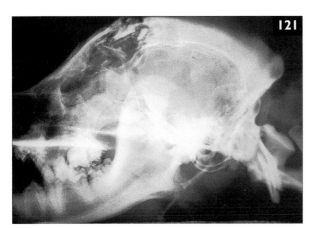

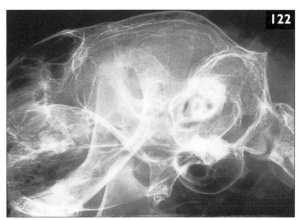

121, 122   Lateral radiographs of the head of a dog (**121**) and a cat (**122**). The bullae are visible but both left and right bullae are superimposed, making interpretation difficult.

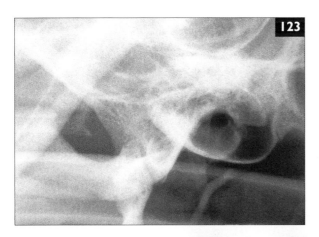

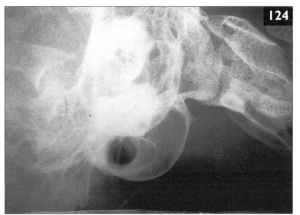

123, 124   Close ups of the tympanic bullae of a dog (**123**) and a cat (**124**) demonstrating the air shadow of the horizontal ear canal.

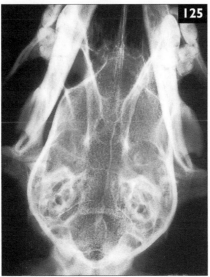

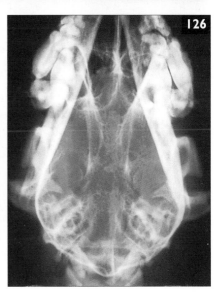

125, 126   Ventrodorsal radiographs of a dog (**125**) and a cat (**126**). Note the appearance of the bullae and the difficulty in visualizing them using this position compared with the lateral oblique and rostrocaudal (open mouth) views.

VISUALIZING THE EXTERNAL EAR CANAL AND ASSESSING THE TYMPANIC MEMBRANE

Radiography is not commonly employed as a means of assessing pathologic changes in the external ear canal. It may be possible to see air shadows (**127, 128**) delineating the external ear canal in some of the standard radiographic views of the ear, particularly the ventrodorsal and rostrocaudal (open mouth) views. In addition, in cases of chronic otitis externa there may be calcification of the cartilages of the external canal (**129–131**). However, it is not possible to assess the integrity of the tympanic membrane or visualize the position of an obstructing luminal neoplasm without using contrast techniques.

Otoscopic and plain radiographic examinations must be performed prior to contrast studies. Significant epidermal hyperplasia or neoplastic proliferation may occlude the lumen to such an extent that adequate distribution of contrast medium is impossible. In addition, the presence of an exudate or mass within the bulla may prevent contrast medium from entering the middle ear. False-negative interpretation may occur if these changes are not identified prior to contrast studies[11].

A standard radiographic contrast medium is used, preferably a non-ionic, water-soluble iodine-based medium rather than an oily medium[11]. The contrast medium may be diluted 50:50 with saline, prior to instilling it into the external ear canal[11]. Care must be taken to ensure that the contrast medium is distributed evenly along the external ear canal and that none contaminates the hair on the surrounding aspects of the head[3, 11]. Gentle massage of the ear canal will ensure an even distribution. Taking care to deliver all the contrast medium into the ear canal, and subsequently plugging the orifice with cotton wool, should prevent soiling of the area around the external ear[3, 11].

Ventrodorsal or, preferably, rostrocaudal (open mouth) radiography will allow evaluation of the lumen of the external ear canal and permit some deductions on the state of the tympanic membrane (**132**)[12]. If contrast medium enters the middle ear (**133**) it is usually visualized as an opacification of the inner wall of the bulla[11], best seen on rostrocaudal (open mouth) views. Failure to detect contrast medium in the bulla should not be interpreted as indicating an intact tympanum.

> It is important to examine the ears otoscopically and radiographically before contrast studies are performed.

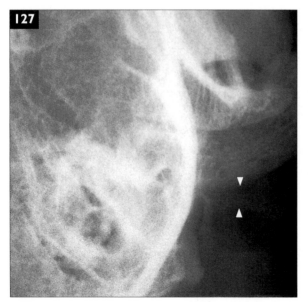

127   Dorsoventral radiograph of a Cairn Terrier with a normal ear. The air shadow within the external ear canal is visible (arrowed).

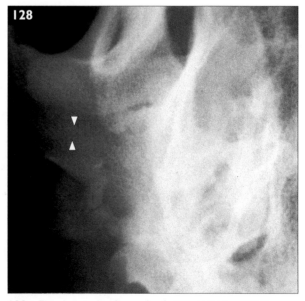

128   Dorsoventral radiograph of a West Highland White Terrier with chronic otitis externa. In this close up of the right side of the skull the narrow ear canal is visible between the thickened walls of the horizontal ear canal (arrowed).

129 Dorsoventral radiograph of an Airedale Terrier showing early signs of calcification of the external ear canal cartilages (arrowed).

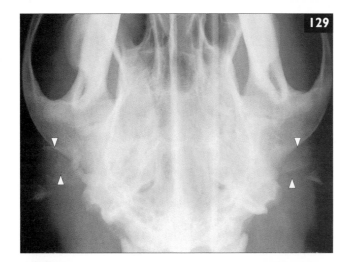

130, 131 Dorsoventral and rostrocaudal open mouth radiographs of a Cocker Spaniel with chronic otitis externa and otitis media. Note the extensive calcification of the ear canal cartilages (arrowheads) and the changes around the left bulla (arrow).

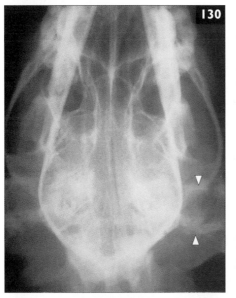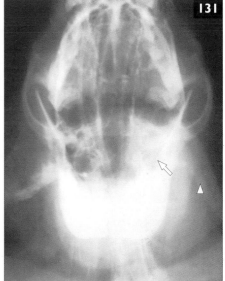

132, 133 Ventrodorsal radiographs demonstrating tympanography. In **132** the tympanum is intact and the concavity is apparent. In **133** the tympanum has been breached and contrast fills the tympanic bulla.

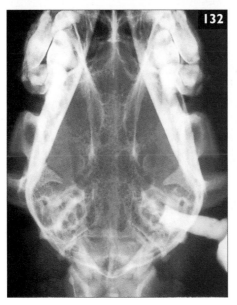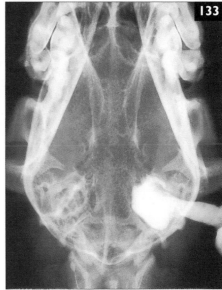

DIAGNOSING OTITIS MEDIA

Although radiography has been shown to be less sensitive than surgery[9] or computed tomography[4] for the diagnosis of otitis media, its importance should not be underestimated. It remains an essential first step in the investigation of ear disease, particularly if surgery is contemplated. Radiography usually underestimates pathologic changes in the middle ear[7], a consequence of the difficulty in interpreting radiographs where superimposition of surrounding tissues takes place and of the minimal radiographic changes associated with early to moderate middle ear pathology.

Radiographs of the normal tympanic bulla show that it has crisp clean lines with no evidence of soft tissue within the bony confines, although air shadow of the external ear canal may be visible in lateral projections (**134**). The radiographic findings associated with otitis media (*Table 5, see page 61*) include[7]:

- Sclerosis and thickening of the wall of the tympanic bulla. Unilateral sclerosis may reflect chronic inflammation or an inflammatory polyp (**135, 136**). Bilateral sclerosis is not uncommon in elderly cats, in bilateral otitis media, in bilateral inflammatory polyps, and in craniomandibular osteoarthropathy.
- Increased soft tissue density within the bulla (**137–140**). This may reflect chronic inflammation, cholesteatoma, or middle ear neoplasia.
- Sclerosis and thickening of the petrous temporal bone.
- Lysis of the wall of the tympanic bulla and petrous temporal bone. This usually reflects inflammation, particularly if predominantly on the ventrocranial aspects of the bulla. Neoplasia must also be a consideration, although it is much less common.

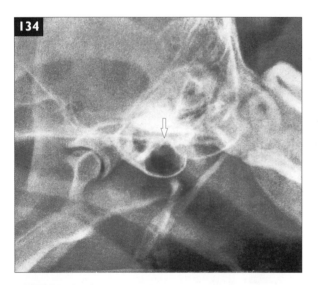

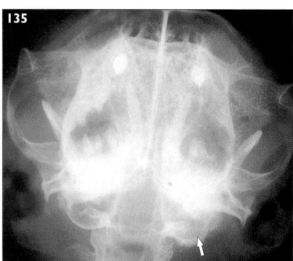

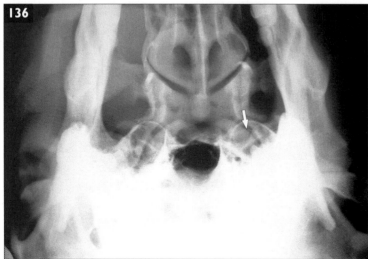

134 Lateral radiograph demonstrating a normal tympanic bulla with air shadow of the external ear canal arrowed.

135 Ten percent ventrodorsal view of a young Himalayan cat with unilateral (left) otitis media. The wall of the affected bulla is thickened (arrow).

136 Rostrocaudal (open mouth) radiograph of a young Hungarian Viszla with unilateral (left) otitis media. Note the increase in thickness in the bony wall of the affected bulla (arrow).

137 Lateral oblique view of the head of a cat with unilateral otitis media secondary to polyp formation. Note the uniform increase in soft tissue density within the bulla.

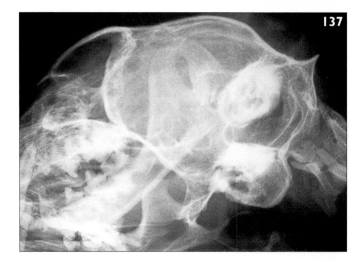

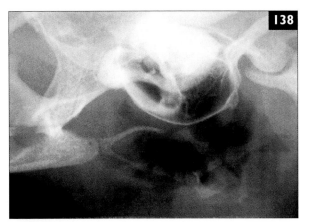 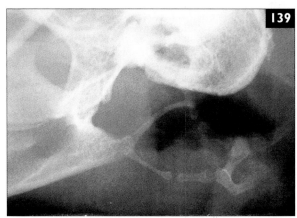

138, 139 Close ups of lateral oblique views of both bullae of the cat radiographed in **137**. Note the clear difference in the density within the bullae.

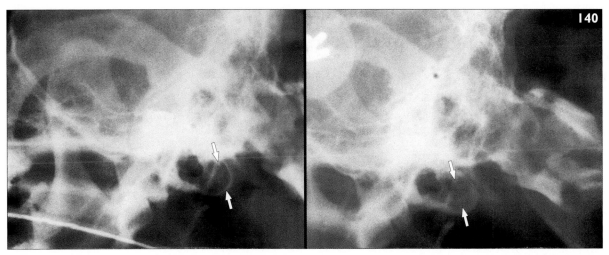

140 Lateral oblique views of the bullae of a Cocker Spaniel with unilateral otitis media. The difference in soft tissue density within the bullae is apparent (arrows).

IMAGING THE MIDDLE AND INNER EARS

KEY POINTS
- Computed tomography (CT) gives better resolution of bony lesions than magnetic resonance imaging (MRI).
- MRI gives better resolution of soft tissue lesions than CT.
- Neither CT nor MRI is likely to replace plain radiography in the diagnosis of external and middle ear disease in clinical practice.

INTRODUCTION
Radiographic examination of the middle ear cannot always demonstrate changes consistent with otitis media, giving false-negative findings compared to surgery in 25–30% of cases[1, 2]. False-positive radiographic findings generally do not occur when compared with surgical diagnosis[1, 2]. In an effort to minimize false-negative results, clinicians and imagers have investigated other techniques, in particular CT and MRI.

COMPUTED TOMOGRAPHY
Computed tomography has a resolution somewhat less than conventional radiography and it takes much longer to perform, in the order of 20–30 minutes[2, 3]. However, by taking repeated, sequential views in the same plane, and then using computed processing, it is possible, digitally, to remove extraneous superimposed structures, permitting visualization of the middle and inner ear[3] (**141, 142**).

Precise positioning and an absolute minimum of movement are prerequisites for CT[3]. Animals are placed in ventral recumbency and they must be under general anesthesia to minimize movement[3]. In one study, which compared CT with radiography in the diagnosis of otitis media[2], CT gave 11% false positives and 17% false negatives (compared to surgical diagnosis), making the technique more sensitive but somewhat less specific than radiography[1]. Neither radiography nor CT was able to detect early changes of otitis media where there was no osseous change.

The authors of one study, which compared radiography with CT in the diagnosis of otitis media, concluded that CT gave too little additional information to justify the additional logistical and financial costs incurred[2].

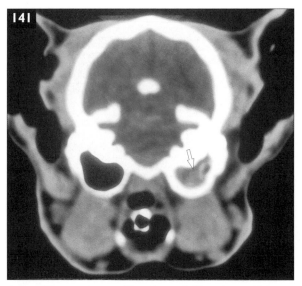

141   CT scan of a cat with otitis media. There is an effusion within the left bulla (arrow).

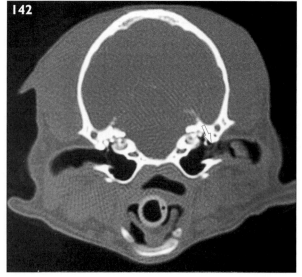

142   CT scan of a dog with a soft tissue mass within the horizontal ear canal. Note that the mass (a neoplasm) has clearly breached the tympanic membrane on the right (arrow).

MAGNETIC RESONANCE IMAGING

Magnetic resonance imaging uses a completely different principle to radiography and CT[4, 5] and the images which result are best regarded as complementary to, rather than replacements for, CT. Thus, CT gives better definition of osseous changes than MRI, whereas the latter gives better definition of soft tissue lesions than CT[6] (**143**).

MRI has been used in the diagnosis of otitis media in dogs, although only one case report exists to date[7]. One experimental study investigated the potential of MRI to assess otitis media in chinchillas and cats[8]. The authors reported superior results using T2-weighted images (requiring a 20 minute scanning/measurement cycle) compared to T1-weighted images (taking about five minutes). In addition, using a contrast agent (gadolinium-diethylenetriaminepentaacetic acid) it was possible to visualize inflamed, swollen middle ear mucosa.

In humans, comparative studies in malignant otitis (a particularly severe *Pseudomonas* spp. infection of the external ear canal) and the fine structure of the temporomandibular joint[6, 9] found that CT was superior for documenting subtle osseous changes whereas MRI was superior in detecting soft tissue aberrations. Furthermore, in a study comparing CT with MRI in detecting osteoid sarcoma it was recommended that MR images should not be interpreted without reference to plain radiographs and CT if serious errors in diagnosis were to be avoided[10].

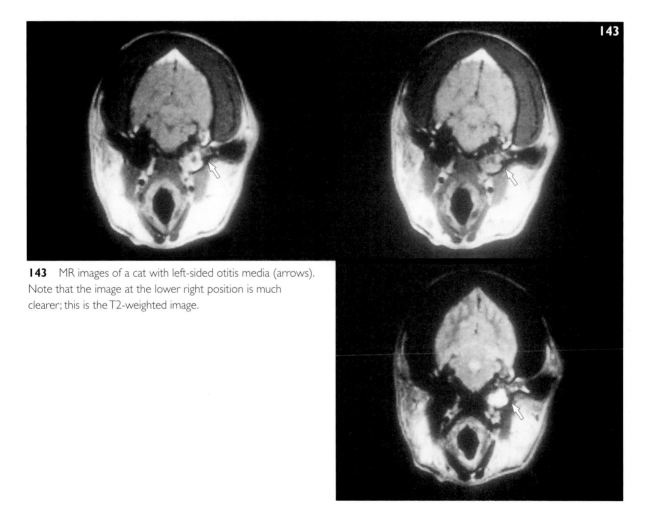

143 MR images of a cat with left-sided otitis media (arrows). Note that the image at the lower right position is much clearer; this is the T2-weighted image.

ELECTROPHYSIOLOGIC PROCEDURES

KEY POINTS
- Electrophysiologic testing is the only objective means of testing the sense of hearing in veterinary species.
- Brainstem auditory evoked response records the neurologic response to sound.
- Tympanometry measures the changes in compliance of the tympanic membrane.

INTRODUCTION
Deafness in a veterinary patient can be frustrating for the clinician because subjective evaluation can be equivocal, particularly when the hearing loss is partial or unilateral. Even bilaterally deaf animals can respond to visual or odoriferous cues, or even vibrations, unbeknown to the person conducting behavioral assessment of the auditory function. For this reason, electrophysiologic testing is the only objective means of testing the sense of hearing in veterinary species.

Both the peripheral and part of the central auditory components can be tested by means of electrophysiologic procedures, including tympanometry, acoustic reflex testing, and auditory evoked responses. These tests are non-invasive and evaluate components of the external ear canal, the middle and inner ear cavities, cranial nerve VIII, and selected areas of the brainstem and cortex. The complete sequence of these procedures will allow differentiation between conductive and sensorineural hearing loss. The great advantage of electrodiagnostic procedures is that they do not require consciousness and they can therefore be performed even in uncooperative animals[1].

BRAINSTEM AUDITORY EVOKED RESPONSE
NB: The physiology of hearing is reviewed in Chapter 8 (Neurologic signs related to inner ear disease).

Theory and technique
Theory
Acoustic stimulation of an ear with a short pulse (click) results in a series of electrical waveforms emanating from structures in the auditory pathways. The wave forms occurring within the first ten minutes after the stimulus are identified as the brainstem auditory evoked response (BAER) or brainstem auditory evoked potential (BAEP), or as short (early) latency auditory potential. This activity can be recorded reliably, with the use of signal-averaging methods, from electrodes attached to various sites on the head. Four or five waves are readily recognized (**144, 145**):
- Wave I reflects activity triggered in the vestibulo-

cochlear nerve in the segment closest to the cochlea.
- Wave II originates from the extramedullary intracranial segment of cranial nerve VIII, with possibly some contribution of the ipsilateral cochlear nucleus.
- Wave III is generated by the dorsal nucleus of the trapezoid body.
- Wave IV originates from the rostral pons by structures of the lateral lemniscus.
- Wave V comes from the caudal colliculus.

The close approximation of these latter generators may explain the overlap between wave IV and wave V[2]. Cochlear microphonics are observed just prior to wave I of the BAER. They are the electrical responses occurring in different parts of the cochlea and are thought to arise from the cuticular surface of the hair cells. They are best seen when the stimulus is a pure tone, and they are affected by the stimulus polarity[3].

A number of non-pathologic factors influence the shape of the potentials obtained. These include mainly the position of the electrodes, the stimulus intensity and its presentation rate and initial phase (rarefaction versus condensation), as well as the subject's body temperature[4]. Body weight and cranium size do not affect wave I but can affect the latency of wave V and the inter-peak latency between waves I and V. It follows that variation in the external auditory canal, middle ear, and inner ear does not significantly contribute to the BAER variability[5]. BAER thresholds are mature by day 20 in both the dog and cat[6]. Other than this, age related changes affecting the BAER are poorly documented.

The amplitude of the waves, measured in V, increases with the stimulus intensity and it is highly variable. The latency of each wave decreases linearly as the acoustic stimulus intensity increases, and decreases in rectal temperature cause a lengthening of the waves' latency[4]. Inter-peak latencies are indicative of conduction time within the brainstem between generator sites and they do not change with the stimulus intensity. They can help to localize the site of deafness along the auditory pathways[2, 7–10]. Normal values for latencies of the peaks and the threshold response have been established for a population of healthy dogs[11].

Whilst the BAER test is non-invasive and painless, some animals are more difficult to restrain than others and chemical restraint may be indicated. However, sedation does not affect any of the BAER parameters and the lack of struggling allows a more precise measurement[11]. Although most anesthetic agents do not affect the characteristic of the BAER components, thiamylal sodium and methoxyflurane have been shown to alter waveform[12] and latencies[13] respectively. Therefore, sedation is preferable to general anesthesia.

Technique

To record the BAER, three small needle electrodes are inserted subcutaneously on the animal's head (**146, 147**). A recording electrode, a reference, and a ground electrode are connected to an amplifying and signal-averaging recording system, ideally coupled with an artefact rejection device. Head phones or ear inserts can be used to produce clicks at various rates of delivery (clicks/second), intensities (dB), and frequencies (Hz)[2, 4]. The acoustic signal which results in the best response is a 'click' with a broad-frequency spectrum in the region of 2–3 kHz. The intensity of the click is most commonly calibrated in decibels (dB) and referred to as the normal hearing level (dB nHL), where 0 dB nHL is the human behavioral hearing threshold in a normal adult population[14].

In animals suspected of suffering from conductive hearing loss, evaluation of the hearing status can be performed with bone-conducted signals. In these cases the BAER is generated with a bone vibrator instead of headphones, in order to bypass the conductive hearing apparatus. However, this technique has limitations. For instance, with bone-conducted BAER the latency of wave V is about 0.5 milliseconds longer at intensities similar to air-conducted BAER, and the maximum acoustic output from a bone vibrator is less than that

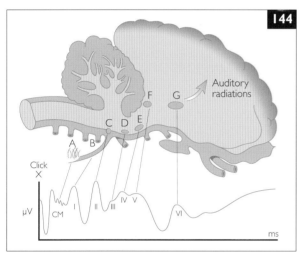

144 Diagram of BAER generators. (Adapted from Mayhew IG and Washbourne JR (1990) A method of assessing auditory function in horses. *British Veterinary Journal* **146**, 509–518, with permission.)

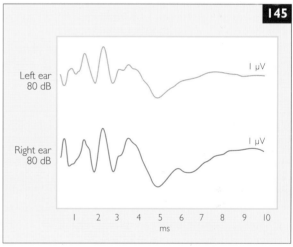

145 Normal BAER in both ears; the wave forms from each ear are similar and both are clearly similar to the stylized diagram in **144**.

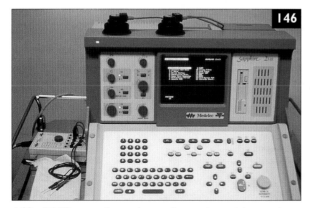

146 BAER generating and recording equipment is complex and bulky.

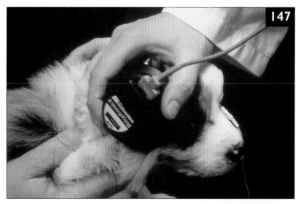

147 Placement of BAER electrodes on a Border Collie pup.

of a click or a tone[15]. In a study by Wolschrijn *et al.*[16] the mean threshold for bone-conducted stimulus was found to vary between 50 and 60 dB whilst the air-conducted threshold in the same population of healthy dogs was 0–10 dB[6]. Bone-conduction thresholds do not just measure inner ear function; sound applied to the skull is transmitted to the cochlea via bone but also via the external auditory canal and the ossicles[16]. Nevertheless, wave forms and inter-peak latencies of the BAER elicited by bone-conducted stimuli and air-conducted stimuli are similar, indicating that the signals have the same origin[16].

Pathologic findings

Reduced hearing/otitis externa and otitis media

In a group of dogs with clinically reduced hearing, no changes in the wave latencies were observed. However, the most striking feature was a decrement in the amplitudes of waves I and II[17]. Following simulation of damage to the external ear canal and tympanic membrane associated with otitis externa, Steiss *et al.*[15] reported that moderate changes, such as stenosis of the ear canal and single puncture of the tympanic membrane, did not alter the BAER thresholds or latencies in a significant manner, nor did more significant damage to the tympanic membrane. Other authors have reported that severe otitis externa and/or otitis media rarely causes complete deafness, but often results in severe conductive hearing loss. This hearing loss can be improved measurably by cleaning the affected ear canal, indicating the profound effect of debris present in the external acoustic meatus[18]. However, if the ossicular chain is interrupted, a more severe loss of 30–40 dB can be expected[15].

BAERs are also used to assess auditory function before and after surgical correction of chronic otitis externa with total ear canal ablation (TECA), with or without ventral or lateral bulla osteotomy (V/LBO). Krahwinkel *et al.*[19] reported that although dogs with severe otitis externa already have greatly compromised auditory function (as reflected by prolonged BAER latencies and low amplitudes), TECA and V/LBO can further decrease auditory function as assessed by BAER.

Presbycusis

In a group of aged cats, peripheral auditory dysfunction was evidenced by consistent elevation in the BAER thresholds to click stimuli. The BAER waveforms were essentially normal, suggesting that the stimulus was effectively transmitted to the appropriate BAER generators. A decreasing trend in the BAER amplitude was observed but was not found to be statistically significant[20].

Deafness

Deafness due to ageing or to a congenital abnormality of the cochlea and/or cranial nerve VIII results in total absence of recognizable recordings (isoelectric tracing)[17] (**148, 149**).

Ototoxicity

Cochlear nerve destruction and aminoglycoside intoxication have been reported to abolish all neural components of the BAER[8, 17]. In the case of neomycin sulphate intoxication, waveform loss is reported to occur between 22 and 50 days after initiation of the treatment and it is permanent[21].

Brainstem lesions

The predominant effect of brainstem lesions on the BAER is an attenuation of the amplitudes of the components and only an occasional increase in their latency[8].

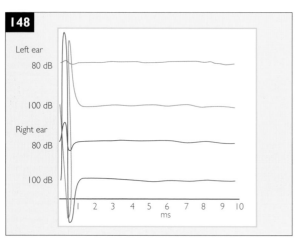

148 BAER trace of a dog with bilateral deafness.

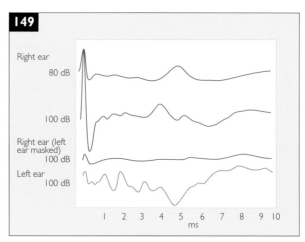

149 BAER trace from a dog with unilateral (right ear) deafness.

TYMPANOMETRY

Tympanometry is the study of changes in compliance of the tympanic membrane which occur as pressure within the external ear canal is changed[22]. Impedance audiometry is based on the principle that the intensity of a sound wave is dependent upon the size of the cavity within which it is generated, and on the compliance or stiffness of the containing walls. Tympanometry, using impedance audiometry, is a non-invasive, objective, reliable method of assessing the integrity of the tympanic membrane[22]. The technique of impedance audiometry can also be used to gain other information; for example, to assess the presence or absence of effusion within the middle ear.

There are no purpose-built veterinary kits for impedance audiometry and the clinician must adapt those designed for humans if tympanometry is to be practised. Essentially, the external ear canal is blocked with an inflatable cuff through which passes a sound probe, a pressure probe, and a microphone. Tympanometry measures the change in compliance of the tympanum as pressure within the occluded external ear canal changes when a sound tone is generated. In a normal ear the rigid sheet of the tympanum behaves differently compared to when there is a ruptured tympanic membrane, and this difference is detected and displayed (**150a–c**).

Tympanometry can be performed in conscious dogs[22] and can provide useful information in terms of indicating whether investigation for otitis media is warranted. Also, tympanometry may impact on the selection of otic medication, since some medications are contraindicated in the presence of a ruptured tympanic membrane[23].

In addition to the logistical problems of sourcing and adapting equipment for canine use, there are some technical problems facing the operator (Dr J Steiss, personal communication):

- The angle between the vertical ear canal and the horizontal ear canal makes aligning the equipment difficult. It is also difficult to achieve a good seal between the cuff and the wall of the vertical canal.
- The sound wave must impact squarely upon the tympanic membrane. Again, the angle between the vertical and the horizontal canal makes this difficult to achieve.

These logistical and technical problems make tympanometry primarily a research tool which is unlikely to be of value to practitioners.

ACOUSTIC (STAPEDIAL) REFLEX TEST AND ACOUSTIC DECAY TEST

When a sufficiently large sound is detected by the ear the stapedius muscle contracts, purportedly to protect the delicate inner ear from the damaging effects of transmitting sound waves of very high amplitude. Using impedance audiometry it is possible to detect this reflex via the sudden contraction of the stapedius muscle, which affects the tension within the tympanum[24]. This information can help to indicate whether one, or both, middle ears are functioning normally.

If the threshold for the acoustic reflex is identified, a signal some 10 dB above the threshold is given for a period of ten seconds[24]. In normal animals, and in animals with cochlear lesions, the reflex should be maintained for the entire test period. In some conditions affecting the function of cranial VIII there is a characteristic decay of the reflex, within the ten-second test period. Reference values for the dog have been published recently.

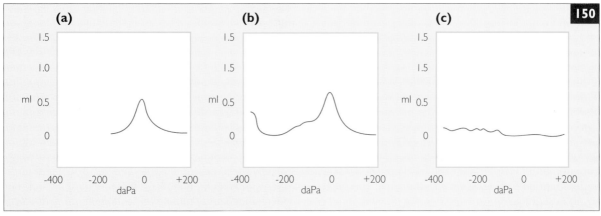

150a–c   Two normal tympanograms (**150a, b**). In both cases the tympanic membrane is intact. Abnormal tympanogram (**150c**) associated with a ruptured tympanic membrane. (Illustrations courtesy Dr J Steiss, Scott Ritchey Research Center, Auburn University, Alabama, USA.)

OTHER INVESTIGATORY PROCEDURES

KEY POINTS
- Myringotomy is the deliberate incision of an intact, though not necessarily healthy, tympanic membrane.
- The process of myringotomy allows assessment of the contents of the tympanic bulla when the tympanum is intact.
- Biopsy of the tissues of the external ear canal is occasionally indicated, particularly if radical excision of neoplasms is contemplated. It may also permit assessment of the degree of fibrosis within mural tissues, helping to elucidate decision making.

MYRINGOTOMY
Surgical incision of the intact tympanum (myringotomy) is indicated in a number of instances:
- To obtain samples of the effusion within the middle ear cavity for microbial culture and sensitivity testing, if otitis media is present.
- To provide a route of access to, or drainage of, accumulated middle ear effusion.
- To provide a means of access to the middle ear cavity to permit flushing, or to facilitate instillation of medication or insertion of a transtympanic ventilation tube.
- Myringotomy must be carried out under direct visual observation.
- The external ear canal must be carefully cleaned and dried before myringotomy is performed.

Needle aspiration
Given that different organisms with different antibacterial sensitivity patterns may exist either side of an intact tympanic membrane[1], it may be necessary to obtain samples from the middle ear by puncturing the intact tympanum and aspirating its contents.

A 22 gauge spinal needle[1] or a pediatric scalp vein catheter are suitable since both are of an appropriate length to be passed through an otoscope. The catheter must be carried to the tympanum by fine-nosed crocodile forceps; this has the advantage of providing a more flexible connection to the 5 ml or 10 ml syringe which is required to aspirate the middle ear contents[1, 2].

There are two disadvantage of simple paracentesis[3]. Firstly, the effusion within the middle ear is often purulent or particulate and narrow needles may become blocked; subsequently, trying to pass even a small swab through the first hole is nigh on impossible. Secondly, the puncture is too small and it heals too quickly to permit adequate drainage of any effusion.

Incisional myringotomy
Greater access may be required for drainage or instillation of medication. Two types of incision are recommended: curvilinear or radial[3]. Both are made into the inferior, caudal quadrant of the tympanum using a Gerzog and Sexton or Buck myringotomy knife. Prior to myringotomy, radiographs of the middle ears should be taken to assess the degree of effusion. Tympanometry may also be helpful as abnormal thickening of the tympanum may be detected and this may have implications in that myringotomy may be more difficult and healing may be compromised. Care must be taken not to incise the tympanum too deeply as structures of the middle and inner ear may be damaged. Similarly, too forceful flushing should be avoided. Postmyringotomy antibacterial cover is indicated until the tympanic defect has healed. Surgical defects in the tympanum of experimental dogs showed evidence of healing by ten days but this was not complete until 21–35 days post surgery[4].

Curvilinear incision provides better drainage than a radial incision[3]. Using a myringotomy knife, a curved incision is made parallel to, but away from, the periphery of the tympanum (**151**).

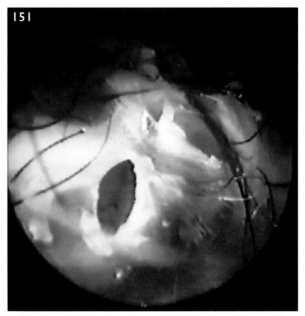

151 Myringotomy. Note the controlled incision avoids both the periphery and the manubrium. (Illustration courtesy Dr LN Gottelf, with permission of *Waltham Focus*.)

Radial incision allows poorer examination of the middle ear than curvilinear incision and makes removal of inspissated material, in particular, difficult[3].

Wire-mounted, small pharyngeal swabs provide an ideal method of collecting samples for microbiology as they are flexible, do not break, and are small enough to permit direct visual manipulation through the otoscope. Once the laboratory sample is collected the effusion may be drained with a blunt needle or washed out with repeated cycles of flushing with a warmed, aqueous solution of an antibacterial agent.

Placement of a transtympanic ventilation tube

Otitis media in the absence of otitis externa and infection is very rare in dogs. In man, particularly in children, otitis media with effusion ('glue ear') is not uncommon. A single case has been reported of apparently 'primary' otitis media with effusion in a young Cocker Spaniel[4]. No bacteriological culture and sensitivity testing was performed on middle ear samples so the true diagnosis in this case must remain unproven. Nonetheless, the dog was successfully treated by placing a flanged transtympanic ventilation tube (a grommet) in the ventral aspect of the tympanic membrane[4].

BIOPSY

Taking 4 mm (0.2 in) punch biopsy samples, under general anesthesia, of the vertical ear canal or of lesions and masses within the external ear canal is an important method of obtaining useful information on the processes underway. Biopsy of the external ear canal has three main indications:

- As a means of providing information on the degree of permanence of epithelial changes. For example, some apparently permanently thickened epithelia will regress dramatically when treated with topical glucocorticoids to suppress the inflammatory reaction. However, fibrosis, in general, will not regress. Biopsy of the luminal wall can yield information on the degree of fibrosis present (see Chapter 1: Microscopic structure of the external ear canal). This information can help decide whether to opt for a surgical or medical approach.

- As a means of providing information on the etiology of ulcerated lesions in the ear canal. Ulcers of the luminal wall may reflect gram-negative bacterial infection particularly, but also auto-immune disease and neoplasia. Biopsy of these lesions can yield information which will influence management.

- As an adjunct to surgery. Neoplastic changes within the ear canal may be fibrogranulomatous, benign, or malignant. Knowing the type of neoplasm and being able to predict its behavior can help the surgeon plan the degree of resection necessary to remove the risk of recurrence.

REFERENCES

OTOSCOPIC APPEARANCE OF THE EXTERNAL EAR CANAL AND TYMPANUM

1 McKeever PJ and Richardson HW (1988) Otitis externa. Part 2: Clinical appearance and diagnostic methods. *Companion Animal Practice* **2**, 25–31.
2 Getty R, Foust HL, Presley ET and Miller ME (1956) Macroscopic anatomy of the ear of the dog. *American Journal of Veterinary Research* **17**, 364–375.
3 Stout-Graham M, Kainer RA, Whalen LR and Macy DW (1990) Morphologic measurements of the external ear canal of dogs. *American Journal of Veterinary Research* **51**, 990–994.
4 Little CJL and Lane JG (1989) An evaluation of tympanometry, otoscopy and palpation for assessment of the canine tympanic membrane. *Veterinary Record* **124**, 5–8.
5 Fraser G, Gregor WW, Mackenzie CP, Spreull JSA and Withers AR (1970) Canine ear disease. *Journal of Small Animal Practice* **10**, 725–754.
6 Neer TM (1982) Otitis media. *Compendium on Continuing Education* **4**, 410–416.
7 Fraser G (1965) Aetiology of otitis externa in the dog. *Journal of Small Animal Practice* **6**, 445–452.
8 Huang HP, Fixter LM and Little CJL (1994) Lipid content of cerumen from normal dogs and otitic canine ears. *Veterinary Record* **134**, 380–381.

CYTOLOGIC CHARACTERISTICS OF NORMAL AND ABNORMAL EARS

1 Griffin CE (1993) Otitis externa and otitis media. In *Current Veterinary Dermatology* (eds CE Griffin, KW Kwochka and JM MacDonald) Mosby, St Louis, pp. 245–262.
2 Rosser EJ (1988) Evaluation of the patient with otitis externa. *Veterinary Clinics of North America* **18**, 765–772.
3 Huang H-P (1993) *Studies of the Microenvironment and Microflora of the Canine External Ear Canal.* PhD Thesis, Glasgow University.
4 Kowalski JJ (1988) The microbial environment of the ear canal in health and disease. *Veterinary Clinics of North America* **18**, 743–754.
5 Chickering WR (1988) Cytologic evaluation of otic exudates. *Veterinary Clinics of North America* **18**, 773–782.
6 Rosychuck RWA (1994) Management of otitis externa. *Veterinary Clinics of North America* **24**, 921–952.
7 Huang H-P (1995) Canine cerumen cytology. *Chinese Society of Veterinary Science* **21**, 18–23.
8 Huang H P and Little CJL (1994) Lipid content of cerumen from normal dogs and otitic canine ears. *Veterinary Record* **134**, 380–381.
9 Rogers KS (1988) Tumors of the ear canal. *Veterinary Clinics of North America* **4**, 859–868.
10 Mansfield PD, Boosinger TR and Attleburger MH (1990) Infectivity of *Malassezia pachydermatis* in the external ear canal of dogs. *Journal of the American Animal Hospital Association* **26**, 97–100.
11 Bond R, Anthony RM, Dodd M and Lloyd DH (1996) Isolation of *Malassezia sympodialis* from feline skin. *Journal of Medical and Veterinary Mycology* **34**, 145–147.
12 Frost CR (1961) Canine otocariasis. *Journal of Small Animal Practice* **2**, 253–256.

NEUROLOGIC EXAMINATION OF THE EAR

1 Whalen L and Kitchell R (1983) Electrophysiologic studies of the cutaneous nerves of the head of the dog. *American Journal of Veterinary Research* **44**, 615–627.
2 Whalen L and Kitchell R (1983) Electrophysiologic and behavioral studies of the cutaneous nerves of the concave surface of the pinna and the external ear canal of the dog. *American Journal of Veterinary Research* **44**, 628–634.
3 Evans HE (1993) *Miller's Anatomy of the Dog.* 3rd edn. (ed HE Evans) WB Saunders, Philadelphia, pp. 988–1008.
4 Oliver JE, Lorenz MD and Kornegay JN (1997) Confirming a diagnosis. In *Handbook of Veterinary Neurology.* 3rd edn. WB Saunders, Philadelphia, pp 89–108.

RADIOGRAPHIC FEATURES OF THE NORMAL AND ABNORMAL EAR

1 Hare WCD (1958) Radiographic anatomy of the canine skull. *Journal of the American Veterinary Medical Association* **133**, 149–157.
2 Gibbs C (1978) Radiological refresher: Part III. The head. *Journal of Small Animal Practice* **19**, 539–545.
3 Rose WR (1977) Small animal clinical otology: radiology. *Veterinary Medicine/Small Animal Clinician* **72**, 1508–1517.
4 Love NE, Kramer RW, Spodnick GJ and Thrall DE (1995) Radiographic and computed tomographic evaluation of otitis media. *Veterinary Radiology and Ultrasound* **36**, 375–379.
5 Douglas SW, Herrtage ME and Williamson HD (1987) Canine radiography: skull. In *Principles of Veterinary Radiography.* Bailliére Tindall, London, pp. 177–192.
6 Sullivan M (1995) The head and neck. In *BSAVA Manual of Small Animal Diagnostic Imaging.* (ed R Lee) British Small Animal Veterinary Association, Cheltenham, pp. 16–22.
7 Hoskinson JJ (1993) Imaging techniques in the diagnosis of middle ear disease. *Seminars in Veterinary Medicine* **8**, 10–16.
8 Smeak DD and Kerpsack SJ (1993) Total ear canal ablation and lateral bulla osteotomy for management of end-stage otitis. *Seminars in Veterinary Medicine* **8**, 30–41.
9 Remedios AM, Fowler JD and Pharr JW (1991) A comparison of radiographic versus surgical diagnosis of otitis media. *Journal of the American Animal Hospital Association* **27**, 183–188.
10 Kealy JK (1987) The skull and vertebral column. In *Diagnostic Radiology of the Dog and Cat.* 2nd edn. (ed JK Kealy) WB Saunders, Philadelphia, pp. 439–441.
11 Trower ND, Gregory SP, Renfrew H and Lamb CR (1998) Evaluation of canine tympanic membrane by positive contrast ear canalography. *Veterinary Record* **142**, 78–81.
12 Eom K-D, Lee H-C and Yoon Y-H (2000) Canalographic evaluation of the external ear canal in dogs. *Veterinary Radiology and Ultrasound* **41**, 231–234.

IMAGING THE MIDDLE AND INNER EARS

1 Remedios AM, Fowler JD and Pharr JW (1991) A comparison of radiographic versus surgical diagnosis of otitis media. *Journal of the American Animal Hospital Association* **27**, 183–188.
2 Love NE, Kramer RW, Spodnick GJ and Thrall DE (1995) Radiographic and computed tomographic evaluation of otitis media. *Veterinary Radiology and Ultrasound* **36**, 375–379.
3 Hoskinson JJ (1993) Imaging techniques in the diagnosis of middle ear disease. *Seminars in Veterinary Medicine* **8**, 10–16.

4 Hendee WR and Morgan CJ (1984) Magnetic resonance imaging. Part 1: Physical principles (medical progress). *Western Journal of Medicine* **141**, 491–500.

5 Scherzinger AL and Hendee WR (1985) Basic principles of magnetic resonance imaging: an update. *Western Journal of Medicine* **143**, 782–792.

6 Westersson P-L, Katzberg RW, Tallents RH, Sanchez-Woodworth RE and Svensson SA (1987) CT and MRI of the temporomandibular joint: comparison with autopsy specimens. *American Journal of Radiology* **148**, 1165–1171.

7 Dvir E, Kirberger RM and Terblanche AG (2000) Magnetic resonance imaging of otitis media in a dog. *Veterinary Radiology and Ultrasound* **41**, 46–49.

8 Chan KH, Swarts D, Doyle WJ and Wolf GL (1991) Assessment of middle ear status during experimental otitis media using magnetic resonance imaging. *Archives of Otolaryngology, Head and Neck Surgery* **117**, 91–95.

9 Grandis JR, Curtin HD and Yu VL (1995) Necrotizing (malignant) external otitis: prospective comparison of CT and MR imaging in diagnosis and follow-up. *Radiology* **196**, 499–504.

10 Assoun J, Richardi G, Railhac J-J et al. (1994) Ostoid osteoma: MR imaging versus CT. *Radiology* **191**, 217–223.

ELECTROPHYSIOLOGIC PROCEDURES

1 Sims MH (1988) Electrodiagnostic evaluation of auditory function. *Veterinary Clinics of North America* **18**, 913–944.

2 Marshall A (1985) Brainstem auditory-evoked response of the nonanesthetized dog. *American Journal of Veterinary Research* **46**, 966–973.

3 Cuddon PA (1988) Electrodiagnostics. In *First Basic Science Course in Veterinary and Comparatve Neurology and Neurosurgery*. (ed PA Cuddon) University of Wisconsin, Madison.

4 Bodenhamer R, Hunter J and Luttgen P (1985) Brainstem auditory-evoked response in the dog. *American Journal of Veterinary Research* **46**, 1787–1792.

5 Pook H and Steiss J (1990) Correlation of brainstem auditory-evoked response with cranium size and body weight. *American Journal of Veterinary Research* **51**, 1779–1783.

6 Strain G, Tedford B and Jackson R (1991) Postnatal development of the brainstem auditory-evoked potential in dogs. *American Journal of Veterinary Research* **52**, 410–414.

7 Achor LJ and Starr A (1980) Auditory brainstem response in the cat. I: Intracranial and extracranial responses. *Electroencephalography and Clinical Neurophysiology* **48**, 155–173.

8 Achor LJ and Starr A (1980) Auditory brainstem response in the cat. II: Effects of lesions. *Electroencephalography and Clinical Neurophysiology* **48**, 174–190.

9 Jewett DL (1970) Volume conducted potentials in response to auditory stimuli as detected by averaging in the cat. *Electroencephalography and Clinical Neurophysiology* **28**, 609–618.

10 Buchwald JS and Huang CM (1975) Far-field acoustic response: origins in the cat. *Science* **189**, 382–384.

11 Venker-vanHaagen AJ, Siemelink RJG and Smoorenburg GF (1989) Auditory brainstem responses in the normal beagle. *Veterinary Quarterly* **11**, 129–137.

12 Sims MH and Moore RE (1984) Auditory evoked response in the clinically normal dog: early latency components. *American Journal of Veterinary Research* **45**, 2019–2017.

13 Myers LF, Redding RW and Wilson S (1985) Reference values of the brainstem auditory evoked response of methoxyflurane anesthetized and nonanesthetized dogs. *Veterinary Research Communications* **9**, 289–294.

14 Shiu J, Munro K and Cox C (1997) Normative auditory brainstem response data for hearing threshold and neuro-otological diagnosis in the dog. *Journal of Small Animal Practice* **38**, 103–107.

15 Steiss JE, Wright JC and Storrs JP (1990) Alteration in the brainstem auditory evoked response threshold and latency-intensity curve associated with conductive hearing loss in dogs. *Progress in Veterinary Neurology* **1**, 205–211.

16 Wolschrijn CF, Venker-vanHaagen AJ and Van-den-Brom WE (1997) Comparison of air- and bone-conducted brainstem auditory evoked responses in young dogs and dogs with bilateral ear canal obstruction. *Veterinary Quarterly* **19**, 158–162.

17 Knowles K, Cash W and Blauch B (1988) Auditory-evoked responses of dogs with different hearing abilities. *Canadian Journal of Veterinary Research* **52**, 394–397.

18 Eger C and Lindsay P (1997) Effects of otitis on hearing in dogs characterised by brainstem auditory evoked response testing. *Journal of Small Animal Practice* **38**, 380–386.

19 Krahwinkel DJ, Pardo AD, Sims MH and Bubb WJ (1993) Effect of total ablation of the external acoustic meatus and bulla osteotomy on auditory function in dogs. *Journal of the American Veterinary Medical Association* **202**, 949–952.

20 Harrison J and Buchwald J (1982) Auditory brainstem response in the aged cat. *Neurobiology of Aging* **3**, 163–171.

21 Morgan JL, Coulter DB, Marshall AE and Goetsch DD (1980) Effects of neomycin on the wave form of auditory evoked brainstem potential in dogs. *American Journal of Veterinary Research* **41**, 1077–1081.

22 Penrod JP and Coulter DB (1980) The diagnostic uses of impedance audiometry in the dog. *Journal of the American Animal Hospital Association* **16**, 941–948.

23 Merchant SR (1994) Ototoxicity. In *Veterinary Clinics of North America* (eds RAW Rosychuck and SR Merchant) **24**, 971–980.

24 Steiss JE, Boosinger TR, Wright JC and Pillai SR (1982) Healing of experimentally perforated tympanic membranes demonstrated by electrodiagnostic testing and histopathology. *Journal of the American Animal Hospital Association* **28**, 307–310.

25 Cole LK, Podell M and Kwochka KW (2000) Impedance audiometric measurements in clinically normal dogs. *American Journal of Veterinary Reasearch* **61**, 442–445.

OTHER INVESTIGATORY PROCEDURES

1 Cole LK, Kwochka KW, Kowalski JJ and Hillier A (1998) Microbial flora and antimicrobial susceptibility patterns of isolated pathogens from the horizontal ear canal and middle ear in dogs with otitis media. *Journal of the American Veterinary Medical Association* **212**, 534–538.

2 Bruyette DS and Lorenz MD (1993) Otitis externa and otitis media: diagnostic and medical aspects. *Seminars in Veterinary Medicine and Surgery (Small Animal)* **8**, 3–9.

3 Rose WR (1977) Surgery. I: Myringotomy. *Veterinary Medicine/Small Animal Clinician* **72**, 1646–1650.

4 Cox CL, Slack RWT and Cox GR (1989) Insertion of a transtympanic ventilation tube for the treatment of otitis media with effusion. *Journal of Small Animal Practice* **30**, 517–519.

Chapter Three

Etiopathogenesis and Classification of Otitis Externa

- **Effects of breed and progressive pathology**

- **Ectoparasitic causes of otitis externa, and antiparasitic agents**

- **Foreign bodies**

- **Nasopharyngeal and middle ear polyps**

- **Otic neoplasia**

- **Underlying disease**

- **The effects of weather on the incidence of otitis externa**

- **References**

EFFECTS OF BREED AND PROGRESSIVE PATHOLOGY

KEY POINTS

- Breeds of dog predisposed to otitis externa, such as Cocker Spaniels, have increased amounts of glandular tissue compared to normal dogs.
- Otitis externa results in increased production of cerumen with a lower lipid content than normal, associated with increased ceruminous gland activity.
- Dogs with pendulous ears are predisposed to otitis externa.
- Pathologic changes within the external ear canal are progressive.
- Changes in structure engender changes in the local microenvironment.
- Surgery is the inevitable consequence of chronic otitis externa.

BREED VARIATION

Fernando[1] observed that the external ear canals of longhaired breeds of dogs and those with fine hair contained more sebaceous and apocrine glandular tissue, which was also better developed, than dogs with short hair. Breeds predisposed to otitis externa also have abnormal morphometric ratios compared to normal dogs[2]. Specifically, they exhibit an increase in the overall amount of soft tissue within the confines of the auricular cartilage, an increase in the area occupied by the apocrine glands, and an increase in the apocrine gland area compared to that of the sebaceous glands.

Overall, the breeds of dog predisposed to otitis externa have increased apocrine tissue[2]. If this increased volume of apocrine tissue is actively secreting, the concentration of lipid within the cerumen will fall[3], humidity within the ear canal will rise, and maceration, followed by infection and otitis externa, will result. Increased moisture and surface maceration creates an environment particularly favorable to gram-negative bacteria. Theoretically, the increased apocrine secretions in the ear canals of these dogs should result in cerumen with a lower pH than normal and an environment not conducive to gram-negative colonization. It may be that the acidifying effect of increased ceruminous gland secretion is not sufficient to overcome the effects of humidity, inflammation, and surface maceration.

RESPONSE TO INSULT AND INJURY

Reactions to inflammation within the external ear canal

The epidermis of the external ear canal reacts to inflammation by increasing its rate of turnover and increasing in thickness, i.e. it becomes hyperplastic[4, 5]. There may be surface erosions and ulceration, particularly with gram-negative infections. The dermis becomes infiltrated with inflammatory cells and fibrosis will follow. In the early stages of otitis externa there is hyperplasia of the sebaceous glands, and their ducts may become dilated[5, 6]. If chronic otitis persists, the apocrine glands become hyperplastic with cystic dilatation of the glands and ducts. Although this may be of such magnitude that the sebaceous glands appear displaced, with very little secretory potential[4, 5], morphometric analysis reveals no significant changes in sebaceous gland size or activity[2]. Papillary proliferation of ceruminous glands and ducts may obliterate the lumen of the external ear canal in some cases[5]. In very chronic cases, ossification of the tissues may take place.

Similar changes take place in the feline ear canal, although the papillary changes in the ceruminous glands may be sufficiently florid that discrete polyps occur[5].

The consequence of these changes is a reduction in luminal cross-section, a result of increasing soft tissue within the bounds of the containing cartilage[2]. The change in nature of the cerumen, the reduction in luminal diameter, and the moisture and warmth which accompany active inflammation contribute to an increase in local humidity[3]. These changes in the otic environment result in surface maceration and the creation of a milieu favorable to microbial multiplication, itself a potent inducer of inflammation (see flow chart right).

Even very early changes in the lining of the external ear canal have the potential to become permanent. This is the reason why the most common surgical procedure practised upon the external ear, the Zepp resection, fails so often. Once any degree of luminal stenosis has occurred, lateral wall resection is not indicated. Vertical ablation is necessary.

It is not clear at which stage these changes become irreversible. Certainly, aggressive medical therapy, initially with antimicrobial agents and then with topical glucocorticoids, can result in significant reduction in soft tissue occlusion of the lumen. However, the structural changes in apocrine ducts and glands are probably irreversible; certainly the progressive changes in glandular architecture correlate with the progression of the otitis externa[2].

Once these permanent changes occur, simple Zepp resection of the lateral wall of the vertical canal is unlikely to be successful[7–9]. Ablation of the canal is indicated.

Influence of breed on otitis externa

Dogs with pendulous ears are predisposed to otitis externa[10, 11] but the low incidence in some breeds with pendulous ears, such as Beagles and Irish Setters, in most studies[12] suggests factors other than conforma-

tion at work. The presence of hair, *per se*, within the ear canal does not correlate with otitis externa[11]. However, Cocker Spaniels have many compound hair follicles throughout the length of the external ear canal whereas non-predisposed breeds typically have fewer, predominantly simple follicles in their ear canals[12]. Certain breeds, such as Cocker Spaniels and Miniature Poodles, appear on every list of affected breeds[10, 12–14]. However, it is now recognized that one of the principal causes of otitis externa is the presence of hypersensitivities, such as atopy, and generalized skin disease, such as defects in keratinization, which predispose to otitis externa. It is the predisposition to these diseases which accounts for the increased relative risk of ear disease rather than the anatomy *per se*.

Only one study[15] has recorded the incidence of otitis externa in cats. In this series of 36 cats, Himalayans and Persian breeds were most commonly affected.

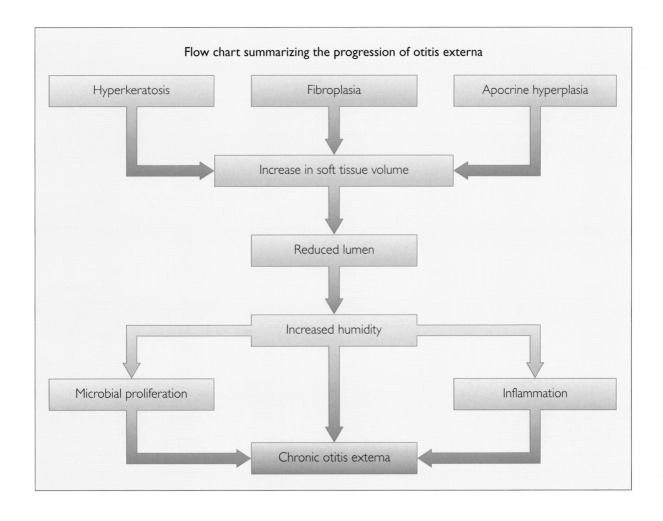

Flow chart summarizing the progression of otitis externa

Influence of progressive pathology

The soft tissues surrounding the lumen of the external ear canal react in a predictable sequence to the inflammation associated with chronic otitis externa[2, 4–6]:

- Epidermal hyperplasia (acanthosis and hyper-keratinization) is an early consequence of otic irritation (**152**). The basal cells of the epidermis respond to inflammation by increasing their rate of division and increasing the transit time of cells moving through the epidermis. In addition, keratinization is affected and a thickened stratum corneum is apparent. This reaction is reversible, provided the initiating cause is alleviated.
- Subepithelial infiltration with inflammatory cells, such as lymphocytes, neutrophils, macrophages, and plasma cells, occurs in response to inflammation. Chronic cellular infiltration results in local release of inflammatory mediators, cutaneous erythema, and edema (**153**). Early cellular infiltration is reversible but the effects of chronic mediator release may engender permanent changes.

- Fibroplasia of the underlying dermis follows chronic inflammatory challenge within the lumen and the epithelium. In long-standing cases the fibrosis may be extensive (**154**) and this contributes considerably to the loss of luminal cross-section.
- Early sebaceous gland hyperplasia is followed by massive ceruminous gland hyperplasia, both of the duct and the glandular portion (**155**). The changes in the ceruminous glands result in gross thickening of the epidermis, particularly in cats.
- Papillary proliferation of the epithelial lining occurs to such an extent that the lumen becomes occluded (**156, 157**). In the external ear canals of cats this papillary proliferation may result in polyp formation with trapping of exudate between the polyp and the tympanum.
- Ossification of the dermis, sometime extending to the auricular cartilage, occurs as a final stage.

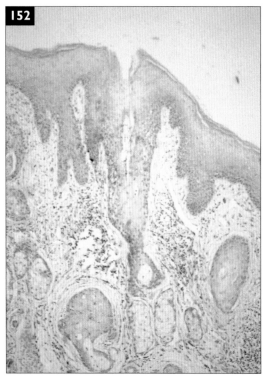

152 Photomicrograph of a section of canine external ear canal demonstrating epidermal hyperplasia.

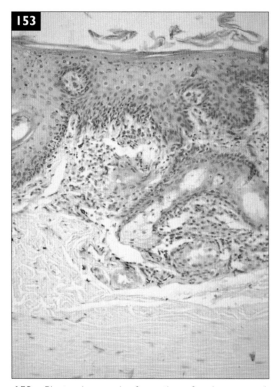

153 Photomicrograph of a section of canine external ear canal demonstrating epidermal hyperplasia, an inflammatory infiltrate, and dermal edema.

154 Photomicrograph of a section of canine external ear canal stained to demonstrate dermal fibrosis, which in this case is extensive.

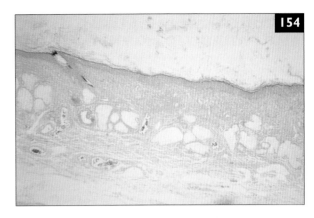

155 Photomicrograph of a section of canine external ear canal demonstrating massive apocrine gland hyperplasia.

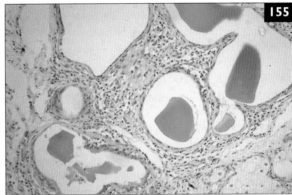

156 Photomicrograph of a section of hyperplastic external ear canal with papillary fronds almost occluding the lumen.

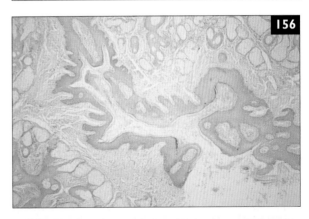

157 Photograph of a section of a chronically hyperplastic external ear canal with almost no lumen.

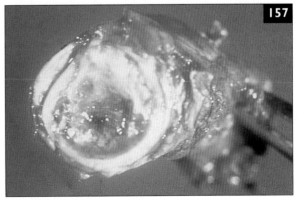

ECTOPARASITIC CAUSES OF OTITIS EXTERNA, AND ANTIPARASITIC AGENTS

KEY POINTS

- *Otodectes cynotis* is the most common ectoparasite involved in otitis externa.
- As few as three otodectic mites have been reported to cause otitis externa.
- Asymptomatic carriage of *O. cynotis* is common in the cat and may occur, though rarely, in the dog.
- *Otodectes cynotis* may, rarely, be zoonotic.
- Other ectoparasitic causes of otitis externa include *Demodex* spp., *Neotrombicula autumnalis* and other harvest mites, and ticks such as *Otobius megnini*.

OTODECTES CYNOTIS

Introduction

Otodectes cynotis is a large (0.3 × 0.4 mm [0.01 × 0.02 in]) mite (**158**) which lives predominantly in the external ear canal of dogs and cats, and perhaps occasionally on the adjacent skin of the head[1]. The mite does not burrow but lives on the skin surface where it feeds on tissue fluid and debris[2]. It has been suggested that otodectic mites can survive within the household, off the host, for weeks if not months[3].

The physical presence of the mite induces a mechanical irritation which accounts for some of the pruritus experienced by infected animals. However, the saliva is both irritant and immunogenic and in the cat the mite stimulates an IgE-like antibody[2], suggesting that hypersensitivity contributes to the pruritus. The mite produces an antibody which cross-reacts with the house dust mite *Dermatophagoides farinae*[3] and may thus play a part in human atopy. Ear mite antigen may play a part in inducing aural hematoma in both the dog and cat and this might have an autoimmune etiology[4, 5].

Zoonotic lesions may occur on in-contact human members of the household[1]. Vesicles, wheals, erythematous papules, and excoriations on the arms and torso have been reported[6].

Lifecycle, transmission, and prevalence

Females lay eggs (**159**) and cement them to the epidermal surface. They hatch to yield six-legged larvae which undergo two moults through eight-legged protonymphs and deutonymphs. The emerging deutonymph is approached by, and attached to, an adult male mite (**160**) and, if it is female, copulation occurs. Although the life cycle of three weeks is confined to the host, it has been suggested that the mite can survive in the environment for long periods[3]. Nevertheless, contact with an infected host is still believed to be the main route of transmission[1].

The prevalence of *O. cynotis* in dogs' ears was assessed as 29.1% in one study of 700 ears, with a significant predisposition in dogs with pendulous and semi-erect pinnae as compared to erect pinnae[7]. This study also reported that there was a highly significant correlation between the presence of mites and otitis externa. In 114 (out of 700 ears) ears, mites were found in the absence of any indication of otitis externa, suggesting that in dogs, asymptomatic carriage is possible. Fewer cases were reported in the summer months. One study[8] suggested a seasonal incidence for the disease; however, a very large study[9] could find no evidence of a seasonal incidence.

Clinical features

Young dogs appear to be more commonly infected than older animals[9]. This probably reflects the fact that infected dogs are easily diagnosed, effectively treated, and not reinfected. The average number of mites per dogs was only 5.6[9].

Otodectes cynotis is typically associated with a pruritic otitis externa[7, 8]. However, Scott[8] considered that in the cat, three syndromes (otitis externa, ectopic infection, and asymptomatic carriage) might be associated with infection with the mite.

Very low numbers of mites, even as low as three[7], may be sufficient to induce clinical signs. This, together with the mite's ability to inhabit the entire external ear canal, can make definitive diagnosis difficult and might make a rule-out of otodectic acariasis, other than by trial therapy, problematic.

Otitis externa

The classic feature of otitis externa due to ear mite infection is moderate to severe otic pruritus. In addition, the external ear canal becomes filled with a crumbly black/brown discharge (**161–163**). Most affected dogs exhibit chronic otic pruritus but Frost[7] reported four dogs out of 200 which had asymptomatic infection. Puppies are most likely to be infected from dams, but in adult dogs the cat is a common cause of contagion[1], particularly since the cat may well be asymptomatic[8, 10].

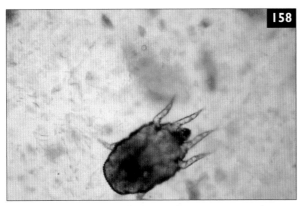

158 Photomicrograph of an adult *Otodectes cynotis* mite.

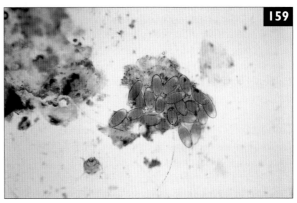

159 Photomicrograph of *Otodectes* ova collected in cerumen.

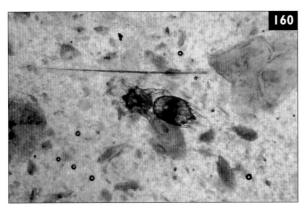

160 Photomicrograph of a deutonymph attached to an adult otodectic mite.

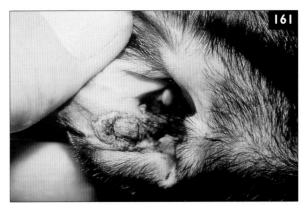

161 Adult cat with *Otodectes cynotis* infestation. Note the typical dark brown color and the dry nature of the cerumen. Note also the lack of self-trauma in this asymptomatic case.

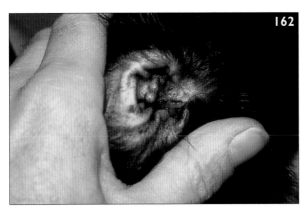

162 Otodectic mange in a pup. Note the presence of the dryish cerumen and evidence of some self-trauma.

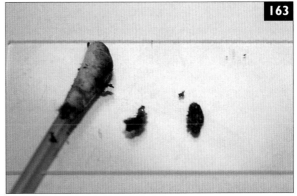

163 Cerumen from an ear infested with *Otodectes cynotis*. Note the crumbly nature of the cerumen and the dark brown color.

In cats the pruritus associated with infection may be associated with moderate to severe self-trauma to the head (**164, 165**). Scott[8] suggested an age predilection in young cats. In cases of chronic infection there may be hyperplastic changes in the lining of the external ear canal and a predisposition to secondary infection.

Ectopic infection

In some cases, perhaps in cats more than in dogs, the mite causes clinical signs distant from the ear. Scott[8] considered that this might be a consequence of cats sleeping in a curled position so that the ear is apposed to the tail-base. Two syndromes may be associated with ectopic infection:

- Crusted papules, i.e. miliary dermatitis.
- Patchy alopecia.

Asymptomatic infection

This may be a feature of older cats where very high numbers of mites may be found with apparently no associated clinical signs[10]. The presence of asymptomatic carriage in dogs has not been considered a major problem in veterinary dermatologic texts, but in light of the discussion above it should be borne in mind, particularly when treatment protocols are discussed.

Diagnosis

The mite is relatively large and may be easily seen in the external ear canal with the aid of an auroscope (**166**). Direct observation may not always result in a diagnosis:

- The degree of discharge may make direct observation difficult.
- There may be so few mites that direct observation is not possible.

In these situations, microscopic examination of discharge may be necessary. Gentle maceration of collected samples in mineral oil will aid diagnosis, and microscopic examination under low power should show evidence of infestation.

Treatment

Topical otic acaricidal preparations are usually sufficient, although ivermectin is also effective. Suitable otic and systemic acaricides include:

- Topical monosulfiram.
- Topical thiabendazole[11, 12].
- Topical rotenone[11, 13].
- Systemic ivermectin (0.2–0.3 mg/kg s/c)[14, 15] or topical ivermectin in mineral oil.
- Topical application of an unidentified component found in a commercial otic preparation (Canaural, Leo Laboratories Limited)[16, 17].
- Topical application (administered via a weight-banded individual dispenser) of a single dose of selamectin at a minimum dose rate of 6mg/kg[18].
- Topical application of fipronil into the ear canal.

Prior cleaning of the ear with ceruminolytics may be beneficial in cases where there is a heavy discharge. In view of the possibility of an ectopic infection with the mite, the body surface of affected animals should also be treated with an appropriate antiparasitic agent such as a carbamate, pyrethrin, dichlorvos/fenitrothion aerosol, pipronyl, or selamectin. In view of the possibility of the mite surviving off the host, within the home, a thorough house clean followed by application of a suitable environmental agent may be indicated in apparently intractable cases.

164   Small area of crust and self-trauma in the entrance to the external ear canal of a cat with otodectic otitis.

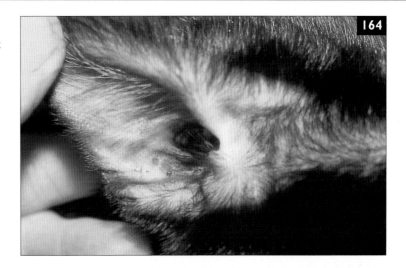

165   Area of erythema and self-trauma associated with otodectic otitis on the lateral aspect of the head of a cat.

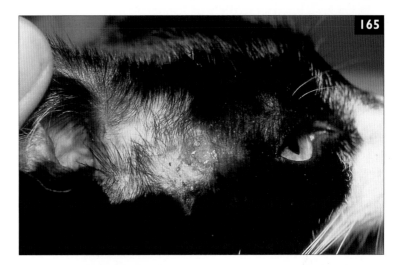

166   Otoscopic view of ceruminous debris and otodectic mites in a feline external ear canal. The mites appear small in this unmagnified view.

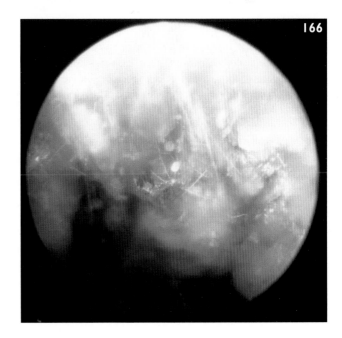

OTHER ECTOPARASITIC CAUSES OF OTITIS EXTERNA

Demodex canis, D. felis and D. gatoi

Demodex canis has been reported as a rare cause of otitis externa in dogs. It may occur as part of a generalized condition, in isolation, or as a long-term complication of juvenile onset generalized demodicosis which has apparently responded to treatment[19]. A history of demodicosis should alert the clinician to the possibility of otodemodicosis but cases arising *de novo* should not be discounted. Typically, otodemodicosis is associated with a ceruminous otitis externa (**167**).

In cats, demodicosis is more usually associated with erythema (**168**) and crusting on the pinnae and head, rather than otitis externa. However, *D. gatoi* may be associated with a ceruminous otitis externa in cats.

Diagnosis is based on recovery of demodecid mites (**169–171**) in skin scrapes and on cotton swabs from the external ear canal. Punch biopsy samples would also give appropriate material for a diagnosis.

Treatment with demodecicidal agents is indicated. The choice of agent will depend on whether the otodemodicosis is in isolation or part of the generalized disease:

- Feline otodemodicosis has been reported to respond to thiabendazole-containing products[11].
- One ml of 19.9% amitraz solution in 30 ml mineral oil[12] or 2 ml of 5% solution in 20 ml mineral oil[19] has been recommended for treatment of both canine and feline otodemodicosis.
- Ivermectin given orally (0.6 mg/kg q24h) might also be successful in canine demodecosis, although clinicians should ensure that the drug is not used in Collie breeds, Collie-crosses, and certain herding breeds.

Harvest mites

Harvest mites such as *Neotrombicula autumnalis* (**172**) and *Euotrombicula alfredugesi* are occasional causes of otitis externa in both dogs and cats. The larvae are parasitic and require a mammalian host; they are not species specific. Larvae hatch in rapid succession and usually tens or hundreds are involved in the parasitic attack. Typically, they cause a pruritic crusting dermatitis on the ventrum and face and in the interdigital areas. Occasional animals exhibit larval clustering and crusting at the base of the pinnae[20] or within the confines of the proximal external ear canal. Close examination usually reveals tiny orange, or orange-red, clusters of larvae.

The parasite is a seasonal threat to the hunting or roaming dog and cat and it is more common on ground composed of well drained, chalky soil. Treatment of the larval infection is relatively easy since simple ectoparasitic treatment is effective[21]. Lime sulfur (2% dip), pyrethrin powder, and dichlorvos/fenitrothion aerosols are good examples which are safe in cats and dogs.

Control of reinfection is much more difficult since the animal must be prevented from traversing infected ground. This is not very practical in most cases. However, dips, sprays, or spot-on formulations of amitraz or fipronil may have a protective effect, and both will aid in removal of larvae from infected hosts[22, 23]. Any residual pruritus may be suppressed with a short course of prednisolone (0.5–1.1 mg/kg p/o q12h).

Ticks

The spinous ear tick, *Otobius megnini*, is most frequently found in the southern and south-western regions of the USA. However, the increased mobility of owners and their pets means that the tick may be found in almost any region of the USA[24, 25]. The larvae (six legs, yellow-pink color) and adults (eight legs, blue-gray color) are parasitic and infest the external ear canal of both dogs and cats to the extent that in some cases the external ear canal is entirely filled with the parasites. Acute otitis externa results. Ixodic, and other hard ticks such as *Demacentor* spp., are usually are found on the pinnae and head, rather than within the external ear canal.

The ticks may be removed with forceps and otic flushing, although this may require sedation or anesthesia. A topical otic preparation containing thiabendazole, neomycin and dexamethasone has also been reported to be curative[25]. Any postinfestation inflammation may be treated with a topical glucocorticoid and antibacterial otic preparation. Reinfestation is a problem as animals will often regularly revisit tick-infested areas. If these are located, the ground can be cleared and, if necessary, treated with an organophosphate such as malathion, chlorpyriphos, or other approved environmental agents[24].

Some protection from reinfestation by ticks may be afforded by amitraz dips and collars or by fipronil preparations, both of which may have some tick-repellent properties:

- Although fipronil is presented in both spray and spot-on formulations, the spray formulation is preferred for the treatment of ticks (and harvest mites) since effective local concentrations on both hair and skin surface may be achieved rapidly. Fipronil has been demonstrated under field conditions to prevent infestation with ticks[23, 26].
- Amitraz dips are useful as a tick repellent[22] and in some countries the chemical is marketed as an amitraz-impregnated collar for tick repellent purposes. Accidental ingestion of amitraz-impregnated collars may prove fatal to the dog and prompt treatment is necessary. Atipamezole (50 mcg/kg i/m) should be followed by oral yohimbine (0.1 mg/kg) every six hours as needed[27].

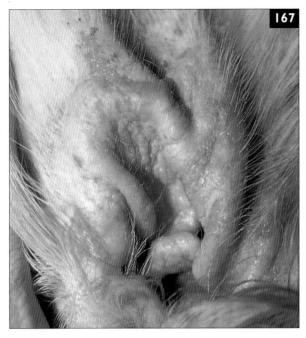

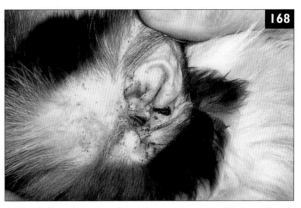

168   Feline demodicosis causing erythematous dermatitis adjacent to the entrance to the external ear canal.

167   Erythematous, ceruminous otitis externa in a Cavalier King Charles Spaniel with otodemodicosis.

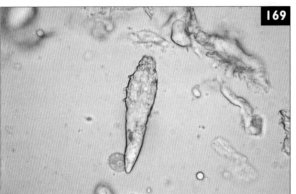

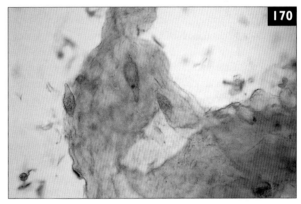

169, 170   Photomicrographs of a juvenile demodectic mite (**169**) and an egg (**170**) in cerumen from the ear of a dog with otodemodectic mange.

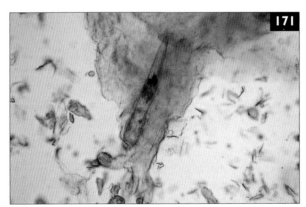

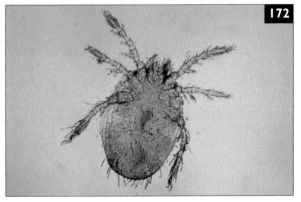

171   Photomicrograph of an adult *Demodex canis* mite in cerumen from the external ear canal of a dog with otodemodectic mange.

172   Larva of *Neotrombicula autumnalis*. Note the red color and six legs.

ECTOPARASITIC AGENTS USED AGAINST OTIC ECTOPARASITES

Monosulfiram (tetraethylthiuran monosulphide)

Indication: *Otodectes cynotis*.

Sulfur has been used for centuries as a scabicide and monosulfiram emulsion has a long history as a topical acaricide[28]. However, it is rarely used in human dermatology as it cross-reacts with alcohol abuse treatments[29]. Monosulfiram also has a fungicidal effect and a 5mg/ml solution is active against malassezial yeast[30].

Thiabendazole (2-(thiazol-4-yl)benzimidazole)

Indications: *Malassezia pachydermatis, Aspergillus* spp., *Otodectes cynotis*, ticks, feline otodemodicosis.

Thiabendazole is an antifungal agent with acaricidal properties[31]. Thiabendazole kills all stages of the mite life cycle[11] and is thus preferred to pyrethrins and rotenone, for example, which have no activity against eggs. Thiabendazole is useful against malassezial yeast and otodectic mites[11, 12] and its lack of toxicity, in standard doses, has made it a popular ingredient in otic polypharmaceutical preparations. A topical otic preparation containing thiabendazole, neomycin, and dexamethasone has also been reported to be curative against *Otobius megnini* ticks[25]. Thiabendazole is also effective in the treatment of feline otodemodicosis[11].

Pyrethrin, pyrethroids, carbamates, and rotenone

Indications: *Otodectes cynotis, Neotrombicula autumnalis, Eurotromicula alfredurgesi*, tick infestation.
These are relatively broad-spectrum insecticides and acaricides. Pyrethrins (natural derivatives of *Chrysanthemum cinerariaefolium*), pyrethroids (synthetic analogues), and rotenone are characterized by quick knock-down and poor persistence. They are thus commonly used in over-the-counter antiparasitic preparations for puppies and kittens. These agents all have similar spectra of activity and a low toxicity potential, although if cats are treated with products marketed for dogs, toxic side-effects may be seen[32, 33]. None of these agents kill the eggs of ear mites and thus repeated treatment is necessary.

Ivermectin

Indications: *Demodex* spp., *Otodectes cynotis, Sarcoptes scabiei, Notoedres cati, Neotrombicula autumnalis*, ticks, *Linognathus setosus*.
Ivermectin is effective against demodectic and sarcoptic mange in dogs, at doses of 0.3 mg/kg body weight[34]. It is given on four occasions at seven-day intervals for scabies, and once daily until remission is achieved for demodicosis[33]. Ivermectin has been advocated for otodectic mange in cats[35] at a dose of 0.2–0.3 mg/kg. Two injections at 10–14 day intervals are curative. Although ivermectin may be administered topically, orally, or by injection, the topical route is least effective[36]. Subcutaneous injections must only be given using the propylene glycol-based presentation[37]. For oral dosing, particularly long-term treatment, it may be more appropriate to use the water-based presentation marketed for oral administration to the horse, although it may prove difficult to measure the exact dose. This will obviate any risk of propylene-glycol toxicity which, although rare, may be noted occasionally (bradycardia and central nervous system and respiratory depression).

Ivermectin should be highly effective against other mites affecting cats and dogs[35]. It has some activity against the sucking louse of dogs (*Linognathus setosus*) and some activity against ticks; it inhibits feeding and the ticks fall off only partially engorged[35].

Certain breeds of dog are susceptible to side-effects when given ivermectin, and great care is warranted when considering its use. Informed, preferably signed, consent may be necessary in some circumstances. Ivermectin toxicity is related to central nervous system effects caused by ivermectin-enhanced gamma-amino butyric acid (GABA) activity[37]. In most canine breeds acute toxicity is seen when a dose in excess of 2.5 mg/kg is given. In cats the maximum dose above which signs of acute toxicity are seen is 0.75 mg/kg orally. Chronic toxicity begins to be noted with doses in excess of 1 mg/kg in dogs and 0.5 mg/kg in cats[37]. There appears to be minimal risk of teratogenic effects following administration of ivermectin to pregnant bitches[37]. Signs of ivermectin toxicity include mydriasis, depression, tremors, ataxia, stupor, emesis, coma, and death[37, 38, 39]. *However, certain breeds of dogs exhibit an idiosyncratic sensitivity to ivermectin, developing side-effects at doses as low as 0.1 mg/kg. Collies, Old English Sheepdogs, and Shetland Sheepdogs are particularly susceptible[37].*

Ivermectin dosages over 0.05 mg/kg will kill *Dirofilaria immitis* larvae. Therefore, in heartworm-endemic areas dogs should be tested for heartworm before receiving ivermectin in acaricidal dosages[37].

Many dogs with ivermectin toxicity will recover, particularly if recognized early and treated adequately. The provision of adequate nursing care is critical[39] and treatment is based on antishock doses of glucocorticoids and intravenous fluids[38, 39]. Specific agents that may antagonize ivermectin include picrotoxin and physostigmine. Clinicians are unlikely to be able to

NB: All use of ivermectin in dogs and cats is off-label. Collies, Collie-crosses, and some herding breeds are very susceptible to central nervous system side-effects when given ivermectin. They may die!

obtain these agents easily or quickly.

The inability to predict with any confidence if an individual dog will exhibit ivermectin toxicity is one of the main problems facing clinicians[38]. A modified dosing schedule has been proposed which provides for a gradually increasing dose, allowing the opportunity to observe the dogs closely for toxic signs[34]. Prompt intervention (and at the subcritical dose stage) increases the chances of recovery from ivermectin toxicity. The modified dosing scheme is as follows[after 34]:

Day 1   0.05 mg/kg
Day 2   0.1 mg/kg
Day 3   0.15 mg/ kg
Day 4   0.2 mg/ kg
Day 5   0.3 mg/ kg

Amitraz

Indications: *Demodex* spp., *Sarcoptes scabiei*, ticks. Amitraz is a monoamine oxidase inhibitor presented in an organic vehicle. Although serious side-effects are rare, owners may report transient lethargy and hypothermia post dipping[40, 41]. Bradycardia, hypertension, and hyperglycaemia may be seen in some animals[27, 40]. Problems are most serious in very small dogs where the hypothermia may be severe. The drug is contraindicated in Chihuahuas, for example. Precautions must be taken to prevent operator exposure[41] and the dipping should be performed in a well-ventilated room. The person carrying out the dipping should wear gloves and waterproof protective clothing.

One ml of 19.9% amitraz solution in 30 ml mineral oil, or 2 ml 5% solution in 20 ml mineral oil, has been recommended for the treatment of canine otodemodicosis[11, 12, 19].

Amitraz is also licensed (in the UK) against scabies, at a dilution of 0.025% (25 ml 5% solution in 5 liters water).

Amitraz dips are useful as a tick repellent[22] and in some countries the chemical is marketed as an amitraz-impregnated collar for this purpose. Accidental ingestion of amitraz-impregnated collars may prove fatal to dogs and prompt treatment is

necessary. Atipamezole (50 mcg/kg i/m) should be followed by oral yohimbine (0.1 mg/kg) every six hours as needed[27].

Fipronil

Indications: *Spilopsyllus cuniculi, Otodectes cynotis, Sarcoptes scabies, Neotrombicula autumnalis*, ticks, lice. Fipronil is primarily marketed as a flea control product and as such it will be effective against *S. cuniculi* (see Chapter 4: Dermatoses characterized by crust and scale). Although presented in both spray and spot-on formulations, the spray formulation is preferred for the treatment of otic parasites since effective local concentrations on both hair and skin surfaces may be achieved rapidly. Fipronil is also effective against lice[42].

Fipronil has been demonstrated under field conditions to prevent infestation with trombiculid mites and ticks[23, 26]. The spray formulation of fipronil is preferred for this indication.

Fipronil spray has also proven effective against scabies[43] and it may be particularly useful when clinicians are faced with scabies in very young puppies, where other topical treatments are inadvisable.

Selamectin

Indications: *Sarcoptes scabiei, Otodectes cynotis*, possibly *Spilopsyllus cuniculi*, lice.
Selamectin is a novel avermectin with considerable advantages over ivermectin:

- It is safe in ivermectin-sensitive Collies[44].
- It is effective against against fleas, roundworms, hookworms, and heartworm[45, 46, 47] in addition to *O. cynotis* and *S. scabiei*.
- It is applied topically.

Selamectin must not be given to animals of less than six weeks of age and it must be applied topically to the back of the neck, even for the treatment of *O. cynotis*.

FOREIGN BODIES

KEY POINTS
- Younger dogs from hunting and working breeds are predisposed.
- Otic foreign bodies usually, but not always, cause acute clinical signs of otitis.
- Grass awns are the most common foreign body entering the external ear canal.
- Always examine both ears as foreign bodies may be bilateral.
- Rupture of the tympanum is a common complication of otic foreign body penetration.
- Otic foreign bodies are most commonly seen in the summer, reflecting the importance of grass awns in the etiology.

There is no sex predisposition to otic foreign body penetration but young dogs are predisposed to grass awn penetration[1, 2]. In general, all breeds of Spaniels and Golden Retrievers are most commonly affected, while German Shepherd Dogs, Miniature Poodles, and Dachshunds are underrepresented[2].

The most common foreign body found in the external ear canal of dogs and cats is the grass awn[1]. In the USA the most common species of plant awn is *Hordeum jubatum*, although other members of the genus, such as *H. murinum*, *H. silvestre*, and genera such as *Stipa*, *Setaria*, *Bromus*, and *Avena*, may be involved in other areas of the world[2]. All have a similar shape (**173**) with wiry barbs which prevent retrograde movement; once in the ear canal they can only move forward (**174**).

Hair shafts, particularly if they contact the tympanum, may also act as foreign bodies (**175**). In one series of 120 cases of otitis externa, 12.6% of the cases were considered to result from matted hair in the external ear canal[3]. Other foreign bodies that may enter, or be put into, the external ear canal include other pieces of vegetation and children's toys. Aggregations of otic, usually proprietary, non-veterinary powders and ointments with cerumen may also induce foreign body reactions.

Foreign body penetration into the ear canal is usually accompanied by acute pain. The dog or cat shakes its head and may attempt to remove the object with a foot. As the object moves down it may induce hyperemia and ulceration followed by the generation of an otic discharge and secondary bacterial proliferation (**176**). If the foreign body penetrates the epithelial lining of the external ear canal, it may become embedded in a pyogranuloma[4]. In one study[2] nearly 20% of cases of otic grass awn penetration were associated with rupture of the tympanum (**177**), suggesting that otitis media should be considered in long-standing cases, even where the tympanum is intact.

The most common bacteria associated with grass awns are streptococci, although *Staphylococcus* spp, *Pasteurella* spp., and *Actinomycetes* spp. may also be cultured[2].

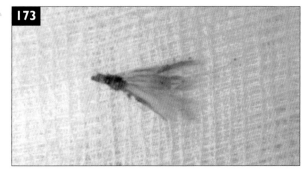

173 Typical shape of a grass awn; this was removed from the external ear canal of a dog.

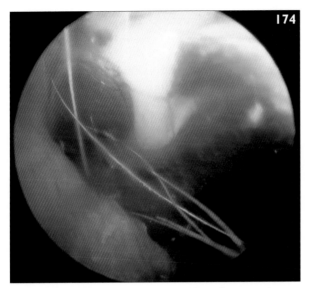

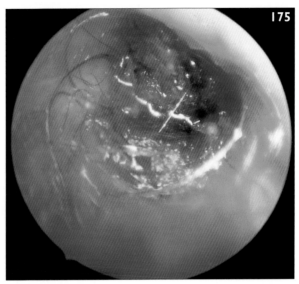

174   Otoscopic picture of grass awn lying adjacent to the tympanic membrane. In this case the grass awn had not punctured the tympanum; however, note the area of erythema and erosion on the tympanic membrane.

175   Accumulation of hair and cerumen obstructing the horizontal ear canal at the level of the tympanum.

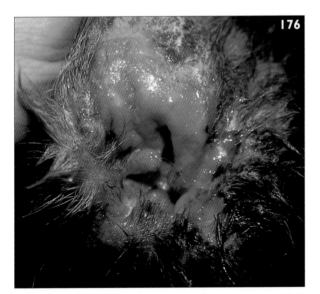

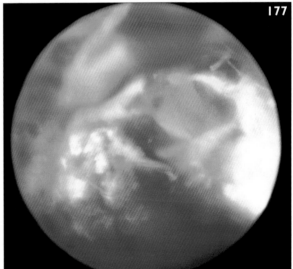

176   Acute, erythematous, ulcerated otitis externa associated with the penetration of a grass awn into the external ear canal.

177   Grass awn penetration of the tympanum. Note the small piece of vegetation still visible on the left, adjacent to the area of hemorrhage.

NASOPHARYNGEAL AND MIDDLE EAR POLYPS

KEY POINTS

- Nasopharyngeal polyps are benign growths which usually arise from the middle ear or distal auditory tube.
- Polyps are extremely rare in the dog and uncommon in the cat.
- Presenting signs may relate to oropharyngeal obstruction, otitis media, or otitis externa.
- Diagnosis is based on clinical signs, radiography, and visual examination at surgery.
- Removing the polyps by traction alone is not advocated as recurrence usually occurs.
- Ventral bulla osteotomy is indicated in most cases.

INTRODUCTION

Inflammatory polyps are non-neoplastic masses arising from the epithelial mucosa of the nasopharynx, auditory tube, or middle ear[1]. The most common sites of origin are within the tympanic bulla or at the distal (tympanic) end of the auditory tube. Polyps are the most common masses arising within the ear system and they are benign in nature[1, 2, 3]. The etiology of these growths is unknown. Polyps are very rare in the dog[4], although they have been reported[5].

CLINICAL FEATURES

There is no breed or age predisposition but most polyps are found in young cats[2, 6]. Most cases are unilateral in presentation[1]. Clinical signs relate to the presence of a mass within the nasopharynx, the middle ear, or the external ear canal:

- Nasopharyngeal polyps protrude from, or through, the proximal oriface of the auditory tube and provoke various signs such as voice change, gagging, a chronic nasal discharge, dysphagia, chronic cough, or severe respiratory embarrassment with cyanosis[2, 3, 6]. Local lymphadenopathy is common[2, 3].
- Polyps confined to the middle ear may produce neurologic signs associated with otitis media such as nystagmus, Horner's syndrome, head tilt, or circling[2, 3, 6].
- Polyps breaching the tympanic membrane may be associated with signs of otitis media but cases may also exhibit a chronic, often malodorous, purulent, occasionally hemorrhagic discharge[2, 3].

In some cases cats may exhibit signs reflecting lesions in one, two, or all three of the areas above. Thus, polyps arising in the middle ear and growing proximally along the auditory tube may provoke signs of respiratory disease without signs of otitis media, provided middle ear drainage is unimpeded and the tympanum is not breached. Alternatively, Horner's syndrome, in association with gagging, may well result from a polyp arising in the middle ear which grows proximally along the auditory tube to protrude into the nasopharynx[6]. Finally, otitis media and chronic otorrhea may result from a polyp arising in the auditory tube, growing distally onto the bulla, provoking otitis media, breaching the tympanum, and resulting in the otic discharge.

DIAGNOSIS

Nasopharyngeal polyps are usually unilateral but typically cause bilateral nasal discharge. There may be local lymphadenopathy. The differential diagnosis of nasopharyngeal polyps includes upper respiratory infection, nasopharyngeal foreign bodies, fungal sinusitis, and neoplasia. In particular, young cats with suspected upper respiratory infection which fail properly to respond to appropriate treatment should be screened for nasopharyngeal polyps[3]. Examination of the pharynx typically reveals a ventrally displaced soft palate (**178**).

Chronic otitis externa mandates otoscopic examination. Bilateral otitis externa in young cats usually reflects *Otodectes cynotis* infestation. Unilateral otitis externa, particularly if chronic in nature, is very suspicious of an otic mass since extraneous otic foreign bodies are rare in cats (**179**). Since most polyps will have passed through, or originated within, the middle ear the tympanum will be ruptured and there may be a detectable mass within the external ear canal (**180**).

> Do not forget to examine the ear canals in cases of nasopharyngeal polyps and the nasopharynx in cases of polyps in the external ear canal.

178 Two nasopharyngeal polyps, identified intraorally after reflecting the soft palate.

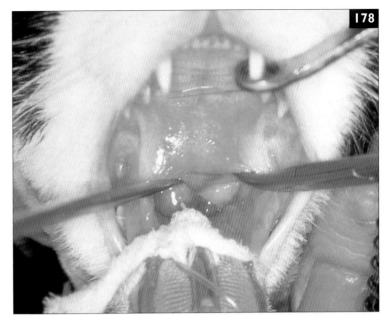

179 An aural polyp at the entrance to the external ear canal.

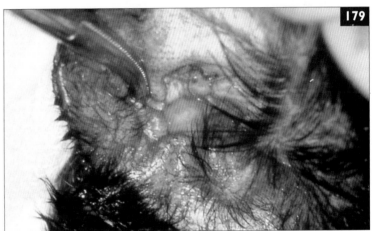

180 Otoscopic view of a polyp within the external ear canal.

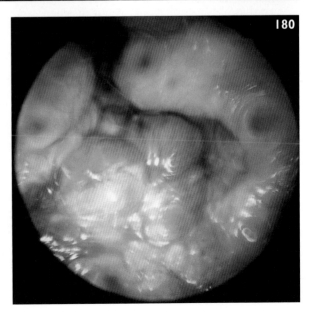

All cats with suspected polyps should be subjected to radiographic examination of the bullae, not only cats with signs referable to the middle ear disease. Signs of otitis media such as thickened walls, soft tissue densities, and fluid lines (**181, 182**) may well indicate that the polyp arises within the middle ear or that there is middle ear pathology. Ventral bull osteotomy and extirpation of the site of origin of the polyp should be performed on these cats.

PATHOLOGIC FEATURES

Polyps are variable in appearance. They may be smooth (**183**), granular, or friable in nature and they often have a pale pinkish-gray coloration[3]. On section they tend to have a pale, rather uniformly dense appearance. Histopathologically the polyps are essentially connective tissue, often containing an inflammatory infiltrate[4], with an epithelial covering. The epithelium is usually thin, one to two layers thick, and it may be ciliated or non-ciliated, columnar or stratified, and squamous non-keratinizing in nature[2, 3, 6]. Some polyps exhibit very ulcerated surfaces. Occasionally, mucus-secreting glands are found beneath the surface[3]. Lymphoid follicles may be found within the stroma[3, 4].

MANAGEMENT

Nasopharyngeal polyps may cause respiratory embarrassment to such an extent that anesthetic induction is potentially complicated[1]. Preanaesthetic oxygenation may allow for an increased safety margin if intubation is difficult because the soft palate is pushed ventrally[1, 3].

Lesions that mimic the appearance of polyps are so rare that presurgical biopsy is not justified[1] and immediate excision should be undertaken. Nasopharyngeal polyps may be removed by transecting the pedicle as close to the opening of the auditory tube as possible. It is usually possible to achieve this without transecting the soft palate; simply maneuver the soft palate rostrally and dorsally to allow the polyp to fall free[1, 3, 6]. Hemorrhage following transection of the pedicle is minimal[1, 3].

Clinicians should note, however, that simply removing the polyp by traction or pedicle section, whether the polyp is pharyngeal or otic, results in recurrence rates of approximately 30%[1, 2, 3]. Therefore, consideration should be given to bulla osteotomy, even in cases where signs of otitis media are not present. This is justified on the basis that the middle ear, or distal auditory tube immediately adjacent to the middle ear, is the most likely site of origin of the polyp[1].

If neurologic and radiographic examination determines that the tympanic bulla is the site of origin, or that there is bulla pathology, ventral bulla osteotomy is indicated[1, 6]. This allows removal of the mucosa from which the polyp arises and permits drainage from the bulla, which alleviates the otitis media. Bacterial infection frequently accompanies polyps which arise from the middle ear, and swabbing for bacterial culture and sensitivity testing is recommended[1, 7].

POSTOPERATIVE COMPLICATIONS

Recurrence will occur if the origin of the polyp is not excised. Removing the polyp by traction has been associated with a recurrence rate of 30%[1, 2]. In contrast, extirpating the mucosal lining of the bulla when polyps originated in the middle ear resulted in no recurrence[1, 6].

181, 182 Lateral (**181**) and rostrocaudal (open mouth) (**182**) radiographs of a cat's skull. Note the increased tissue density within the right bulla and external ear canal (arrows).

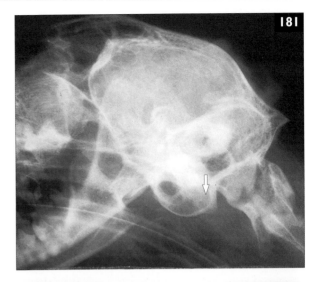

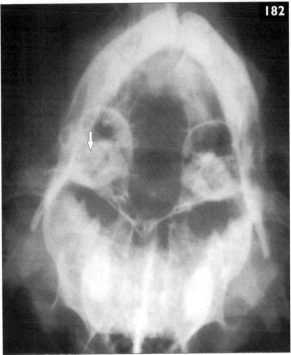

183 A resected nasopharyngeal polyp removed from a cat's bulla via ventral bulla osteotomy. The stump of stalk, which originated within the auditory tube, is visible on the right.

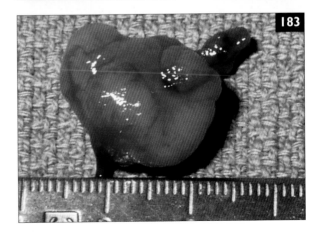

OTIC NEOPLASIA

KEY POINTS

- Otic neoplasia is uncommon.
- Not all growths within the external ear canal are neoplastic; polyps and inflammatory granulomas can occur.
- In the dog most conchal neoplasia is benign, whereas in the cat it is malignant.
- The most common sign of conchal neoplasia is chronic otitis externa, often associated with malodour.
- Radical excision is indicated, usually associated with lateral wall resection or ablation of the external ear canal.

INTRODUCTION

Neoplasia of the external ear canal is generally agreed to be uncommon in dogs and cats[1–4]. Pinnal neoplasms are somewhat more common. Thus, in a study of 340 cats with skin neoplasia, 8.7% of basal cell tumors, 8% of fibrosarcomas, 13.8% of mast cell tumors, and 40% of squamous cell carcinomas occurred on the pinna[5]. The pinna is the most common site for canine cutaneous histiocytoma, the most common canine tumor[6]. Pinnal neoplasia is more commonly encountered in dogs and cats in tropical and subtropical areas, a consequence of prolonged exposure to actinic radiation inducing squamous cell carcinomas[7, 8]. Neoplasia of the middle ear is rare[9].

PINNAL NEOPLASIA

Pinnal neoplasia in dogs tends to be benign, with the exception of mast cell tumors (*Table 6*). Pinnal neoplasia in cats tends to be malignant. Numerous tumor types are reported, as might be expected from an organ composed of skin, connective tissue, and cartilage, but only the most frequently recognized types will be discussed here.

Papilloma

Cutaneous papillomas (**184**) are almost exclusively confined to dogs[10, 11]. Cocker Spaniels, Kerry Blue Terriers, and male dogs in general are predisposed[10, 12]. The lesions are usually well-demarcated, superficial, occasionally pedunculated papules (i.e. <1 cm [<0.4 in] diameter) which tend to bleed if traumatized[13]. Many papillomas exhibit a frond-like appearance[10]. The virus is related to, but is a subtype of, the papovavirus which causes canine oral papillomatosis[14]. Cutaneous papillomas are not considered transmissible in the clinical setting[15]. Papillomas sometimes occur in the external ear canal[3].

Diagnosis is generally made on clinical grounds, although sebaceous adenomas may have a similar clinical appearance. Diagnosis may be confirmed by histopathologic examination of excised tissue. Cutaneous papillomas rarely undergo spontaneous regression. Since they are benign they generally do not warrant surgical excision, unless the papilloma becomes traumatized. However, many owners find them esthetically displeasing and request excision. After excision a good prognosis may be given[13].

Table 6: Most common pinnal neoplasms of dogs and cats[2, 6].

Dogs	Cats
Benign	*Benign*
Pinnal histiocytoma	Basal cell tumor
Papilloma	
Malignant	*Malignant*
Rare	Mast cell neoplasia
	Sqaumous cell carcinoma
	Fibrosarcoma

Canine cutaneous histiocytoma

Canine cutaneous histiocytomas (**185**) are most likely of Langerhans cell origin[16]. These are the most common neoplasms of the dog and 50% of cases occur in dogs under two years of age[17]. Pedigree dogs are predisposed, particularly Boxers, English Bulldogs, Greyhounds, and Scottish Terriers[6, 17]. The most common site for the tumor is the dorsal pinna, often toward the base[2, 6, 17]. These are solitary, elevated, domed, erythematous, well-demarcated, minimally pruritic lesions which are often reported to show rapid growth. Occasionally they are ulcerated and very rarely they have been reported to be multiple[17].

A tentative diagnosis is generally made on clinical grounds but because of the difficulty in ruling out mast cell tumor, in particular, further work up is indicated. A granulomatous lesion would be the other most likely differential. Microscopic examination of aspirated cytologic samples will usually allow differentiation of histiocytoma (**186**) from mast cell tumor[2, 18, 19], but histopathologic examination of excised tissue is necessary to rule out granuloma and to obtain a definitive diagnosis. Canine cutaneous histiocytomas are benign lesions and the response to surgery is close to 100%[17]. A good prognosis may be given.

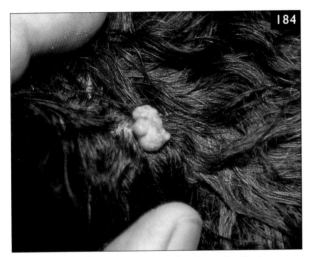

184 Flesh-colored papilloma on the pinna of a Cocker Spaniel.

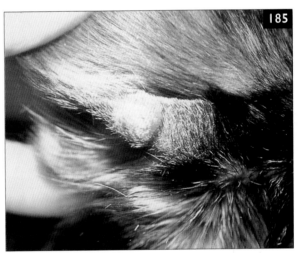

185 Discrete, erythematous histiocytoma on the rostral edge of the pinna.

186 Photomicrograph of a needle cytologic sample from the lesion in **185**. Note the discrete, large, round cells with an absence of granules in the cytoplasm.

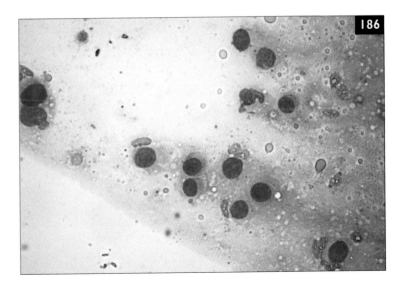

Squamous cell carcinoma

Squamous cell carcinoma is the most common malignant neoplasm of the cat and the pinna is a predilection site [2, 5, 20, 21]. Squamous cell carcinoma rarely affects the canine pinna[13]. In one study the mean age of affected cats was 12 years[5]. Early lesions of actinic dermatitis may precede neoplastic transformation; this is related to long-term exposure to actinic radiation[22]. Consequently the disease is more common in tropical regions. Squamous cell carcinoma may also be seen in temperate regions, particularly on the tips of the pinnae of white ears[20]. White cats with blue eyes are generally predisposed[21]. The earliest clinical sign is hyperemia (**187**), which may wax and wane for a number of years in temperate climates. Malignant transformation is characterized by a thickened, folded pinnal margin, ulceration, and crust (**188, 189**).

Squamous cell carcinoma of the feline pinna has low metastatic potential[21] and it may remain *in situ* for some considerable time[23]. Local invasion and spread to the regional lymph nodes and, ultimately, the lung fields may be seen[2]. Surgical excision of the pinnal margin is curative in most cases (**190, 191**); a 5 mm (0.2 in) margin must be achieved[2, 20]. In cats with white pinnae the tips of the pinnae may be excised as a prophylactic measure at the earliest sign of actinic damage. Cryotherapy achieves good cosmetic results[20] but local recurrence is quite common[24], perhaps because the margin of affected tissue is not well delineated[25]. In a study comparing surgical excision, cryotherapy, and radiotherapy[26], it was found that although all modalities were effective, surgical excision achieved the longest disease-free interval (*Table 7*).

Table 7: A comparison of the disease-free intervals and survival times for various treatments of feline squamous cell carcinoma of the nasal planum and pinna[27].

Treatment modality	Disease-free interval (median)	Survival time (median)
Surgical excision (n = 39)	594 days	673 days
Cryosurgery (n = 11)	254 days	682 days
Radiotherapy (n = 11)	361 days	383 days

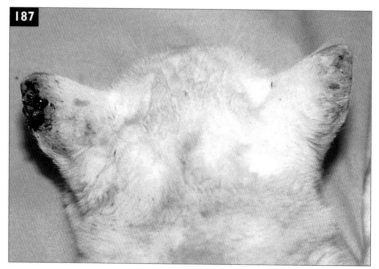

187   White haired cat with erythematous lesions of early squamous cell carcinoma on the right pinna. More advanced disease is apparent on the left pinna.

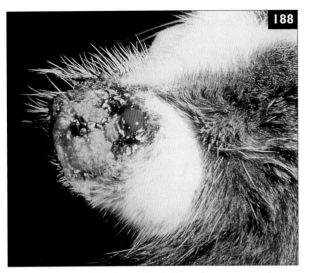

188   Crusted and early erosive lesions of squamous cell carcinoma on the distal pinna of a cat.

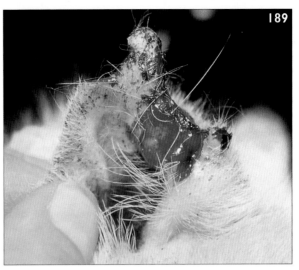

189   Advanced stage of squamous cell carcinoma of the pinna of a cat. The ulceration is well advanced.

190   This cat has had the distal pinna amputated to well below the hair line.

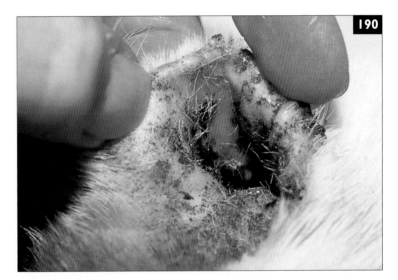

191   This cat has had bilateral pinnal ablation to remove active lesions.

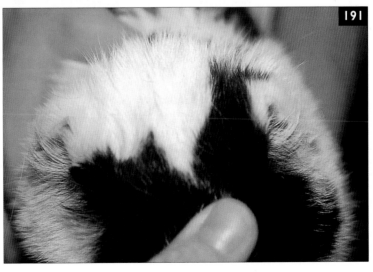

Canine mast cell tumor

Mast cell tumors are common in the dog[18, 19]. Although mast cell tumors may occur in young dogs (hence the inclusion of canine cutaneous histiocytoma as a differential diagnosis), the incidence increases with age, peaking at eight or nine years of age[18, 19]. Boxers, and other breeds with Bulldog ancestry, are predisposed but mast cell tumors may occur in any dog[18, 19]. The predilection site for mast cell neoplasia varies from breed to breed[19]. Thus in the Boxer it is the hindlimb which is predisposed, whereas in the Rhodesian Ridgeback it is the tail[19].

The clinical appearance of the tumor is very variable but single cutaneous lesions less than 3 cm (1.2 in) in diameter (**192**) are the most common presentation. The diagnosis of mast cell tumor is made by a combination of cytologic and histopathologic examination of aspirated or excised material. However, clinical management of all but single nodules (treated by wide surgical excision) will mandate clinical staging prior to initiation of treatment (*Table 8*). Note, however, that with regard to the pinna, the advised 3 cm (1.2 in) margin rule is clearly impractical[18]. Given that most mast cells extend laterally rather than deeper, it may be best to amputate the pinna at the first presentation[18].

The selection of various treatment modalities for extensive or recurrent canine mast cell tumors is beyond the scope of this book, and readers are referred to specialist texts. Clinicians may well have to consider referral to institutions offering radiotherapy and chemotherapy.

Feline mast cell tumor

The skin of the convex surface of the feline pinna has a higher concentration of mast cells than skin in other areas[27], although whether this relates to the relatively high incidence of feline mast cell tumors which occur on the pinna and head[3, 25] is not known. There is no sex predisposition but Siamese cats appear to be at risk[3, 19]. Mast cell tumors of the pinna tend to occur toward the base[5]. Feline mast cell tumors present and behave in a different way to canine mast cell tumors. They may appear as slow or rapidly growing intracutaneous papules or nodules, which may have a pink coloration and may ulcerate. Some animals present with multiple small papules, often closely grouped[19, 28]. Feline mast cell tumors tend to behave in a benign manner[5, 19], with a low rate of visceral metastasis compared to the canine form of the disease[28, 29, 30]. They tend to recur locally and the relatively benign nature should not preclude aggressive management. Furthermore, mast cell tumors may arise, *de novo*, at distant sites[19].

Basal cell tumor

Canine basal cell tumors tend to be solitary, slow growing, well-defined, occasionally ulcerated nodules, 1–5 cm (0.4–2.0 in) in diameter, which are benign in behavior[13, 31]. Feline basal cell tumors are much more variable at presentation; they may be rounded or intradermal and they may be cystic[5, 31]. Although feline basal cell tumors are benign, with an excellent prognosis[5, 31], they may undergo malignant transformation to basal cell carcinoma. These malignant tumors may be multicentric, tend to occur on the rostral end of the body, are intradermal, and often ulcerate[5, 31]. Given that clinically it is not possible to differentiate a benign neoplasm from a malignant one, wide surgical margin is advocated[31]. Basal cell tumors may sometimes occur in the external ear canal[3].

Fibrosarcoma

Fibrosarcomas are more common in the cat than in the dog[32]. The most common presentation is of a solitary, domed, rarely ulcerated, well-demarcated neoplasm[5, 32]. Solitary fibrosarcomas usually occur in older cats and it is this type (rather than the viral-associated multiple presentation sometimes seen in younger cats) which is usually found on the pinna[5, 32]. Feline fibrosarcomas tend to recur after surgery[21, 32] and a wide margin is advised. Again, in practice this implies a degree of pinnal amputation. Postsurgical radiotherapy may be beneficial[21, 32]. Fibrosarcomas are rarely found on the canine pinna[2, 32].

Table 8: Summary of the diagnosis, staging, and management of canine mast cell neoplasia (based on Goldschmidt and Shofer[19]).

Clinical work up of canine mast cell neoplasia
- Cytologic examination of aspirates or touch impressions of lesion and regional lymph node.
- Histopathologic examination of excised material.
- Full hematology and biochemistry.
- Buffy coat examination.
- Bone marrow biopsy.

Consider results and stage tumor
- One tumor, confined to the dermis, no lymph node involvement (Stage 1):
  (a) without systemic signs;
  (b) with clinical signs.
- One tumor, confined to the dermis, regional lymph nodes involved (Stage 2):
  (a) without systemic signs;
  (b) with clinical signs.
- Multiple dermal tumors, or large infiltrating tumors with or without lymph node involvement (Stage 3):
  (a) without systemic signs;
  (b) with clinical signs.
- Any tumor, or recurrence, with metastasis (Stage 4).

Treatment plans
- Stage 1 (a and b): local excision with 3 cm (1.2 in) margins on all sides.
- Stage 2 (a and b): local excision of tumor, radiotherapy of surgical site and regional lymph node. In addition, Stage 2b receives systemic prednisolone. **NB:** No radiotherapy of perineal or genital lesions.
- Stages 3 and 4: Local debulking if possible, chemotherapy, consider radiotherapy.

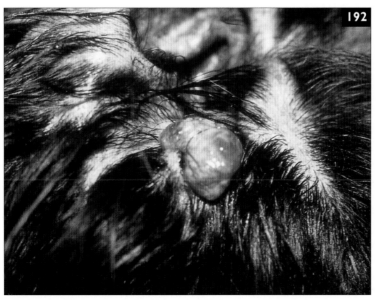

192 Mast cell tumor. Solitary, well-demarcated, rapidly growing ulcerated nodule at the base of the pinna of a dog.

CONCHAL NEOPLASIA

Neoplasia of the external ear canal is rare[3]. In general, otic neoplasia in cats tends to be malignant[1, 3] and is likely to be found in either the vertical or the horizontal canal with equal frequency[3]. Otic discharge, pruritus, and pain are common, whereas neurologic signs are rare[3]. Canine conchal neoplasia is more likely to be benign than feline conchal neoplasia, but distribution and clinical signs are similar[1, 3]. Most benign tumors do not affect the bullae[3]. Although the malignant tumors, particularly in the cat, tend to invade locally, it appears that distant metastasis is the exception rather than the rule[3]. When nervous signs accompany otic neoplasia, a generally poor prognosis is necessary since this usually indicates middle ear involvement and squamous cell carcinoma; altogether a more malignant tumor than ceruminous gland adenocarcinoma of the external ear canal[3]. Indeed, when squamous cell carcinoma is found in the external ear canal it usually has its origins in the middle ear.

Papillomas, basal cell tumors, and ceruminous gland adenomas are the most commonly found benign tumors in dogs, while in cats ceruminous gland adenomas are most common (*Table 9*)[3]. Carcinomas, adenocarcinomas, and squamous cell carcinomas are the most common malignant tumors

> Malignant conchal neoplasia must be identified and treated radically. Lateral wall resection is not adequate; total ablation of the ear canal and lateral bulla osteotomy is indicated.

in both dogs and cats. The clinical appearance of these neoplasms is usually that of a raised, frequently ulcerated mass which may occlude the lumen[3].

Ceruminous gland adenoma

Benign ceruminous gland neoplasia tends to present with signs of obstructive otitis externa (**193**): pruritus, head shaking, malodor, otorrhea, and occasional hemorrhage[20, 33]. Ceruminous gland adenomas are most commonly seen in middle-aged to elderly animals[2, 33]. These benign tumors tend to be raised and occasionally pedunculated (**194**) and they may occlude the external ear canal[32]. They may have a melanotic appearance (**195**) and may be multiple[2]. Aggressive surgical management is usually curative and lateral wall resection, vertical wall ablation, or total ablation of the external ear canal is indicated, as dictated by the extent of the tumor.

Table 9: The most common tumors of the external ear canal of dogs and cats[5].

Dogs	Cats
Benign	*Benign*
Papilloma	Ceruminous gland adenoma
Basal cell tumor	
Ceruminous gland adenoma	
Sebaceous gland adenoma	
Malignant	*Malignant*
Ceruminous gland adenocarcinoma	Ceruminous gland adenocarcinoma
Other carcinomas	Squamous cell carcinoma
Squamous cell carcinoma	Other carcinoma

193 Obstructive otitis secondary to ceruminous gland neoplasia in a cat.

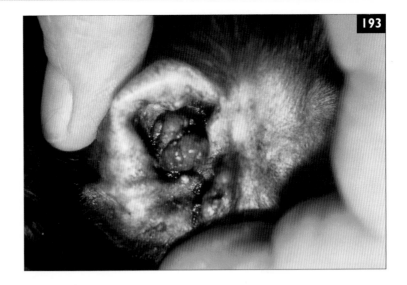

194 Large, pedunculated ceruminous gland adenoma protruding from the external ear canal of a dog.

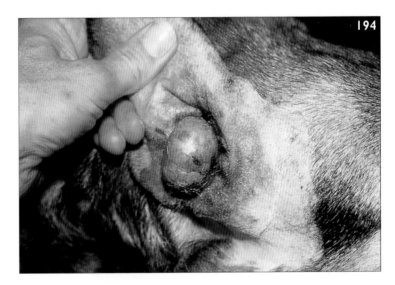

195 Multiple, melanotic ceruminous gland adenomas in the external ear canal of a cat.

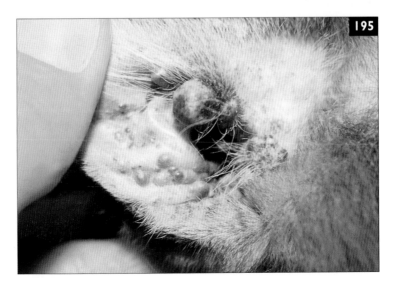

Ceruminous gland adenocarcinoma

Malignant ceruminous gland tumors tend to be ulcerative and infiltrating rather than occlusive[2, 33]. Most cases tend to occur in old animals – cats: mean age 12 years; dogs: mean age nine years[34, 35]. Otoscopically they are pinkish in color (**196**), ulcerated, and friable in nature[34, 35]. Most dogs and cats exhibit an otic discharge which is commonly malodorous, purulent (**197**), and blood stained[34, 35]. Otic pruritus and ipsilateral mandibular lymphadenopathy is also commonly noted[34, 35]. Bulla involvement was demonstrated in nearly half the cats and dogs in recent studies[34, 35]. This tendency to involve the bulla (**198, 199**) is reflected in the response to surgery; radical, total ear canal ablation and bulla osteotomy results in a longer disease-free interval, a lower recurrence rate, and longer postoperative survival time than simple lateral wall resection[34, 35]. If the tumor has extended through the external ear canal into surrounding soft tissue, adjunctive radiotherapy is indicated[33, 36].

Squamous cell carcinoma

In cats, squamous cell carcinoma appears to be as common as ceruminous gland adenocarcinoma[3]. The tumors are proliferative and ulcerated (**200**) and they have a tendency to grow rapidly[2]. Most conchal tumors with otoscopically visible evidence of extensive spread and histopathologic evidence of local infiltration are squamous cell carcinomas[3]. Radical resection is necessary and presurgical biopsy may be advantageous.

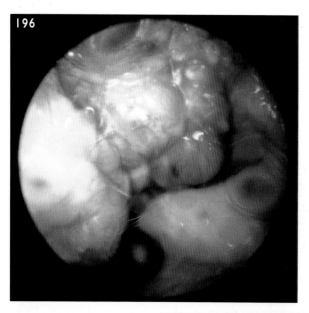

196 Pinkish, nodular appearance of a ceruminous gland adenocarcinoma in the external ear canal of a cat.

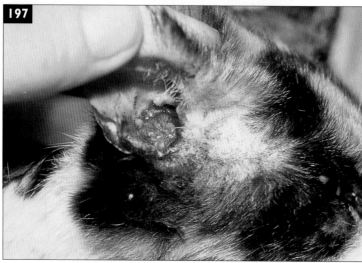

197 Malodorous, hemorrhagic obstructive otitis secondary to ceruminous gland adenocarcinoma in a cat. The ulcerated mass of tumor may be seen protruding into the lumen at the entrance to the external ear canal.

198   CT scan of a 13-year-old cat. There is increased soft tissue opacity in the right external ear canal extending up to, and perhaps across, the tympanic membrane. This is a ceruminous gland adenocarcinoma. Note that the right bulla appears as normal as the left. The bony septum dividing the feline bulla into lateral and medial compartments is clearly visible with this imaging modality.

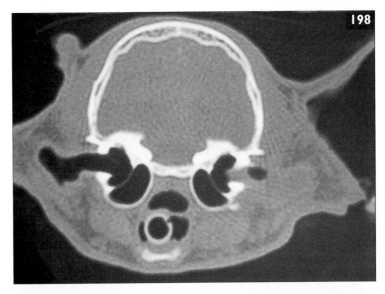

199   CT scan of a ten-year-old Cocker Spaniel. The left-hand side exhibits an irregular, imprecise outline to the bulla, increased density within the bulla, loss of air within the external ear canal, mineralization of soft tissue in the external ear canal, and a homogenous soft tissue mass on the ventral aspect of the skull. This is a ceruminous gland adenocarcinoma.

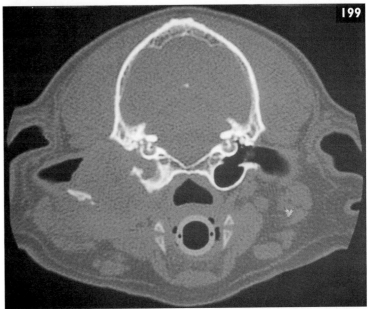

200   Ulcerated, poorly defined squamous cell carcinoma at the entrance to the external ear canal of a dog.

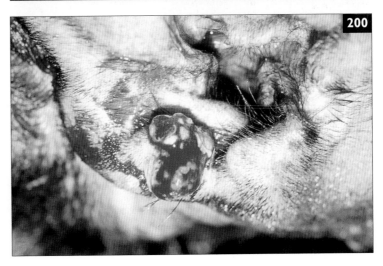

Non-neoplastic growths

Pyogenic granulomas

These have been reported to occur within the external ear canal of cats[37]. Clinically the granulomas appear as fleshy masses that may be covered in epithelium. However, the epithelial surface is usually ulcerated[37]. The prognosis for pyogenic granuloma is much better than for overt neoplasia. However, histopathologic examination of biopsy samples is essential to distinguish the two.

Eosinophilic granulomas

Eosinophilic granuloma of the external ear canal has been reported in four dogs[38]. These dogs presented with chronic otitis externa. Otoscopic examination revealed a solitary, friable mass occluding the vertical canal. Surgical excision was curative.

Cryptococcosis

Cryptococcosis and other fungal disease may occasionally cause granulomatous lesions near the external ear canal (**201**). Histopathologic examination of biopsy samples will identify these lesions. Cryptococcosis has a better prognosis that squamous cell carcinoma, thereby justifying biopsy.

MIDDLE EAR NEOPLASIA

Neoplastic transformation within the middle ear is rare, accounting for only 2.6% of cases referred to the authors of a review of ten years of referral surgery[9]: in total 11 dogs comprising three cases of ceruminous gland adenocarcinoma, two basal cell tumors, two sebaceous adenocarcinomas, two papillary adenomas, one squamous papilloma, and one anaplastic tumor. (However, one report stated that squamous cell carcinoma is the most common tumor of the middle and inner ear of dogs[39].)

Only one of the 11 dogs was less than six years old and there was no sex bias. Persistent otorrhea and otic irritation or pain was the most common clinical sign. Rarely, signs referable to a pharyngeal mass or to neurologic lesions occured[9]. In six dogs there was a visible mass within the external ear canal and in two there was para-aural abscessation. All the animals were examined radiographically and in all cases there was increased radiopacity within the middle ear[9].

Of the eleven dogs in this study only five were amenable to surgery, typically total ablation of the external ear canal combined with bulla osteotomy. Of the five dogs treated surgically four survived for more than eight months after surgery[6].

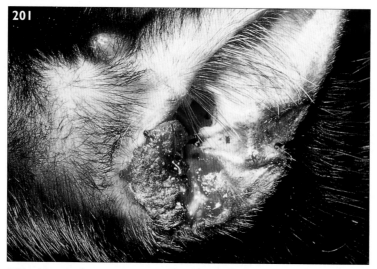

201   Ulcerated granulomatous lesions due to cryptococcosis should be considered in the differential diagnosis of conchal neoplasia.

UNDERLYING DISEASE

KEY POINTS

- Underlying disease is an important cause of chronic otitis externa.
- Atopy is by far the most common underlying disease in chronic otitis externa.
- Unless the underlying disease is recognized and treated, the otitis will continue.
- Corrective surgery, such as Zepp resection, will not be successful if the underlying disease is not treated.

INTRODUCTION

Underlying disease as a cause of otitis externa is important[1]. Most underlying diseases were classified as primary causes of otitis externa by August[1], i.e. they may directly result in otitis externa without the presence of predisposing factors (such as conformation) or perpetuating factors (such as microorganisms). Failure to recognize that atopy is present, for example, may condemn the dog to a lifetime of symptomatic otic therapy and surgery which will fail to elicit a cure.

> Whenever a case of bilateral otitis externa is presented the clinician should consider the possibility of otodectic mange or underlying disease before initiating symptomatic therapy.

HYPERSENSITIVITIES

Atopy

Atopy is an inherited predisposition to develop IgE to environmental allergens resulting in disease[2]. Affected dogs exhibit pruritus and otitis externa[2-4]. Atopy has been stated to be the most common cause of chronic otitis externa in dogs[4]. The incidence of otitis externa in atopic dogs has been estimated at 55% and in 3% of atopic dogs otitis externa was the only clinical sign[3]. Although atopy does exist in cats, it is not usually associated with otitis externa in this species, possibly reflecting differences in otic microclimate.

Otitis externa in atopic dogs often begins as erythema at the base of the concave aspects of the pinnae and on the vertical portions of the external ear canals (**202, 203**)[2]. The horizontal portion of the external ear canal is minimally affected in early cases. Scott[3] reported that otitis externa associated with atopy often flared in association with the skin disease. This is a valuable clue that an alert clinician should spot when taking a history.

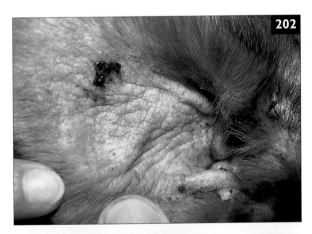

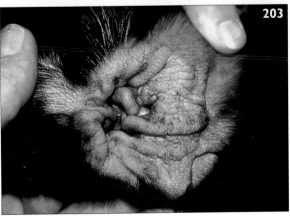

202, 203   Classic signs of a hypersensitivity affecting the proximal aspect of the concave side of the pinna (**202**) and the upper portions of the external ear canal (**203**). There is erythema and hyperplasia in both areas.

Atopy is associated with erythema and edema of the ear canal but there is usually little exudation[3]. Secondary changes and microbial proliferation result in extension of these early clinical signs to the horizontal canal and hyperplasia of the epithelial lining (**204**). Malassezial proliferation may be particularly troublesome (**205**). Although chronic otitis externa is commonly due to atopy, it rarely results in gram-negative bacterial infection.

Lateral wall resection or vertical canal ablation should not be carried out on an atopic ear, in an attempt to alleviate the otitis externa, without an appreciation of the underlying disease. The inflammation will continue to affect the medial and lateral walls of the residual canal and the proximal aspect of the pinna (**206, 207**).

Dietary intolerance

Dietary intolerance is a dermatosis which is much less common than atopy. However, when it occurs there may be concurrent otitis externa. Although otitis externa may, on rare occasions[5], be the only sign of dietary intolerance, it is commonly associated with other signs, typically pruritus[5, 6, 7]. The otitis associated with dietary intolerance appears to be more severe that that seen in atopy and it exhibits a rapid progression. Otitis externa is also associated with dietary intolerance in cats[7, 8].

Contact dermatitis

Allergic contact dermatitis is a rare dermatosis in dogs and almost unknown in cats[9]. In dogs with very extensive or generalized allergic contact dermatitis the concave aspects of the pinnae and upper portion of the vertical ear canals may exhibit lesions (**208**)[10].

More commonly, allergic contact dermatitis or irritant contact dermatitis may occur due to exposure to any of the components of an otic preparation, provided it is used for long enough. Irritant contact dermatitis within the confines of the external ear canal may be due to exposure to one of the common vehicles, propylene glycol[11]. However, the most commonly implicated component is neomycin, although documented, published reports are very rare. Bilateral, erythematous otitis externa would be anticipated (**209**). The classic history is a cat or dog with chronic, relapsing otitis externa, which had previously responded well to a certain medication only to deteriorate when exposed to the medicant again.

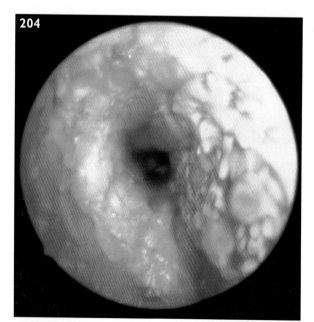

204 Otoscopic picture of the lower portion of the vertical ear canal of a dog with atopy. Note the erythema and hyperplasia.

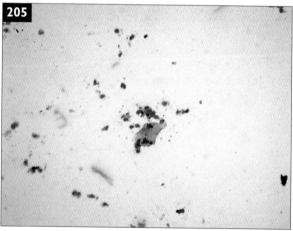

205 Photomicrograph of a cytologic sample taken from an atopic dog's external ear canal. There are a few squames, no inflammatory cells, but many yeast.

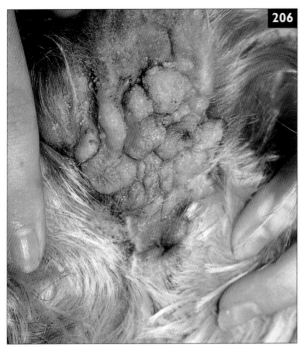

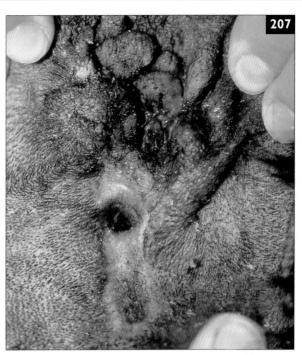

206 Failed lateral wall resection in an atopic West Highland White Terrier. Persistent erythema and hyperplasia continue to affect the residual medial wall of the external ear canal.

207 Only partially successful vertical canal ablation in an atopic dog. Erythema and hyperplasia still affect the proximal aspect of the pinna and the residual portion of the medial wall of the external ear canal.

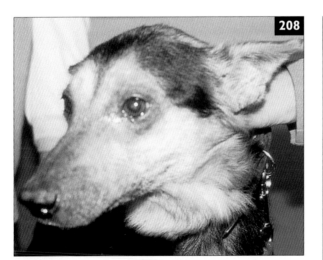

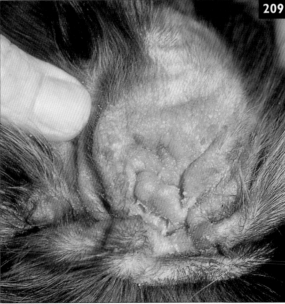

208 Allergic contact dermatitis. Note the hyperpigmentation affecting the perioral, periocular regions in addition to the concave aspect of the pinna and the upper portion of the vertical ear canal.

209 Allergic contact dermatitis following neomycin therapy. Erythematous, hyperplastic otitis externa. Note the lack of lesions on the concave aspect of the pinna, a pointer to this not being atopy, even though the changes in the external ear canal are indistinguishable on clinical grounds.

DEFECTS IN KERATINIZATION

Defects in keratinization may be primary or be secondary to another disease. By far the most common causes of scaling and crusting dermatoses are secondary causes such as ectoparasites, infectious agents, hypersensitivities, and endocrinopathies[12]. Otitis externa may be anticipated with these disorders only if the underlying disease is itself a cause of ear disease. Superficial pyoderma, dermatophytosis, or demodicosis are common causes of crust and scale on the trunk or limbs, but they rarely cause otitis externa. In contrast, the inflammation caused by atopy is generalized, as are the aberrations in cutaneous homeostasis which accompany an endocrinopathy. Thus, these diseases are often associated with otitis externa.

Similarly, some, but not all, of the primary defects in keratinization (idiopathic seborrhea) may be associated with otitis externa. Examples include idiopathic seborrhea in Cocker Spaniels[13] and epidermal dysplasia in West Highland White Terriers[14]. The relationship between epidermal dysplasia and the yeast *Malassezia pachydermatis* in West Highland White Terriers is complex and poorly understood[14, 15]. Basset Hounds also suffer from a dermatosis which used to be classified as idiopathic seborrhea. Many of these dogs suffer from *M. pachydermatis* dermatitis and they show a spectacular response to antimalassezial therapy[16]. Whatever the exact nature of these two disorders, or their relationship, they are both associated with severe otitis externa[14, 16].

The otitis externa associated with primary seborrhea in Cocker Spaniels is initially ceruminous (**210**), but epidermal hyperplasia (**211**) soon follows. The otic discharge is typically thick and oleaginous (**212**). Otoscopic examination of early cases reveals hyperplasia, a moister appearance than in an atopic ear canal (compare with **204**), and a tendency to bleed easily (**213**). Cytologic examination from many cases will reveal plenty of cerumen and cellular debris but only a few inflammatory cells (**214**). Indeed, subsequent bacterial culture from these ears may fail to record any significant bacterial growth at all, illustrating the value of otic cytology. However, in contrast to the otitis associated with atopy, the disease in Cocker Spaniels is often complicated by gram-negative infection (**215**), perhaps a reflection of differences in glandular secretion.

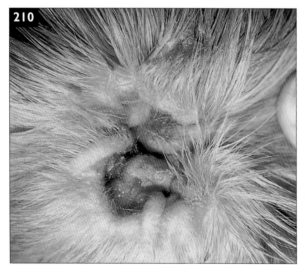

210 Early changes associated with chronic otitis externa in a Cocker Spaniel. Ceruminous otitis with early hyperplasia.

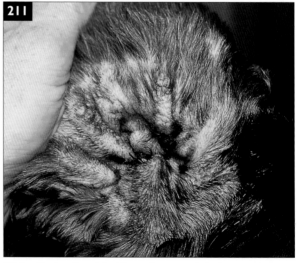

211 Cocker Spaniel with an almost occluded external ear canal, a consequence of chronic otitis externa.

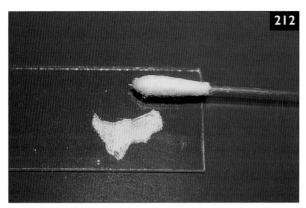

212   Unstained cytology smear. Note the thick, oleaginous nature of the cerumen.

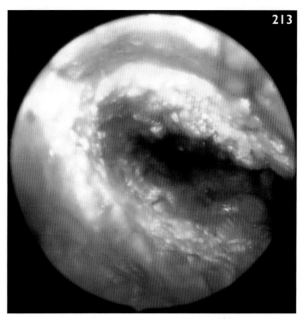

213   Otoscopic picture of the external ear canal of a Cocker Spaniel with early changes associated with chronic otitis externa. There is erythema and the ear canal has a moister appearance than the atopic ear (compare with **204**). Note that the ear canal has been plucked to facilitate cleaning.

214   Photomicrograph of a stained cytologic smear from a Cocker Spaniel. Note the increased numbers of squames, the amount of cerumen, the lack of microorganisms, and the absence of inflammatory cells.

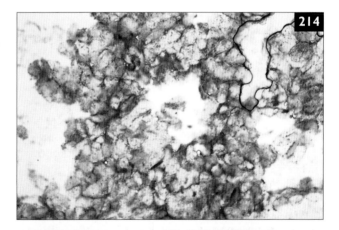

215   Ulcerated external ear canal due to gram-negative bacterial infection in a Cocker Spaniel.

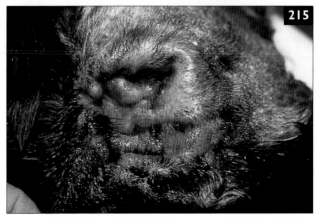

M. pachydermatis is a common cause of otitis externa in West Highland White Terriers and Basset Hounds. In these animals the ears are erythematous, malodorous, and hyperplastic (**216, 217**). Cerumen may be thick and oleaginous and vast numbers of yeast may be detected when smears are stained and examined microscopically (**218**).

Hereditary defects in keratinization have been reported in cats[17]. Persian cats are most commonly affected (**219**), although the condition may occur in other breeds. Affected animals show signs from a very early age and either sex may be affected. The ears develop a ceruminous otitis externa and greasy scale may accumulate on the pinnae. The entire trunk is also affected with scale, grease, and malodor. Because of the severity of the disease, many cases are euthanased at an early age as there is no effective treatment.

ENDOCRINOPATHIES

Endocrinopathies are often cited as underlying causes of chronic ceruminous otitis externa. However, neither hypothyroidism nor hyperadrenocorticism are commonly associated with otitis externa[18, 19, 20]. Gonadal hormone changes (e.g. Sertoli cell tumors), in contrast, may have a profound effect on cutaneous glandular function and may therefore be associated with ceruminous otitis (**220**) in association with other signs[21].

AUTOIMMUNE AND IMMUNE-MEDIATED DISEASES

Pemphigus foliaceus, pemphigus erythematosus, vasculitis, and systemic lupus erythematosus commonly affect the pinnae but they very rarely cause otitis externa[22–25]. However, if vesicles, blisters, erosions, or ulcers are found on the concave aspect of the pinna and in the external ear canal (**221**), these diseases should be considered, particularly if bacteriology and cytology suggest minimal microbial involvement. Cytological examination of vesicular contents may reveal acanthocytes and neutrophils, a combination suggestive of pemphigus foliaceus (see **96**).

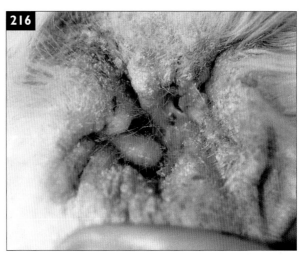

216   Hyperplastic otic epithelium occluding the external ear canal of a West Highland White Terrier.

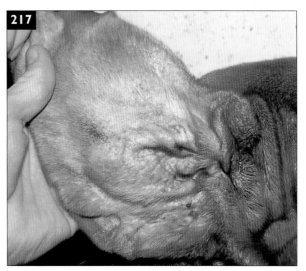

217   Greasy, erythematous, malodorous, hyperplastic otitis externa in a Bassett Hound. Note the extension of the lesions on the pinna.

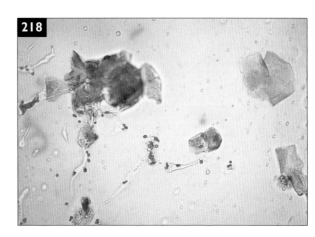

218   Cytologic smear demonstrating cerumen, squames, and many yeast.

219   Persian cat with an hereditary defect in keratinization. There is a greasy otitis externa and greasy tags are apparent on the adjacent skin and hair of the pinna. (Illustration courtesy Dr Manon Paradis.)

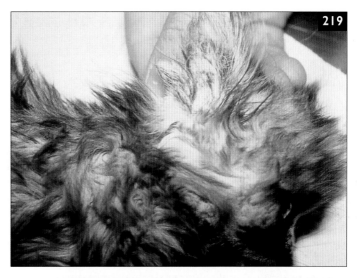

220   Otitis externa associated with a Sertoli cell tumor. Note the ceruminous discharge adhering to the concave aspect of the pinna.

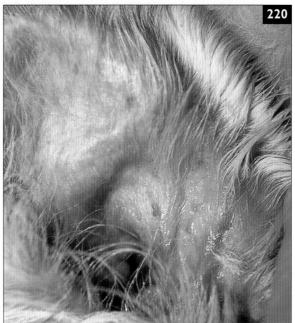

221   Primary lesions of pemphigus foliaceus at the entrance to the external ear canal and on the concave aspect of the pinna.

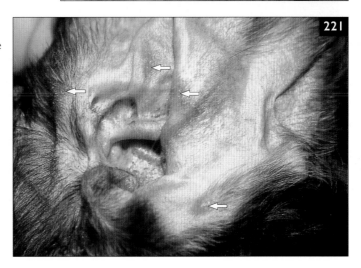

THE EFFECTS OF WEATHER ON THE INCIDENCE OF OTITIS EXTERNA

KEY POINTS
- Increases in environmental temperature and humidity are reflected in the external ear canal.
- The incidence of otitis externa peaks in late summer and early autumn.
- Gram-negative infections of the external ear canal are more common in humid and warm environments.

CLIMATE AND WEATHER

The three main components of weather which impact on external ear disease are temperature, humidity, and rainfall. All three factors interact with each other and affect the internal environment of the external ear canal[1, 2]. Thus, increasing environmental temperature or relative humidity is reflected in a small but measurable increase in temperature or relative humidity within the external ear canal[1]. The incidence of otitis externa increases as environmental temperature, relative humidity, and rainfall increases, although there is a lag effect of 1–2 months[3]. This results in a peak incidence of otitis externa, in dogs, in late summer and early autumn[3].

Variations in climate, commensurate upon geographic location, affect both the incidence and type of otitis externa. Thus, although temperature, relative humidity, and rainfall all affect the incidence of otitis externa, the local climate also exerts its effect[3] (*Table 10*).

The local climate will also affect the microbial flora of the external ear canal. In hot and humid environments there are fewer ear canals from which no bacterial growth can be cultured[4]. In man the incidence of gram-negative bacterial complication of otitis externa increases in hot humid environments[5] and there is evidence that this is also the case in dogs[4].

Finally, in man it has been demonstrated that the incidence of asthma increases after thunderstorms[6]. Thunderstorms are associated with a decrease in temperature and an increase in humidity and rainfall and, more significantly, a significant rise in the concentration of pollen allergen in the air, secondary to osmotic rupture of pollen grains[7]. Given that a high proportion of cases of otitis externa are a consequence of atopy, it may be that some cases of acute otitis externa may also be related to thunderstorms.

Table 10: Illustration of how the peak incidence of otitis externa in dogs varies with climate, although the effect of one particular component of the climate may be delayed by up to two months. (After Hayes, Pickle, and Wilson[3])

Region	Temperature	Relative humidity	Rainfall
Missouri	2 month lag	current month	1 month lag
Minnesota	2 month lag	current month	1 month lag
Georgia	2 month lag	current month	1 month lag
California	2 month lag	1 month lag	current month
Ohio	1 month lag	2 month lag	current month
Illinois	1 month lag	2 month lag	current month
Brisbane	1 month lag	2 month lag	data not available

REFERENCES

EFFECTS OF BREED AND PROGRESSIVE PATHOLOGY

1 Fernando SDA (1966) A histological and histochemical study of the glands of the external auditory canal of the dog. *Research in Veterinary Science* **7**, 116–119.

2 Stout-Graham M, Kainer RA, Whalen LR and Macy DW (1990) Morphologic measurements of the external ear canal of dogs. *American Journal of Veterinary Research* **51**, 990–994.

3 Huang HP, Fixter LM and Little CJL (1994) Lipid content of cerumen from normal dogs and otitic canine ears. *Veterinary Record* **134**, 380–381.

4 Fernando SDA (1966) Certain histopathological features of the external auditory meatus of the cat and dog with otitis externa. *American Journal of Veterinary Research* **28**, 278–282.

5 van der Gagg I (1986) The pathology of the external ear canal in dogs and cats. *Veterinary Quarterly* **8**, 307–317.

6 Fraser G (1961) The histopathology of the external auditory meatus of the dog. *Journal of Comparative Pathology* **71**, 253–258.

7 Grono LR (1970) Studies of the microclimate of the external auditory canal in the dog. III: Relative humidity within the external auditory meatus. *Research in Veterinary Science* **11**, 316–319.

8 Fraser G, Gregor WW, Mackenzie CP, Spreull JSA and Withers AR (1970) Canine ear disease. *Journal of Small Animal Practice* **10**, 725–754.

9 Lane JG and Little CJL (1986) Surgery of the external auditory meatus: a review of failures. *Journal of Small Animal Practice* **27**, 247–254.

10 Baxter M and Lawler DC (1972) The incidence and microbiology of otitis externa of dogs and cats in New Zealand. *New Zealand Veterinary Journal* **20**, 29–32.

11 Hayes HM, Pickle LW and Wilson GP (1987) Effects of ear type and weather on the prevalence of canine otitis externa. *Research in Veterinary Science* **42**, 294–298.

12 Fraser G (1965) Aetiology of otitis externa in the dog. *Journal of Small Animal Practice* **6**, 445–452.

13 Fraser G, Withers AR and Spreull JSA (1961) Otitis externa in the dog. *Journal of Small Animal Practice* **2**, 32–47.

14 Rycroft AK and Saban HS (1977) A clinical study of otitis externa in the dog. *Canadian Veterinary Journal* **18**, 64–70.

15 Baba E, Fukata T and Saito M (1981) Incidence of otitis externa in dogs and cats in Japan. *Veterinary Record* **108**, 393–395.

ECTOPARASITIC CAUSES OF OTITIS EXTERNA, AND ANTIPARASITIC AGENTS

1 Scott DW and Horn RT (1987) Zoonotic dermatoses of dogs and cats. *Veterinary Clinics of North America* **17**, 117–144.

2 Powell MB, Weisbroth SH, Roth L and Wilhelmsen C (1980) Reaginic hypersensitivity in *Otodectes cynotis* infestation of cats and mode of mite feeding. *American Journal of Veterinary Research* **6**, 877–881.

3 Larkin AD and Gaillard GE (1981) Mites in cats' ears: a source of cross antigenicity with house dust mites. *Annals of Allergy* **46**, 301–304.

4 Kuwahara J (1986) Canine and feline aural hematoma: clinical, experimental, and clinicopathologic observations. *American Journal of Veterinary Research* **47**, 2300–2308.

5 Kuwahara J (1986) Canine and feline aural hematomas: results of treatment with corticosteroids. *Journal of the American Animal Hospital Association* **22**, 641–647.

6 Hewitt M, Walton GS and Waterhouse M (1971) Pet animal infestations and skin lesions. *British Journal of Dermatology* **85**, 215–255.

7 Frost CR (1961) Canine otocariasis. *Journal of Small Animal Practice* **2**, 253–256.

8 Scott DW (1980) Feline dermatology 1900–1978. A monograph. *Journal of the American Animal Hospital Association* **16**, 331–459.

9 Park G-S, Park J-S, Cho B-K, Lee W-K and Cho J-H (1996) Mite infestation rate of pet dogs with ear dermatoses. *Korean Journal of Parasitology* **34**, 143–150.

10 Grono LR (1969) Studies of the ear mite, *Otodectes cynotis*. *Veterinary Record* **85**, 6–8.

11 Chester DK (1988) Medical management of otitis externa. In *Veterinary Clinics of North America* (ed JR August) **18**, 799–812.

12 White SD (1992) Otitis externa. *Waltham Focus* **2**, 2–9.

13 McKeever PJ and Richardson HW (1988) Otitis externa. Part 3: Ear cleaning and medical treatment. *Companion Animal Practice* **2**, 24–29.

14 Schneck G (1988) Use of ivermectin against ear mites in cats. *Veterinary Record* **123**, 599.

15 Medleau L (1994) Using ivermectin to treat parasitic dermatoses in small animals. *Veterinary Medicine* **August**, 770–774.

16 Pott JM and Riley CJ (1979) The efficacy of a topical ear preparation against *Otodectes cynotis* infection in dogs and cats. *Veterinary Record* **104**, 579.

17 Scherk-Nixon M, Baker B, Pauling GE and Hare JE (1997) Treatment of feline otoacariasis with two otic preparations not containing miticidal active ingredients. *Canadian Veterinary Journal* **38**, 229–230.

18 Thomas CA, Shanks DJ, Six RH et al. (1999) Efficacy of selamectin against natural infestations of *Sarcoptes scabiei* and *Otodectes cynotis* in dogs and cats. *Proceedings of the American Association of Veterinary Parasitology*. New Orleans, p. 58.

19 Knottenbelt MK (1994) Chronic otitis externa due to *Demodex canis* in a Tibetan Spaniel. *Veterinary Record* **135**, 409–410.

20 Greene RT, Scheidt VJ and Moncol DJ (1986) Trombiculiasis in a cat. *Journal of the American Veterinary Medical Association* **188**, 1054–1055.

21 Scheidt VJ (1987) Common feline ectoparasites. Part 3: Chigger mites, cat fur mites, ticks, lice, bot fly larvae, and fleas. *Companion Animal Practice* **1**, 5–15.

22 Folz SD, Ash KA, Conder GA and Rector DL (1986) Amitraz: a tick and flea repellent and tick detachment drug. *Journal of Veterinary Pharmacology and Therapeutics* **9**, 150–156.

23 Famose F (1995) Efficacy of fipronil (Frontline) spray in the prevention of natural infestation by *Trombicula autumnalis* in dogs. *Proceedings of The Royal Veterinary College Seminar: Ectoparasites and Their Control* pp. 28–30.

24 Moriello KA (1987) Common ectoparasites of the dog. Part 1: Fleas and ticks. *Canine Practice* **14**, 6–18.

25 White SD, Scott KV and Cheney JM (1995) *Otobius megnini* infestation in three dogs. *Veterinary Dermatology* **6**, 33–35.

26 Hunter JS, Keister DM and Jeannin P (1996) A comparison of the tick control efficacy of Frontline Spray against the American dog tick and brown dog tick. *Proceedings of the 41st Annual Meeting of the American Association of Veterinary Parasitologists*, Louisville, p. 51.

27 Hugnet C, Buronfosse F, Pineau X, Cadoré J-L, Lorgue G and Berny PJ (1996) Toxicity and kinetics of amitraz. *American Journal of Veterinary Research* **57**, 1506–1510.

28 Clayton TM (1943) Treatment of scabies by T.E.T.S. *British Medical Journal* **1**, 443–445.

29 Gold S (1966) A skin full of alcohol. *Lancet* **ii**, 1417.

30 Evans JM and Jemmett JE (1978) Otitis externa: the case for polypharmacy. *New Zealand Veterinary Journal* **26**, 280–283.

31 Wilcke JB (1988) Otopharmacology. *Veterinary Clinics of North America* **18**, 783–797.

32 Hansen SR (1995) Management of adverse reactions to pyrethrins and pyrethroid insecticides. In *Current Veterinary Therapy XII*. (ed JD Bonagura) WB Saunders, Philadelphia, pp. 242–245.

33 Hansen SR (1995) Management of organophosphate and carbamate toxicoses. In *Current Veterinary Therapy XII*. (ed JD Bonagura) WB Saunders, Philadelphia, pp. 245–248.

34 Mueller RD and Bettenay SV (1999) A proposed new therapeutic protocol for the treatment of canine mange with ivermectin. *Journal of the American Animal Hospital Association* **35**, 77–80.

35 Schneck G (1988) Use of ivermectin against ear mites in cats. *Veterinary Record* **123**, 599.

36 Gram D (1991) Treatment of ear mites (*Otodectes cynotis*) in cats: comparison of subcutaneous and topical ivermectin. *Proceedings 7th Annual Meeting AAVD/ACVD*, Scottsdale, p. 26.

37 Paradis M (1998) Ivermectin in small animal dermatology. Part I: Pharmacology and toxicology. *Compendium on Continuing Education* **20**, 193–199.

38 Dorman DC (1995) Neurotoxic drugs in dogs and cats. In *Current Veterinary Therapy XII*. (ed JD Bonagura) WB Saunders, Philadelphia, pp. 1140–1145.

39 Paul AJ, Tranquilli WJ, Seward RL, Todd KS jnr and DiPietro JA (1987) Clinical observations in Collies given ivermectin orally. *American Journal of Veterinary Research* **48**, 684–685.

40 Hsu WH and Schaffer DD (1988) Effects of topical application of amitraz on plasma glucose and insulin concentrations in dogs. *American Journal of Veterinary Research* **49**, 130–131.

41 Medleau L and Willemse T (1995) Efficacy of daily amitraz on generalised demodicosis in dogs. *Journal of Small Animal Practice* **36**, 3–6.

42 Cooper PR and Penaliggon EJ (1996) Use of fipronil to eliminate recurrent infestation by *Trichodectes canis* in a pack of Bloodhounds. *Veterinary Record* **139**, 95.

43 Curtis CF (1996) Use of 0.25% fipronil spray to treat sarcoptic mange in a litter of five-week-old puppies. *Veterinary Record* **139**, 43–44.

44 Novotny MJ, Krautmann MJ, Ehrhart J et al. (1999) Clinical safety of selamectin in dogs. *Proceedings of the American Association of Veterinary Parasitology*. New Orleans, p. 61.

45 McTier TL, McCall JW, Jernigan AD et al. (1998) Efficacy of UK-124, 114, a novel avermectin for the prevention of heartworms in dogs and cats. *Recent Advances in Heartworm Disease Symposium*. Tampa, pp. 187–192.

46 Wren JA, McTier TL, Thomas CA, Bowman DD and Jernigan AD (1999) Efficacy of selamectin against *Toxacara canis* in dogs. *Proceedings of the American Association of Veterinary Parasitology*. New Orleans, p. 60.

47 Six RH, McTier TL and Shanks DJ (1999) Efficacy of selamectin against induced and natural infections of *Toxocara cati* and *Ancylostoma tubaeformis* in cats. *Proceedings of the American Association of Veterinary Parasitology*. New Orleans, p. 60.

FOREIGN BODIES

1 McKeever PJ and Torres S (1988) Otitis externa. Part 1: The ear and predisposing factors to otitis externa. *Companion Animal Practice* **2**, 7–14.

2 Brennan KE and Ihrke PJ (1983) Grass awn migration in dogs and cats: a retrospective study of 182 cases. *Journal of the American Veterinary Medical Association* **182**, 1201–1204.

3 Rycroft AK and Saben HS (1977) A clinical study of otitis externa in the dog. *Canadian Veterinary Journal* **18**, 64–70.

4 Roth L (1988) Pathologic changes in otitis externa. *Veterinary Clinics of North America* **14**, 755–764.

NASOPHARYNGEAL AND MIDDLE EAR POLYPS

1 Pope ER (1995) Feline inflammatory polyps. *Seminars in Veterinary Medicine and Surgery* **10**, 87–93.

2 Harvey CE and Goldschmidt MH (1978) Inflammatory polypoid growths in the ear canals of cats. *Journal of Small Animal Practice* **19**, 669–677.

3 Lane JG, Orr CM, Lucke VM and Gruffydd-Jones TJ (1981) Nasopharyngeal polyps arising in the middle ear of the cat. *Journal of Small Animal Practice* **22**, 511–522.

4 van der Gaag I (1986) The pathology of the external ear canal in dogs and cats. *Veterinary Quarterly* **8**, 307–317.

5 Pollock S (1971) Nasopharyngeal polyp in a dog. *Veterinary Medicine/Small Animal Clinician* **66**, 705–706.

6 Bradley RL, Noone KE, Saunders GK and Patnaik AK (1985) Nasopharyngeal and middle ear poylpoid masses in five cats. *Veterinary Surgery* **14**, 141–144.

7 Kirpenstein J (1993) Aural neoplasms. *Seminars in Veterinary Medicine and Surgery* **8**, 17–23.

OTIC NEOPLASIA

1 van der Gaag I (1986) The pathology of the external ear canal in dogs and cats. *Veterinary Quarterly* **8**, 307–317.

2 Kirpenstein J (1993) Aural neoplasms. *Seminars in Veterinary Medicine and Surgery (Small Animal)* **8,** 17–23.

3 London CA, Dubilzieg RR, Vail DM et al. (1996) Evaluation of dogs and cats with tumors of the ear canal: 145 cases (1978–1992). *Journal of the American Veterinary Medical Association* **208**, 1413–1418.

4 Scott DW (1980) External ear disorders. *Journal of the American Animal Hospital Association* **16**, 426–433.

5 Miller MA, Nelson SL, Turk JR et al. (1991) Cutaneous neoplasia in 340 cats. *Veterinary Pathology* **28**, 389–395.

6 Goldschmidt MH and Shofer FS (1992) Canine cutaneous histiocytoma. In *Skin Tumors of the Dog and Cat*. (eds MH Goldschmidt and FS Shofer) Pergammon Press, New York, pp. 222–230.

7 Mueller RA (1996) Tropical and subtropical dermatoses. *Waltham Focus* **6**, 16–23.

8 Kwa RE, Campana K and Moy RL (1992) Biology of cutaneous cell carcinoma. *Journal of the American Academy of Dermatology* **26**, 1–26.

9 Little CJL, Pearson GR and Lane JG (1989) Neoplasia involving the middle ear cavity of dogs. *Veterinary Record* **124**, 54–57.

10 Goldschmidt MH and Shofer FS (1992) Cutaneous papilloma. In *Skin Tumors of the Dog and Cat*. (eds MH Goldschmidt and FS Shofer) Pergammon Press, New York, pp. 11–15.

11 Lozano-Alarcon F, Lewis TP, Clarke EG, Bradley GA, Shupe MR and Hargis AM (1996) Persistent papilloma infection in a cat. *Journal of the American Animal Hospital Association* **32**, 392–396.

12 Scott DW, Miller WH jnr and Griffen CE (199) Neoplastic and non-neoplastic tumors. In *Muller and Kirk's Small Animal*

Dermatology. 5th edn. (eds DW Scott, WH Miller jnr and CE Griffin) WB Saunders, Philadelphia, pp. 994–999.

13 Bevier DE and Goldschmidt MH (1981) Skin tumors in the dog. Part I: Epithelial tumors and tumor-like lesions. *Compendium on Continuing Education* **3**, 389–400.

14 Watrach AM (1969) The ultrastructure of canine cutaneous papilloma. *Cancer Research* **29**, 2079–2084.

15 Calvert CA (1990) Canine viral papillomatosis. In *Infectious Diseases of the Dog and Cat*. 2nd edn. (ed CE Greene) WB Saunders, Philadelphia, pp. 288–290.

16 Moore PF and Schrenzel MD (1991) Canine cutaneous histiocytoma represents a Langerhans cell proliferative disorder based on an immunophenotypic analysis. *Proceedings of the American College of Veterinary Pathology* **42**, 119.

17 Goldschmidt MH and Bevier DE (1981) Skin tumors in the dog. Part III: Lymphohystiocytic and melanocytic tumors. *Compendium on Continuing Education* **3**, 588–594.

18 Macy DW (1986) Canine and feline mast cell tumors: biologic behavior, diagnosis, and therapy. *Seminars in Veterinary Medicine and Surgery* **1**, 72–83.

19 Goldschmidt MH and Shofer FS (1992) Mast cell tumors. In *Skin Tumors of the Dog and Cat*. (eds MH Goldschmidt and FS Shofer) Pergammon Press, New York, pp. 231–251.

20 Legendre AM and Krahwinkel AJ (1981) Feline ear tumours. *Journal of the American Animal Hospital Association* **17**, 1035–1037.

21 Goldschmidt MH and Shofer FS (1992) Squamous cell carcinoma. In *Skin Tumors of the Dog and Cat*. (eds MH Goldschmidt and FS Shofer) Pergammon Press, New York, pp. 37–49.

22 Kwa RE, Campana K and Moy RL (1992) Biology of cutaneous squamous cell carcinoma. *Journal of the American Academy of Dermatology* **26**, 1–26.

23 Miller WH, Affolter V, Scott DW and Suter MM (1992) Multicentric squamous cell carcinomas *in situ* resembling Bowen's disease in five cats. *Veterinary Dermatology* **3**, 177–182.

24 Atwater SW, Powers BE, Straw RC et al. (1991) Squamous cell carcinoma of the pinna and nasal planum. 54 cats (1980–1991). *Proceedings of the Veterinary Cancer Society* **11**, 35–36.

25 Macy DW and Reynolds HA (1981) The incidence, characteristics, and clinical management of skin tumors of cats. *Journal of the American Animal Hospital Association* **17**, 1026–1034.

26 Lana Se, Ogilvie GK, Withrow SJ, Straw RC and Rogers KS (1997) Feline cutaneous squamous cell carcinoma of the nasal planum and the pinnae: 61 cases. *Journal of the American Animal Hospital Association* **33**, 329–332.

27 Foster AP (1994) A study of the number and distribution of cutaneous mast cells in cats with disease not affecting the skin. *Veterinary Dermatology* **5**, 17–20.

28 Chastain CB, Turk MA and O'Brian D (1988) Benign cutaneous mastocytosis in two litters of Siamese kittens. *Journal of the American Veterinary Medical Association* **193**, 959–960.

29 Wilcock BP, Yager JA and Zink MC (1986) The morphology and behaviour of feline cutaneous mastocytomas. *Veterinary Pathology* **23**, 320–324.

30 Buerger RG and Scott DW (1987) Cutaneous mast cell neoplasia in cats: 14 cases (1975–1985). *Journal of the American Veterinary Medical Association* **190**, 1440–1444.

31 Goldschmidt MH and Shofer FS (1992) Basal cell tumors. In *Skin Tumors of the Dog and Cat*. (eds MH Goldschmidt and FS Shofer) Pergammon Press, New York, pp. 16–28.

32 Goldschmidt MH and Shofer FS (1992) Cutaneous

fibrosarcoma. In *Skin Tumors of the Dog and Cat*. (eds MH Goldschmidt and FS Shofer) Pergammon Press, New York, pp. 158–167.

33 Goldschmidt MH and Shofer FS (1992). Ceruminous gland tumors. In *Skin Tumors of the Dog and Cat*. (eds MH Goldschmidt and FS Shofer) Pergammon Press, New York, pp. 96–102.

34 Marino DJ, MacDonald JM, Matthiesen DT and Patnaik AK (1994) Results of surgery in cats with ceruminous gland adenocarcinoma. *Journal of the American Animal Hospital Association* **30**, 54–58.

35 Marino DJ, MacDonald JM, Matthiesen DT, Salmeri KR and Patnaik AK (1993). Results of surgery and long-term follow-up in dogs with ceruminous gland adenocarcinoma. *Journal of the American Animal Hospital Association* **29**, 560–563.

36 Theon AP, Barthez PY, Madewell BR and Griffey SM (1994) Radiation therapy of ceruminous gland carcinomas in dogs and cats. *Journal of the American Veterinary Medical Association* **205**, 566–569.

37 Howlett CR and Allan GS (1974) Tumours of the feline ear canal. *Australian Veterinary Practitioner* **4**, 56–57.

38 Poulet FM, Valentine BA and Scott DW (1991) Focal proliferative eosinophilic dermatitis of the external ear canal in four dogs. *Veterinary Pathology* **28**, 171–173.

39 Rogers KS (1988) Tumors of the ear canal. *Veterinary Clinics of North America* **18**, 859–868.

UNDERLYING DISEASE

1 August JR (1988) Otitis externa. A disease of multifactorial etiology. *Veterinary Clinics of North America* **18**, 731–742.

2 Halliwell REW and Gorman NT (1989) Atopic disease. In *Veterinary Clinical Immunology*. (eds REW Halliwell and NT Gorman) WB Saunders, Philadelphia, pp. 232–252.

3 Scott DW (1981) Observations on canine atopy. *Journal of the American Animal Hospital Association* **17**, 91–100.

4 Griffin CE (1993) Canine atopic disease. In *Current Veterinary Dermatology*. (eds CE Griffin, KW Kwochka and JM MacDonald) Mosby, St Louis, pp. 99–120.

5 Harvey RG (1993) Food allergy and dietary intolerance in dogs: a report of 25 cases. *Journal of Small Animal Practice* **34**, 175–179.

6 Rosser EJ (1993) Diagnosis of food allergy in dogs. *Journal of the American Veterinary Medical Association* **203**, 259–262.

7 Carlotti DN, Remy I and Prost C (1990) Food allergy in dogs and cats: a review and report of 43 cases. *Veterinary Dermatology* **1**, 55–62.

8 White SD and Sequoia D (1989) Food hypersensitivity in cats: 14 cases (1982–1987). *Journal of the American Veterinary Medical Association* **194**, 692–695.

9 Walder EJ and Conroy JD (1994) Contact dermatitis in dogs and cats: pathogenesis, histopathology, experimental induction, and case reports. *Veterinary Dermatology* **5**, 149–162.

10 Nesbitt GH and Schmitz JA (1977) Contact dermatitis in the dog: a review of 35 cases. *Journal of the American Animal Hospital Association* **13**, 155–163.

11 Griffin CE (1993) Otitis externa and otitis media. In *Current Veterinary Dermatology*. (eds CE Griffin, KW Kwochka and JM MacDonald) Mosby, St Louis, pp. 245–262.

12 Kwochka KW (1993) Overview of normal keratinization and cutaneous scaling disorders of dogs. In *Current Veterinary Dermatology*. (eds CE Griffin, KW Kwochka and JM MacDonald) Mosby, St Louis pp. 167–175.

13 Kwochka KW and Rademakers AM (1989) Cell proliferation

kinetics of epidermis, hair follicles, and sebaceous glands of Cocker Spaniels with idiopathic seborrhea. *American Journal of Veterinary Research* **50**, 1918–1922.

14 Scott DW and Miller WH jnr (1989) Epidermal dysplasia and *Malassezia pachydermatis* infection in West Highland White Terriers. *Veterinary Dermatology* **1**, 25–36.

15 Maudlin EA, Scott DW, Miller WH jnr and Smith CA (1997) *Malassezia* dermatitis in the dog: a retrospective histopathological and immunopathological study of 86 cases (1990–95). *Veterinary Dermatology* **8**, 183–190.

16 Bond R, Rose JF, Ellis JW and Lloyd DH (1995) Comparison of two shampoos for treatment of *Malassezia pachydermatis*-associated seborrhoeic dermatitis in Basset Hounds. *Journal of Small Animal Practice* **36**, 99–104.

17 Paradis M and Scott DW (1990) Hereditary primary seborrhoea in Persian cats. *Feline Practice* **18**, 17–20.

18 Pancierra DL (1994) Hypothyroidism in dogs: 66 cases (1987–1992). *Journal of the American Veterinary Medical Association* **204**, 761–767.

19 Ling GV, Stabenfeldt GH, Comer KM, Gribble DH and Schechter RD (1979) Canine hyperadrenocorticism: pretreatment clinical and laboratory evaluation of 117 cases. *Journal of the American Veterinary Medical Association* **174**, 1211–1215.

20 White SD, Ceragioli KL, Bullock LP and Mason GD (1989) Cutaneous markers of canine hyperadrenocorticism. *Compendium on Continuing Education* **11**, 446–464.

21 Schmeitzel LP and Lothrop CD (1990) Sex hormones and skin disease. *Veterinary Medicine Report* **2**, 28–41.

22 Scott DW, Miller WJ jnr, Lewis RM, Manning TO and Smith CA (1980) Pemphigus erythematosus in the dog and cat. *Journal of the American Animal Hospital Association* **16**, 815–823.

23 Manning TO, Scott DW, Smith CA and Lewis RM (1982) Pemphigus diseases in the feline: seven case reports and discussion. *Journal of the American Animal Hospital Association* **18**, 433–443.

24 Scott DW, Walton DK, Manning TO, Smith CA and Lewis RM (1983) Canine lupus erythematosus. I: Systemic lupus erythematosus. *Journal of the American Animal Hospital Association* **19**, 561–579.

25 Ihrke PJ, Stannard AA, Ardans AA and Griffin CE (1985) Pemphigus foliaceus in dogs: a review of 37 cases. *Journal of the American Veterinary Medical Association* **186**, 59–66.

THE EFFECTS OF WEATHER ON THE INCIDENCE OF OTITIS EXTERNA

1 Grono LR (1970) Studies of the microclimate of the external auditory canal in the dog. I: Aural temperature. *Research in Veterinary Science* **11**, 307–311.

2 Grono LR (1970) Studies of the microclimate of the external auditory canal in the dog. III: Relative humidity within the external ear auditory meatus. *Research in Veterinary Science* **11**, 316–319.

3 Hayes HM, Pickle LW and Wilson GP (1987) Effects of ear type and weather on the prevalence of canine otitis externa. *Research in Veterinary Science* **42**, 294–298.

4 Grono LR and Frost AJ (1969) Otitis externa in the dog. *Australian Veterinary Journal* **45**, 420–422.

5 Wilkinson JD (1992) The external ear. In *Textbook of Dermatology*. 4th edn. (eds RH Champion, JL Burton and FJG Ebling) Blackwell Scientific Publications, Oxford, pp. 2671–2688.

6 Pack GE and Ayres JG (1985) Asthma outbreaks during a thunderstorm. *Lancet* **2**, 199–203.

7 Knox RB (1993) Grass pollen, thunderstorms and asthma. *Clinical and Experimental Allergy* **23**, 345–359.

Chapter Four

Diseases of the Pinna

INTRODUCTION

KEY POINTS

- Dermatoses other than neoplasia are rarely confined to the pinna.
- The most common dermatoses affecting the pinnae cause crust and scale, and many are ectoparasitic in origin.
- Pinnal pruritus, other than that associated with otitis externa, is not common and usually represents scabies or pediculosis.
- Papules and nodules are quite common presenting signs.
- Histopathologic examination of biopsy samples may be needed to define a diagnosis before surgery is attempted, since achieving adequate margins is not easy.

Dermatoses other than neoplasia are rarely confined to the pinna, an exception being aural hematoma, which is discussed in Chapter 10 (Aural hematoma, and other pinnal surgery). Some diseases, such as scabies and dermatophytosis, may initially present with lesions on the pinna before spreading elsewhere. Other diseases, such as atopy, initially may affect the pinna and then the external ear canal. Finally, the pinna may be involved as part of a generalized condition; for example, endocrinopathy, defects in keratinization, or pemphigus foliaceus.

In common with skin elsewhere on the body, the pinnal skin responds with a range of primary and secondary lesions. However, primary lesions, other than nodules, are rare. Papules and pustules are most commonly associated with pemphigus foliaceus, itself a rare condition. Scale, crust, self-excoriation, and alopecia are the most common secondary lesions. It is rare to see lichenification, for example.

In combination with the history and a physical examination of the pinna, and with the results of appropriate laboratory tests, a differential diagnosis and ultimately a definitive diagnosis will follow.

PINNAL TRAUMA

Trauma to the pinna, particularly in cats, is relatively common. Fight wounds result in torn pinnae (222) and, often, prolific bleeding. Surprisingly, postbite infection is uncommon. In dogs, pinnal trauma more often results from head shaking than fighting. Otodectic mange, otic foreign bodies, otitis media, and facial pruritus may all result in damage to the pinna, typically trauma to the periphery (223).

Many texts ascribe aural hematoma (224) to trauma. However, the relationship is unclear and currently the etiology of aural hematoma is unknown (see Chapter 10: Aural hematoma, and other pinnal surgery).

DERMATOSES CHARACTERIZED BY CRUST AND SCALE

ECTOPARASITES

Sarcoptes scabiei and *Notoedres cati*

Scabies is an intensely pruritic disease of dogs which results from infestation with the mite *Sarcoptes scabiei*. The mite exhibits a typical distribution pattern with early lesions usually appearing on the distal pinna, the elbows, and the hocks – 'launch points'[1]. An erythematous papular dermatitis is usually present on the elbows and hocks, whereas the pinnal lesions are typically crust and scale (225). With time these lesions spread along the periphery of the pinna, but accompanying pruritus may result in crust, scale, alopecia, and self-excoriation on the dorsum of the pinna (226). Rubbing the tip of the pinna between finger tip and thumbnail usually evokes an intense scratching action from the ipsilateral hindlimb – a pinnal scratch reflex.

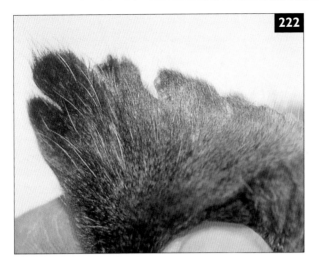

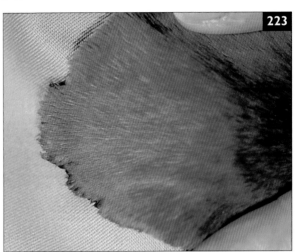

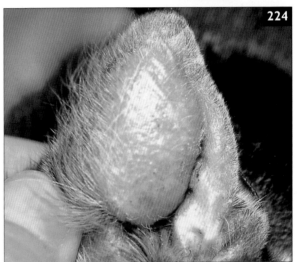

222 Lacerations to the periphery of the pinna of a cat due to fight wounds.

223 Traumatic lesions on the tip of the pinna of a Hungarian Viszla with otitis media. Head shaking had resulted in repeated damage.

224 Aural hematoma on the pinna of a dog. Although commonly assumed to be associated with trauma, it has so far proved impossible to demonstrate a relationship between trauma and hematoma.

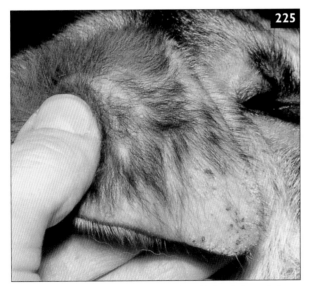

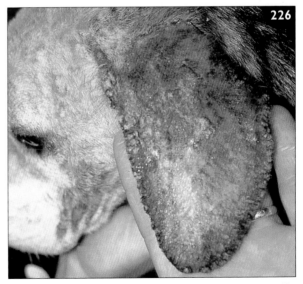

225 Classic lesions of scabies. Peripheral pinnal alopecia in association with fine crust and scale.

226 Severe self-trauma has resulted in alopecia, scale, and self-excoriation in this Beagle with scabies.

Scabies is one of the few dermatoses which can induce steroid-resistant pruritus (*Table 11*).

Microscopic examination of multiple skin scrapes may reveal the typical shape of a sarcoptic mite (**227**). Clinicians can maximize recovery of mites by taking care to collect skin scrapes from lesions which are not heavily traumatized, or from the periphery of the pinna.

Feline scabies is caused by *Notoedres cati*. This mite also exhibits a preference for the pinnae, although in contrast to *S. scabiei* infestation, the early lesions are typically on the anterior periphery of the pinna, rather than the tip. Notoedric mange is often restricted to the pinnae and head (**228**) and generalized infections are

Table 11: Causes of steroid resistant pruritus in dogs.

- Scabies.
- Dietary intolerance and food allergy.
- Allergic contact dermatitis.
- Mycosis fungoides.
- Metabolic epidermal necrosis.
- Calcinosis cutis
- *Malassezia pachydermatis* dermatitis

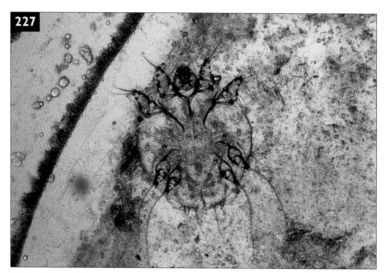

227 Photomicrograph of an adult *Sarcoptes scabiei* mite.

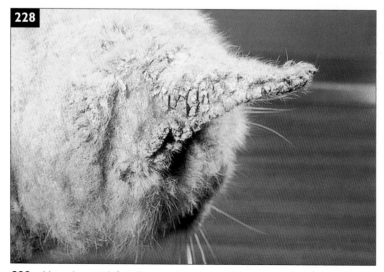

228 *Notoedres cati* infestation causing spectacular crust on the pinna and adjacent areas of the head of a cat.

unusual[2]. Mites are usually plentiful and easily found on microscopic examination of skin scrapes.

The treatment of scabies and other ectoparasitic diseases is discussed in Chapter 3 (Ectoparasitic causes of otitis externa, and antiparasitic agents).

Pediculosis

Pediculosis in dogs and cats causes variable pruritus and variable secondary lesions such as scale, knotted hair, alopecia, and serohemorrhagic crust, particularly on the pinnae (**229**) but also on the trunk. The lice are quite large (**230**) and they may be seen with the naked eye. Egg cases on the hair shafts (nits) may also be seen on gross examination or microscopic examination of hair. However, diagnosis of pediculosis may be difficult as *Trichodectes canis* (the biting louse of dogs) can move surprisingly quickly. Furthermore, because of the supposition that the parasite is easily killed, a diagnosis of pediculosis is often not considered. Treatment of pediculosis is not difficult in individual animals, since the insect is confined to the host and is easily killed by most insecticides. Infection in groups of animals may be more difficult to control[3].

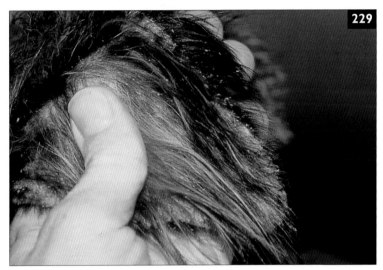

229 Pediculosis resulting in traumatic alopecia to the pinna.

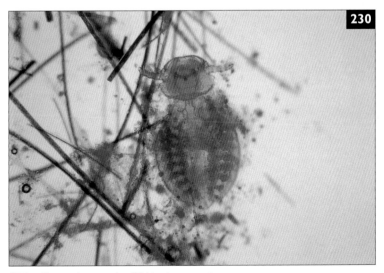

230 Photomicrograph of *Trichodectes canis*.

Demodicosis

Demodicosis is an uncommon cause of pinnal alopecia in dogs. It is usually seen in association with more extensive lesions of generalized demodicosis (**231**) rather than with the localized form. Demodicosis is rare in cats, although the pinnae and head are sites of predisposition[4, 5]. Diagnosis of demodicosis is made by microscopic examination of skin scrapings (**232**).

Harvest mite infestation

Trombiculidiasis results from infestation with the parasitic larval stage of free living mites[6]. The most common infestation results from contact with larvae of *Neotrombicula autumnalis* and *Eutrombicula alfredugesi*, typically in the late summer; hence the name harvest mite. Clusters of mites gather on the tip of the pinna or within the deep folds of skin covering the cartilage at the entrance to the vertical portion of the external ear canal. Moderate to severe pruritus results and this, together with dried serous exudate, may result in crust formation. Diagnosis is straightforward as the six-legged larva is unmistakable (**233**).

Insect bite dermatitis

The rabbit flea, *Spilopsyllus cuniculi*, is a seasonal cause of pinnal dermatitis that has been reported in hunting cats in the UK and Australia[7, 8]. The flea times its maximum activity to coincide with the rabbit's parturition, thus the seasonality can be predicted. Small, dark brown fleas may be seen attached to the tips of the pinnae. Focal alopecia (**234**) may be associated with these fleas. In some cases there is marked alopecia and crusting (**235**).

Stable flies (*Stomoxys calcitrans*) may cause a serosanguinous, crusted dermatitis which may progress to a granulomatous dermatitis. Lesions are principally confined to the tips of the pinnae (**236**) and they are usually confined to dogs with erect pinnae and access to stables[9]. Black flies (*Simulium* spp.) and other small biting flies may cause a papular dermatitis on the dorsal aspect of the pinna which may be accompanied by focal alopecia (**237**)[9]. These lesions may look very similar to those associated with *Spilopsyllus cuniculi* but no parasites will be found.

Mosquito bites may cause a seasonal dermatitis in cats[10]. The lesions are a result of hypersensitivity[11] and they consist of papules, erythematous erosions, alopecia, and occasionally hypopigmentation on the dorsum of the face and pinnae. Affected animals may also exhibit moderate polylymphadenopathy, mild pyrexia and symmetrical erythema, fissuring, and hyperkeratosis of the footpads. Lesions resolve with the onset of winter or with effective screening to prevent exposure to mosquitoes.

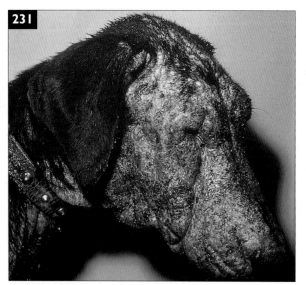

231   Adult onset generalized demodicosis in a Doberman Pinscher resulting in scale, crust, and alopecia.

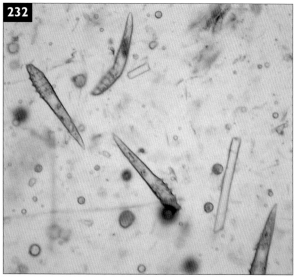

232   Photomicrograph of canine demodectic mites illustrating the unmistakable shape of the mite.

233 Photomicrograph of a harvest mite (*Neotrombicula autumnalis*).

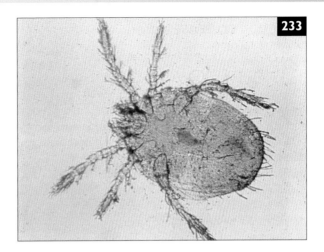

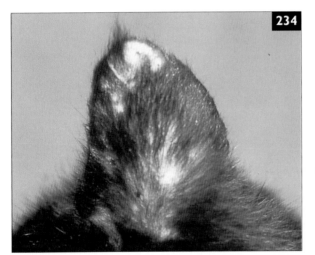

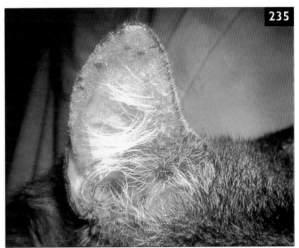

234, 235 *Spilopsyllus cuniculi* infestation in cats. The tiny fleas can be seen at the tip of the pinna (**234**). The associated crust and alopecia which follows prolonged infestation (**235**).

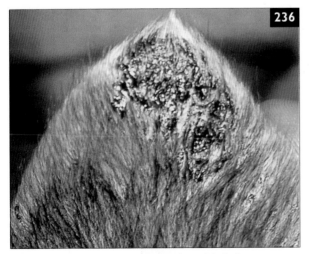

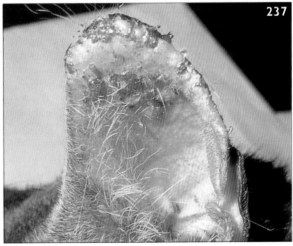

236 Fly bite dermatitis caused by the stable fly *Stomoxys calcitrans*. Relatively focal, tightly adherent crust at the tip of the pinna.

237 More extensive alopecia with a papulocrustous dermatitis on the pinna of a cat.

INFECTIOUS DISEASES

Leishmaniasis

Canine leishmaniasis is a severe, often fatal disease of dogs caused by parasites of the genus *Leishmania*[12]. Classically, leishmaniasis is characterized by chronic wasting and systemic signs such as intermittent pyrexia, anemia, and polylymphadenopathy. Cutaneous lesions often accompany the systemic signs; the most common sign is alopecia, which is often symmetrical and accompanied by a fine dry scale (**238**). The diagnosis and management of leishmaniasis is beyond the scope of this book and readers are referred to current texts for details of up-to-date treatment recommendations.

Malassezia pachydermatis

Dermatitis caused by the yeast *Malassezia pachydermatis* is frequently found as a secondary complication in many chronic dermatoses; atopy and idiopathic defects in keratinization, for example. Malassezzial dermatitis may also occur in the absence of discernible underlying disease.

The clinical signs consist of erythematous dermatitis, occasionally papular, associated with a variable, typically yellowish gray, greasy scale (**239**). In some dogs the dermatitis may affect the concave aspect of the pinna only as an extension of otitis externa, but in some breeds, notably the Basset Hound and West Highland White Terrier, both sides of the pinna, as well as adjacent areas of the head and neck, may be affected. Pruritus is often intense and it may be steroid resistant.

Diagnosis is based on demonstrating the yeast in tape strips, skin scrapes, or on contact plate cultures[13]. The approach to treatment is based on identifying the underlying disease and removing the yeast with either topical shampoos (miconazole, ketoconazole, chlorhexidine) or systemic ketoconazole (5–10 mg/kg q12h). Some animals, particularly Basset Hounds, require regular shampoo therapy to maintain remission.

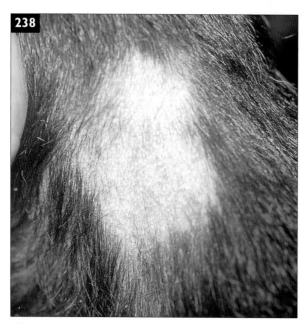

238   Alopecia and fine scale on the base of the pinna of a dog with leishmaniasis.

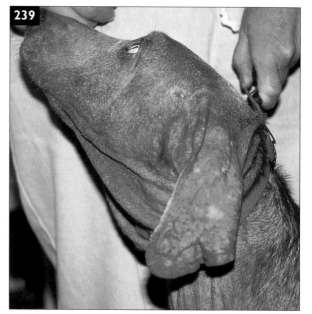

239   Severe *Malassezia pachydermatis* dermatitis in a Weimaraner. Note the erythema, alopecia, and scale. The dog exhibited severe steroid-refractory pruritus.

IMMUNE MEDIATED AND AUTOIMMUNE DISEASE

Pemphigus foliaceus

This is the most common of this rare group of diseases[14, 15]. Lesions in the dog are usually symmetrical and they are often generalized[15]. Pinnal lesions may appear first and they may be very severe with pruritus, crusting, and alopecia (**240**). In the cat the disease is often confined to the face and pinnae[15] and spectacular crusting may be seen (**241**). Pruritus is variable in the cat. Careful examination of these cases may reveal primary lesions, tiny papules, and pustules (**242**). Other dematoses in this group which may affect the pinnae include pemphigus erythematosus and systemic lupus erythematosus (SLE). Both of these conditions are extremely rare and SLE is notoriously difficult to diagnose[16].

Diagnosis is based on cytology and on histopathologic examination of biopsy samples, although other tests will be necessary for the definitive diagnosis of SLE. Management is based on immunosuppressive doses of systemic glucocorticoids. Details of this is beyond the scope of this book and clinicians are referred to specialist texts.

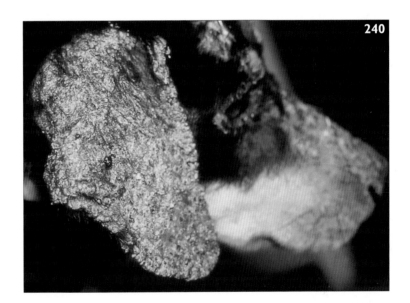

240 Crusting and alopecia on the pinna, periorbital region, and face of a dog with pemphigus foliaceus.

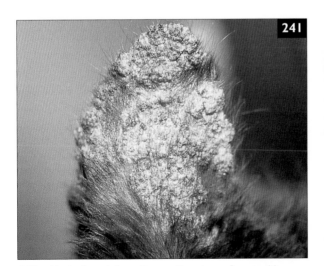

241 Marked crust formation on the pinna of a cat with pemphigus foliaceus.

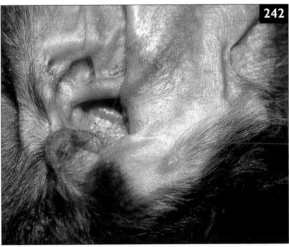

242 Erythematous papules and pustules on the concave aspect of a pinna. These are primary lesions of pemphigus foliaceus.

Vasculitis

Vasculitis is usually an inflammatory process in which cell-mediated (neutrophils, lymphocytes, or macrophages) damage occurs within the walls of blood vessels[17]. The cellular infiltrate may occur in response to antigen-antibody complex deposition in the vascular endothelium. This immune complex deposition may be associated with an underlying disease such as SLE or drug eruption. More commonly the underlying cause remains unidentified[18]. The damaged endothelium results in extravasation of erythrocytes and underperfusion of the tissue served by the blood vessel. There is erythema, edema, and sloughing of necrosed tissue producing 'punched out' ulcers (**243**). Initial investigations should try to identify an underlying disease, such as SLE, which may dictate therapy. In idiopathic cases immunosuppressive doses of prednisolone (1.1–2.2 mg/kg q12–24h) may be necessary, although pentoxyphylline may also be helpful.

ENVIRONMENTAL DERMATOSES

Actinic dermatitis

Actinic dermatitis results from exposure to ultraviolet B radiation and it is most commonly seen on the tips of the pinnae of white haired cats[19, 20]. Early lesions consist of erythema, fine scale, and alopecia which may be bilateral. With continued exposure there is preneoplastic and finally neoplastic transformation to squamous cell carcinoma[19, 20, 21]. These lesions are erosive and crusted and may be hemorrhagic (**244, 245**). If exposure cannot be prevented, tattooing may be helpful, although amputation of the pinnal tip to below the hair line is the most effective prophylactic, and the most effective treatment once neoplastic transformation has occurred[19, 20, 21].

Dermatoses associated with cold temperatures

Frost bite, cold agglutinin disease, and cryoglobulinemia/cryofibrinogenemia may affect the tips of the pinnae, in addition to the tip of the tail and the digits.

Frost-bitten pinnae

Frost-bitten pinnae may appear pale or cyanosed and they are cold to the touch. Lesions of frostbite are best treated with gentle warming.

Cold agglutinin disease

Cold agglutinin disease is an immune-mediated disease in which autoagglutination of erythrocytes occurs in distal extremities when the temperature within the tissue falls to a critical level[17]. Microthromboses occur in small end-arterioles and capillaries, with ischemic necrosis ensuing. Early lesions consist of edema and erythema and this may be followed by the appearance of crust and even ulceration. Cold agglutinin disease is managed by immunosuppressive doses of prednisolone (1.1–2.2 mg/kg q12–24h).

Cryoglobulins and cryofibrinogins

Cryoglobulins and cryofibrinogins are proteins which precipitate out of cold serum, only to redissolve when the serum is warmed[22]. The precipitating proteins induce microthrombi and vasculitis. The clinical signs in one case were limited to well-demarcated areas of necrosis at the distal end of the pinnae (**246**)[22]. The only treatment required was to keep the dog indoors during the winter months.

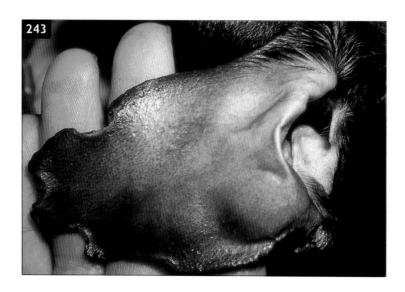

243

243 Punched out ulcers on the periphery of the pinna of a dog with vasculitis.

244, 245 Advanced actinic dermatitis on the pinnae of a cat (**244**), and advanced neoplastic transformation on another cat (**245**).

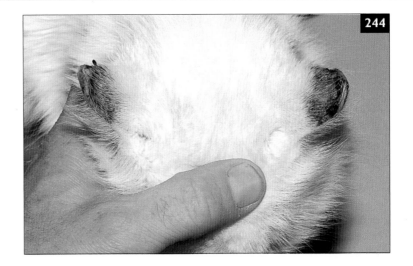

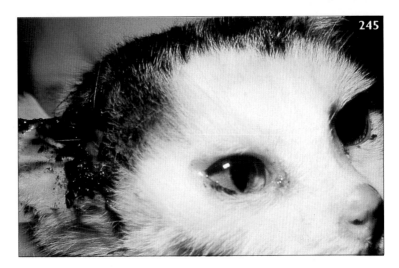

246 Distal pinnal necrosis due to precipitation of cryoglobulins and cryofibrinogins in small blood vessels at the tip of the pinna, induced by exposure to cold weather. (Illustration from Nagata M, Nanko H, Hashimoto K, Ogawa M and Sakashita E (1998) Cryoglobulinaemia and cryofibronogenaemia: a comparison of canine and human cases. *Veterinary Dermatology* **9**, 277–281, with permission.)

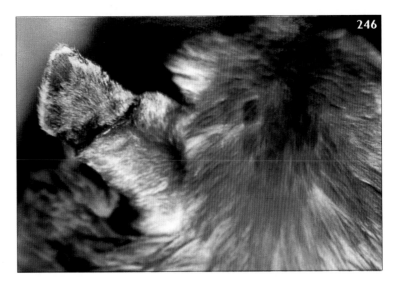

HYPERKERATOSES
Idiopathic defects in keratinization
A defect in keratinization may be primary or secondary (*Table 12*). Primary defects in keratinization reflect inherent errors in the control of the various processes associated with epidermal turnover, sebaceous gland function, and the production of hair. The disease is best documented in American Cocker Spaniels[23, 24] but other breeds such as Basset Hounds, West Highland White Terriers, Labrador Retrievers, Doberman Pinschers, and Springer Spaniels may also be affected. An hereditary seborrhea oleosa has been described in Persian cats[25].

Affected animals show varying degrees of papules, scale, crust, and alopecia (**247, 248**). The scale may be very greasy or dry. Affected animals frequently have chronic otitis externa and a greasy, ceruminous exudate often coats the hairs on the concave aspect of the pinna (**247**). Diagnosis is based on ruling out the differential diagnoses and on histopathologic findings. Management is based on the individual and involves control of secondary infection (*Staphylocccus intermedius* and *Malassezia pachydermatis* in particular), suppressing exuberant keratinization (retinoids, Vitamin A, for example) and degreasing the skin with shampoos. Clinicians are referred to specialist texts for detailed discussion of these conditions[24, 26].

Peripheral hyperkeratosis
Peripheral hyperkeratosis is regarded as a primary keratinization defect and it affects principally the Miniature Dachshund[26]. Mild lesions are confined to the pinnal periphery and consist of non-pruritic, greasy or scaly plugs attached to the pinnal margin (**249**). Severe cases may affect the body of the pinna. Treatment consists of keratolytic and keratoplastic shampoos such as tar, sulphur and salicyclic acid, benzoyl peroxide, or selenium sulphide.

Sebaceous adenitis
Sebaceous adenitis is a disease of unknown etiology characterized by an inflammatory response against the sebaceous glands[27, 28]. The lack of sebum results in follicular disruption, alopecia, and surface scale (**250, 251**). In some breeds, particularly shorthaired breeds, there may be a granulomatous response. Astute owners may notice that the crimp and nature of the coat changes before alopecia is apparent. Affected animals exhibit progressive loss of hair associated with prominent follicular casts. The pinnae and dorsal trunk are usually the first places to be affected. Diagnosis is based on clinical suspicion but it must be confirmed by histopathologic examination of multiple (>3) biopsy samples. There is no effective treatment once the sebaceous glands are destroyed. Early treatment with essential fatty acids, humectants, and anti-inflammatory doses of prednisolone may suppress the inflammation and help to preserve some function. Retinoids may be useful in the granulomatous presentation.

Idiopathic benign lichenoid keratosis
Idiopathic benign lichenoid keratosis affecting the pinnae has been reported in four dogs[29]. Affected animals present with multiple, wart-like papules, or hyperkeratotic plaques. Histologically the lesions are distinct. Complete surgical excision is curative.

Table 12: Classification of the defects in keratinization which may affect the pinnae.

Primary defects	Secondary defects
Idiopathic seborrhea	Ectoparasite infestation
Follicular dystrophy	Dermatophytosis
Epidermal dysplasia of West Highland White Terriers	Hypersensitivities
	Immune-mediated dermatoses
Icthyosis	Endocrinopathies
Zinc responsive dermatosis	Neoplasia
Sebaceous adenitis	Low humidity
Ear margin dermatosis	
Lichenoid-psoriasiform dermatosis	
Lupoid dermatosis of Pointers	

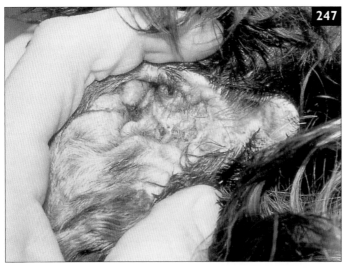

247, 248 Otitis externa (**247**) and pinnal crust, scale, and alopecia (**248**) in a Cocker Spaniel with an idiopathic defect in keratinization.

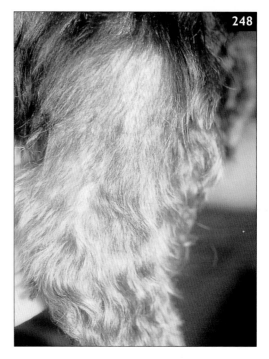

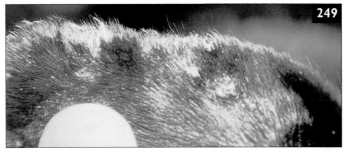

249 Peripheral hyperkeratosis resulting in crust and scale in a Miniature Dachshund.

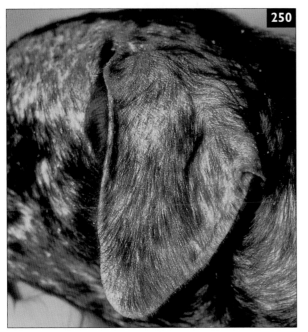

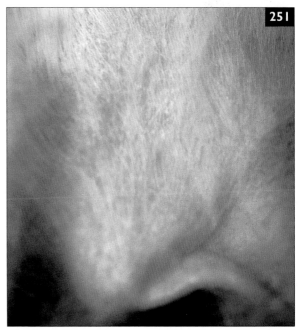

250 Labrador Retriever with advanced sebaceous adenitis. Note the surface scale and alopecia.

251 Standard Poodle with sebaceous adenitis. Note the tightly adherent surface scale and alopecia on this pinna.

Lichenoid psoriasiform dermatosis

Lichenoid psoriasiform dermatosis is an extremely rare dermatosis which has only been reported in young Springer Spaniels in the USA[30], raising the possibility that it is a genodermatosis. Affected animals exhibit erythematous papules and lichenoid plaques on the concave aspects of the pinnae, external ear canals, and other, predominantly ventral, parts of the head and trunk. Diagnosis is based on the almost pathognomonic signalment and clinical signs and confirmed by histopathologic examination of biopsy samples. The condition is frustrating to treat, requiring combinations of topical antimicrobial shampoo and systemic antibacterial agents, usually with systemic glucocorticoids, to effect even a modicum of control.

Lupoid dermatosis

Lupoid dermatosis is a rare heritable disease of German Shorthaired Pointers[31]. The disease is characterized by progressive, non-pruritic scale and alopecia of the face, pinnae (**252**), and trunk. There is no effective treatment.

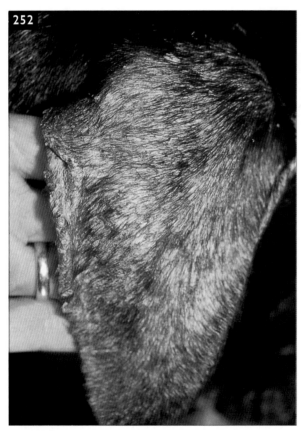

252 Shorthaired Pointer with lupoid dermatosis. Not the surface scale and alopecia.

NUTRITIONAL DERMATOSES

Zinc deficiency

Zinc deficiency occurs as two clinical syndromes in the dog[32] but has not been reported in the cat. Occasional clusters of cases, affecting any breed of dog, may occur when a deficient diet is fed. Some breeds, for example Alaskans, may manifest a physiologic inability to absorb zinc. The major clinical sign in such cases is crusting of the pinnae and perioral, periorbital, perianal, and perivulval sites, as well as crusting over pressure points[32].

Food allergy

Dietary intolerance and food allergy are rare conditions which may be associated with any combination of clinical signs, and therefore they should always be included in differential diagnoses for animals with chronic pinnal dermatosis. Approximately half of affected animals will have a history of steroid-resistant pruritus[33, 34] (*Table 11*). Clinical signs will almost always reflect pruritus, although the degree and duration of the pruritus will dictate the changes: erythema, alopecia, crust and scale and, ultimately, hyperpigmentation and lichenification. There are no primary or pathognomic lesions. Diagnosis of dietary intolerance and food allergy depends on eliminating diagnoses from the working differential and then instituting dietary testing. The formulation of an exclusion diet and demonstrating that the clinical signs resolve when it is fed, relapse when the normal diet or the offending component is subsequently fed, and resolve upon refeeding the exclusion diet is diagnostic[33–35]. The diet should be fed for a minimum period of six weeks, and in some cases it may need to be fed for 12 weeks. This procedure should not be undertaken lightly.

FOCAL LESIONS PRINCIPALLY AFFECTING THE DORSAL PINNA

DERMATOPHYTOSIS

Dermatophytosis is one of the most common conditions affecting the pinnae of cats but it is much less common in dogs. Dermatophytosis is more common in young cats than in mature individuals, unless their immune system is compromised by ill health. The most common lesions consist of broken, dull-looking hairs and a thin, often silvery scale (**253**)[1]. However, dermatophytosis may also cause a papular dermatitis, erythematous dermatitis (**254**) and, in some cases, a granulomatous reaction, although these are much less common on the pinnae than on the trunk or limbs. Diagnosis is by examination of skin scrapes, examination of the affected area under Wood's light, and ultimately by culture. 'Spot' treatment, even of localized lesions, is not advised and current treatment recommendations advocate principally systemic medication (griseofulvin or ketoconazole) and topical dips with, for example, enilconazole[2, 3].

FELINE POXVIRUS

Feline poxvirus infection (synonym: cowpox) is caused by an Orthopoxvirus, presumably transmitted by bites from small rodents[4]. Primary lesions appear as transient erythematous papules or erosions, usually on the anterior part of the body. Some 10–14 days later secondary lesions appear as papules, which rapidly crust and become alopecic erosions (**255**). The disease has zoonotic potential and suitable precautions against infection should be taken. Supportive treatment with systemic antibacterial agents is usually sufficient. Glucocorticoids should be avoided as they may predispose to systemic infection and severe complications, even death, may ensue.

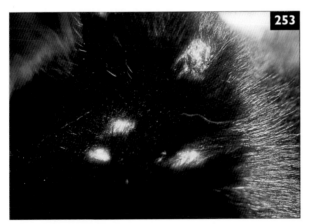

253 Dermatophytosis causing patchy alopecia on the head and pinnae of a cat.

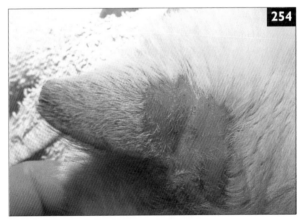

254 Erythematous patch caused by dermatophytosis in a cat.

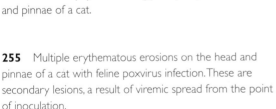

255 Multiple erythematous erosions on the head and pinnae of a cat with feline poxvirus infection. These are secondary lesions, a result of viremic spread from the point of inoculation.

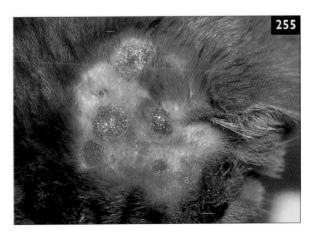

DERMATOSES CAUSING PAPULES AND NODULES

Nodules on the pinnae may reflect many etiologies. It is almost impossible to distinguish between them with confidence on the basis of clinical appearance. Cytologic examination may be helpful but punch or excision biopsy is indicated in all cases in which the etiology is unknown.

TICK INFESTATION

Owners often mistakenly identify ticks as tumors. The most common ticks found on the pinnae of dogs are the American dog tick (*Dermacentor variablis*), the lone star tick (*Amblyomma americanum*), the brown dog tick (*Rhipicephalus sanguinus*), and *Ixodes* spp. (**256**). The latter are the species least likely to be found on the pinnae and head[1, 2]. It has been speculated that the prevalence of ticks on the head and pinnae simply reflects the inability of the host to remove them easily from this area of the body[2].

In addition to causing local irritation and occasionally postbite granulomas (**257**), ticks are frequently associated with vectoring infectious disease. Viral (e.g. louping ill in dogs), bacterial (e.g. tularemia in cats), rickettsial (e.g. ehrlichiosis) and protozoal (e.g. babesiosis) diseases may all be transmitted by various species of tick.

Ticks may be removed with gentle traction. Removal is more easily accomplished if the ticks are killed first, for example by application of vegetable or mineral oil, or a specific agent such as amitraz or fipronil[3–5] (see Chapter 3: Ectoparasitic causes of otitis externa, and antiparasitic agents).

NEOPLASTIC LESIONS

Papilloma

Cocker Spaniels, Kerry Blue Terriers, and male dogs in general are predisposed[6, 7]. Papillomas are usually well-demarcated (**258**), superficial, occasionally pedunculated papules (i.e. <1 cm [<0.4 in] diameter) which tend to bleed if traumatized[7]. Many papillomas exhibit a frond-like appearance[6].

Canine cutaneous histiocytoma

Canine cutaneous histiocytomas are most likely of Langerhans cell origin[8]. These are the most common neoplasms of the dog and 50% of cases occur in dogs under two years of age[9]. Pedigree dogs are predisposed, particularly the Boxer, English Bulldog, and Scottish Terrier[10]. The most common site for the tumor is the dorsal pinna[10]. These are solitary, elevated, domed, erythematous, well-demarcated, minimally pruritic lesions (**259**) which are often reported to show rapid growth. Occasionally they are ulcerated and very rarely they have been reported to be multiple. Canine cutaneous histiocytomas are benign lesions and response to surgery is close to 100%[10]. The principal differential diagnoses are mast cell tumors and granulomas.

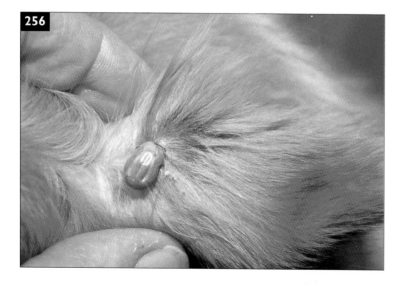

256

256   *Ixodes ricinus* on a cat.

257 Post tick-bite granuloma on the pinna of a dog.

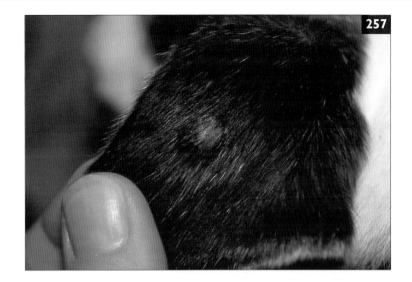

258 Well-demarcated, flesh-colored papilloma on the pinna of a Cocker Spaniel.

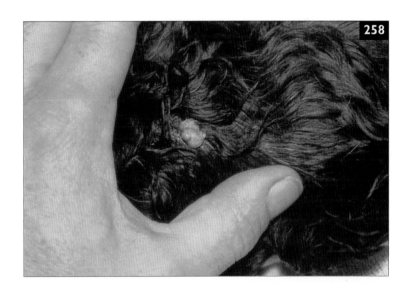

259 Erythematous nodule on the pinna of a dog – histiocytoma.

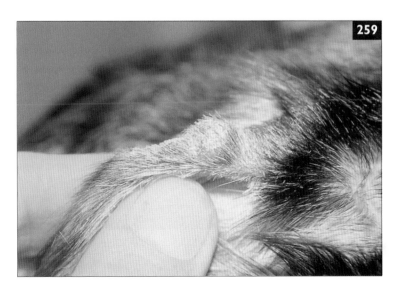

Mast cell tumor

Mast cell tumors are common in the dog[11, 12]. Although mast cell tumors may occur in young dogs (hence the inclusion of canine cutaneous histiocytoma as a differential diagnosis) the incidence increases with age, peaking at eight or nine years old[11, 12]. Boxers and other breeds with Bulldog ancestry are predisposed but mast cell tumors may occur in any dog[11]. The clinical appearance of the tumor is very variable but single cutaneous lesions less than 3 cm (1.2 in) in diameter are the most common presentation (**260**)[12]. The diagnosis of mast cell tumor is made by a combination of cytology and histopathology. However, clinical management of all but single nodules (treated by simple surgical excision) will mandate clinical staging prior to initiation of treatment[12, 13]. The selection of various treatment modalities for extensive canine mast cell neoplasia is beyond the scope of this book and readers are referred to references.

GRANULOMATOUS LESIONS

Staphylococci, *Nocardia* spp, *Actinomycetes* spp., mycobacteria, atypical mycobacteria, dermatophytes, subcutaneous mycoses, deep mycoses, algae, ticks, *Leishmania* spp., and foreign bodies are all potential causes of granulomatous dermatitis[14]. Clinically these are usually nodular in appearance, slowly growing, and domed in appearance (**261**). Granulomas may be solitary or multiple (**262**), exudative, or ulcerated. They are usually non-pruritic. The management of these nodules is primarily aimed at defining the etiology so that specific treatment may be provided. The clinical approach may therefore include aspiration cytology, serology, histology, microbiology, and fungal culture.

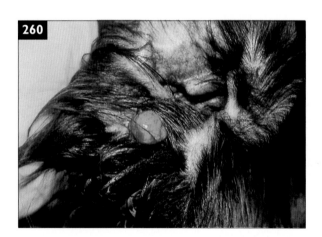

260   Large, erythematous, eroded mast cell tumor at the base of the pinna of a Newfoundland dog.

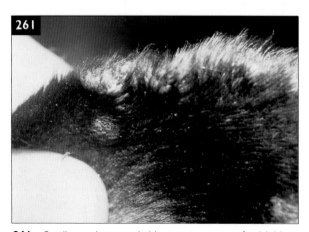

261   Small granuloma, probably a consequence of a tick bite, on the pinna of a dog.

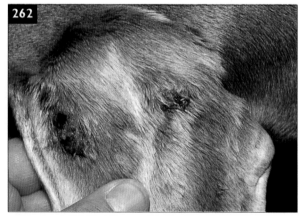

262   Eosinophilic furunculosis/granulomas on the pinna of a Weimaraner recently bitten by a bee. These lesions are intensely pruritic.

DERMATOSES PRINCIPALLY AFFECTING THE CONCAVE ASPECT OF THE PINNA

ATOPY

Atopy is possibly the most common cause of recurrent otitis externa and lesions are often found on the concave aspect of the pinnae as well as within the external ear canal (**263, 264**). In early cases of atopy, where the otitis externa has not yet become fully established, astute clinicians may note erythema and hyperplasia on the concave aspect of the pinnae and in the upper portions only of the vertical part of the external ear canal. With time a chronic, recurrent, erythematous, ceruminous otitis externa results. Although most dogs with atopy exhibit otitis externa in association with other signs, in about 3% of atopic dogs otitis externa is the only clinical sign[1].

> The importance of recognizing atopy early cannot be overemphasized since the association with recurrent chronic otitis externa is well documented.

ALLERGIC CONTACT DERMATITIS

Allergic contact dermatitis is rare. Most commonly it affects middle-aged animals since the induction period is long[2, 3]. If the allergen is contained within something on which the animal lies, the pinnae may be involved. Since the convex aspect of the pinna is haired it is usually the glabrous concave surfaces which exhibit lesions first. The glabrous ventral aspect of the pinna may also be involved in allergic contact dermatitis to topical otic medications such as neomycin and propylene glycol (**265**). The management of allergic contact dermatitis is based upon identifying the allergen with exclusion/provocative or closed patch testing, neither of which is easy. Failure to identify the allergen, and avoiding contact, condemns the animal to systemic glucocorticoid therapy, usually in such high dosages that side-effects become apparent.

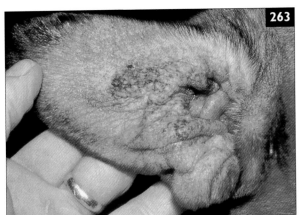

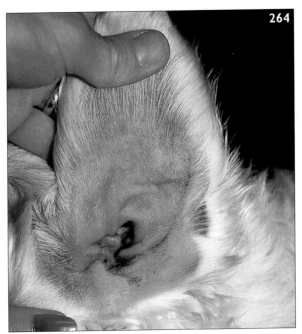

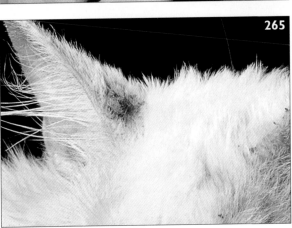

263, 264 Hyperplasia and lichenification on the concave aspect of the pinnae of an atopic dog (**263**) often accompanies erythema of the vertical ear canal (**264**).

265 Erythematous pinna as a result of allergic contact dermatitis to topical application of Vaseline.

DEFECTS IN KERATINIZATION, HYPOTHYROIDISM, AND SEX HORMONE ABERRATIONS

Defects in keratinization, hypothyroidism, and sex hormone aberrations are often associated with excessive sebaceous gland activity, and a greasy, hyperkeratotic dermatosis results on the concave aspect of the pinna (**266–268**). Diagnosis, in the absence of demonstrable gonadal neoplasia, is difficult and may require ACTH testing combined with pre- and postadrenal sex hormone assay. This may be very expensive and difficult to justify in practice. Clinicians should consult a specialist if sex hormone aberrations are suspected.

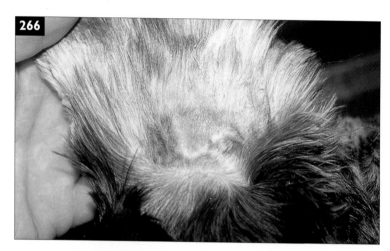

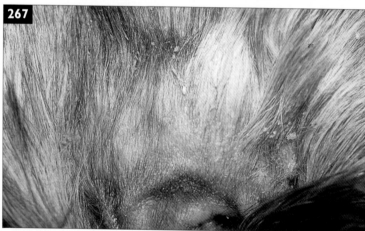

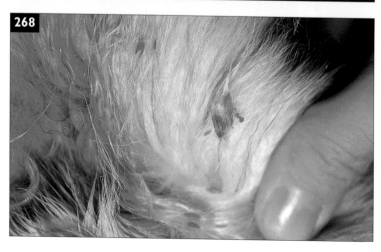

266–268 Greasy scale on the concave aspect of the pinna in a Cocker Spaniel with a defect in keratinization, even after vertical ear canal ablation has been performed (**266**); in a Cocker Spaniel with hypothyroidism (**267**); and in a German Shepherd Dog with Sertoli cell tumor (**268**).

DERMATOSES PRINCIPALLY CAUSING SYMMETRICAL PINNAL ALOPECIA

ENDOCRINOPATHY

Hypothyroidism, feline hyperthyroidism, and sex hormone aberrations are the endocrine diseases most likely to be associated with alopecia. Hypothyroidism is the most common endocrinopathy affecting dogs but it is extremely rare in cats. Hypothyroidism occurs most commonly in middle-aged dogs and is characterized by an insidious onset and a plethora of clinical signs. Bilateral symmetrical alopecia of the trunk is one of the most common cutaneous signs. On rare occasions the pinnae may be affected (**269**).

Hypothyroidism in the cat may follow thyroidectomy, and alopecia may be noted. However, more commonly, alopecia occurs with feline hyperthyroidism, a consequence of overgrooming (**270**). Diagnosis of thyroid disease in the dog is based on documenting subnormal serum total T4 concentrations, elevated serum TSH concentrations, or a blunted response to the TSH stimulation test[1]. In the cat the diagnosis is based on clinical examination and elevated serum total T4 concentration.

DRUG ERUPTION

Drug eruption may result in unpredictable clinical signs, occasionally even very localized lesions. However, in many cases the lesions are symmetrical and alopecia may be part of the clinical syndrome displayed (**271**).

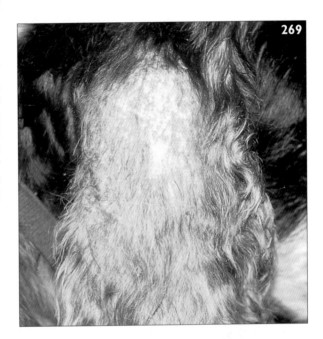

269 Alopecia of the pinna of a hypothyroid Cocker Spaniel.

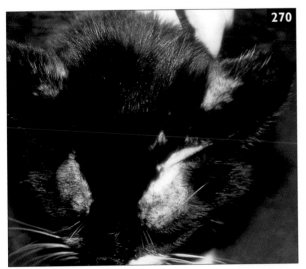

270 Symmetrical alopecia at the base of the pinnae in a cat with hyperthyroidism. The alopecia is a result of overgrooming rather than telogen arrest.

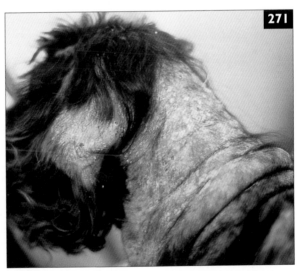

271 Cocker Spaniel with drug eruption. There is marked alopecia, scale, and crust formation.

FOLLICULAR DYSPLASIA

Follicular dysplasia occurs when the hair follicle cannot produce a normal hair shaft[2, 3]. Color dilute alopecia is a type of follicular dysplasia[3]. The result of the follicular defects in these animals is symmetrical alopecia, typically affecting the dorsal and lateral trunk, although the convex aspects of the pinnae may also become alopecic (**272**). There are occasional papules or comedones and there may be a variable epidermal scale. Generally the dermatosis is non-pruritic, unless secondary pyoderma ensues. Doberman Pinschers and Dachshunds, in particular, are affected, although it has been reported in many other breeds[4]. Diagnosis is based on ruling out the differential diagnoses (endocrinopathy in particular) and on histopathologic findings. Treatment is palliative.

PATTERN BALDNESS

Pattern baldness is an uncommon dermatosis in which animals display symmetrical alopecia, or hypotrichosis, of the pinnae, ventrum, and caudal medial thighs. Miniature Dachshunds and Staffordshire Bull Terriers appear to be predisposed. Diagnosis is based on ruling out the differential diagnoses and on histopathologic findings.

PINNAL HYPERPIGMENTATION AND ALOPECIA

Pinnal hyperpigmentation and alopecia has been recognized in Yorkshire Terriers (**273**) and occasionally other breeds, such as the Doberman Pinscher. The etiology of the condition is unknown. There is no effective treatment.

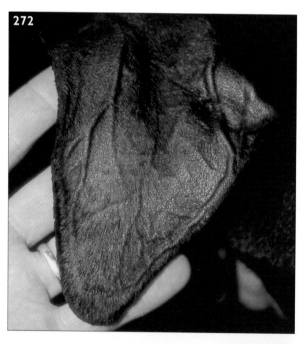

272 Pinnal alopecia in a Doberman Pinscher with a follicular defect.

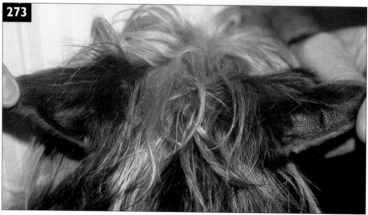

273 Pinnal alopecia and hyperpigmentation in a Yorkshire Terrier.

REFERENCES

DERMATOSES CHARACTERIZED BY CRUST AND SCALE

1 August JR (1986) Taking a dermatologic history. *Compendium on Continuing Education* **8**, 510–518.

2 Scheidt VJ (1987) Common feline ectoparasites. Part 2: *Notoedres cati, Demodex cati, Cheyletiella* spp., and *Otodectes cynotis. Feline Practice* **17**, 13–23.

3 Cooper PR and Penaliggon J (196) Use of fipronil to eliminate recurrent infestation by *Trichodectes canis* in a pack of Bloodhounds. *Veterinary Record* **139**, 95.

4 Chesney CJ (1989) Demodicosis in the cat. *Journal of Small Animal Practice* **30**, 689–695.

5 Wilkinson GT (1983) Demodicosis in a cat due to a new mite species. *Feline Practice* **13**, 32–36.

6 Greene RT, Scheidt VJ and Moncol DJ (1986) Trombiculiasis in a cat. *Journal of the American Veterinary Medical Association* **188**, 1054–1055.

7 Studdert VP and Arundel JH (1988) Dermatitis of the pinnae of cats in Australia associated with the European rabbit flea (*Spilopsyllus cuniculi*). *Veterinary Record* **123**, 624–625.

8 Harvey RG (1990) Dermatitis in a cat associated with *Spilopsyllus cuniculi. Veterinary Record* **126**, 89–90.

9 Angarano DW (1988) Diseases of the pinnae. In *Veterinary Clinics of North America.* (ed JR August) **18**, 869–884.

10 Mason KV and Evans AG (1991) Mosquito bite-caused eosinophilic dermatitis in cats. *Journal of the American Veterinary Medical Association* **198**, 2086–2088.

11 Nagata M and Takuo I (1997) Cutaneous reactivity to mosquito bites and its antigens in cats. *Veterinary Dermatology* **8**, 19–26.

12 Ferrer L, Rabanal R, Fondevila D, Ramos JA and Domingo M (1988) Skin lesions in canine leishmaniasis. *Journal of Small Animal Practice* **29**, 381–388.

13 Bond R, Collin NS and Lloyd DH (1994) Use of contact plates for the quantitative culture of *Malassezia pachydermatis* from canine skin. *Journal of Small Animal Practice* **35**, 68–72.

14 Ihrke PJ, Stannard AA, Ardans AA and Griffin CE (1985) Pemphigus foliaceus in the dog: a review of 37 cases. *Journal of the American Veterinary Medical Association* **186**, 59–66.

15 Manning TO, Scott DW, Smith CA and Lewis RM (1982) Pemphigus diseases in the feline: seven case reports and discussion. *Journal of the American Animal Hospital Association* **18**, 433–443.

16 Scott DW, Walton DK, Manning TO, Smith CA and Lewis RM (1983) Canine lupus erythematosus. I: Systemic lupus erythematosus. *Journal of the American Animal Hospital Association* **19**, 461–479.

17 Halliwell REW and Gorman NT (1989) Autoimmune blood diseases. In *Veterinary Clinical Immunology.* (eds REW Halliwell and NT Gorman) WB Saunders, Philadelphia, pp. 308–336.

18 Parker WM and Foster RA (1989) Cutaneous vasculitis in five Jack Russell Terriers. *Veterinary Dermatology* **7**, 109–115.

19 Lana Se, Ogilvie GK, Withrow SJ, Straw RC and Rogers KS (1997) Feline cutaneous squamous cell carcinoma of the nasal planum and the pinnae: 61 cases. *Journal of the American Animal Hospital Association* **33**, 329–332.

20 Goldschmidt MH and Shofer FS (1992) Squamous cell carcinoma. In *Skin Tumors of the Dog and Cat.* (eds MH Goldschmidt and FS Shofer) Pergammon Press, New York, pp. 37–49.

21 Atwater SW, Powers BE, Straw RC *et al.* (1991) Squamous cell carcinoma of the pinna and nasal planum: 54 cats (1980–1991). *Proceedings of the Veterinary Cancer Society* **11**, 35–36.

22 Nagata M, Nanko H, Hashimoto K, Ogawa M and Sakashita E (1998) Cryoglobulinemia and cryofibronogenemia: a comparison of canine and human cases. *Veterinary Dermatology* **9**, 277–281.

23 Kwochka KW and Rademakers AM (1989) Cell proliferation kinetics of epidermis, hair follicles, and sebaceous glands of Cocker Spaniels with idiopathic seborrhea. *American Journal of Veterinary Research* **50**, 1918–1922.

24 Kwochka KW (1993) Primary keratinization disorders of dogs. In *Current Veterinary Dermatology* (eds CE Griffin, KW Kwochka and JM MacDonald) WB Saunders, Philadelphia, pp. 176–190.

25 Paradis M and Scott DW (1990) Hereditary primary seborrhea oleosa in Persian cats. *Feline Practice* **18**, 17–20.

26 Kwochka KW (1993) Overview of normal keratinization and cutaneous scaling disorders. In *Current Veterinary Dermatology* (eds CE Griffin, KW Kwochka and JM MacDonald) WB Saunders, Philadelphia, pp. 167–175.

27 Rosser EJ, Dunstan RW, Breen PT and Johnson GR (1987) Sebaceous adenitis with hyperkeratosis in the standard poodle: a discussion of 10 cases. *Journal of the American Animal Hospital Association* **23**, 341–345.

28 Scott DW (1986) Granulomatous sebaceous adenitis in dogs. *Journal of the American Animal Hospital Association* **22**, 631–634.

29 Anderson WI, Scott DW, and Luther PB (1989) Idiopathic benign lichenoid keratosis on the pinna of the ear in four dogs. *Cornell Veterinarian* **79**, 179–184.

30 Mason KV, Halliwell REW and McDougal BJ (1986) Characterization of lichenoid-psoriasiform dermatosis of Springer Spaniels. *Journal of the American Veterinary Medical Association* **189**, 897–901.

31 Theaker AJ and Rest JR (1992) Lupoid dermatosis in a German Shorthaired Pointer. *Veterinary Record* **131**, 495.

32 Willemse T (1992) Zinc-related cutaneous disorders of dogs. In *Current Veterinary Therapy XI.* (eds RW Kirk and JD Bonagura) WB Saunders, Philadelphia, pp. 532–534.

33 Rosser EJ jnr (1993) Diagnosis of food allergy in dogs. *Journal of the American Veterinary Medical Association* **203**, 259–262.

34 Harvey RG (1993) Food allergy and dietary intolerance in dogs: a report of 25 cases. *Journal of Small Animal Practice* **34**, 175–179.

35 Wills JM and Harvey RG (1994) Diagnosis and management of food allergy and dietary intolerance in dogs and cats. *Australian Veterinary Journal* **71**, 322–326.

FOCAL LESIONS PRINCIPALLY AFFECTING THE DORSAL PINNA

1 Wright AI (1989) Ringworm in dogs and cats. *Journal of Small Animal Practice* **30**, 242–249.

2 Moriello KA (1995) Treatment of feline dermatophytosis: revised recommendations. *Feline Practice* **24**, 32–36.

3 White-Weithers MS and Medleau L (1995) Evaluation of topical therapies for the treatment of dermatophyte-infected hairs from dogs and cats. *Journal of the American Animal Hospital Association* **31**, 250–253.

4 Bennett M, Gaskell CJ, Gaskell RM, Baxby D and Gruffyd-Jones TJ (1986) Poxvirus infection in the domestic cat: some clinical and epidemiological investigations. *Veterinary Record* **118**, 387–390.

DERMATOSES CAUSING PAPULES AND NODULES

1 Koch HG (1982) Seasonal incidence and attachment sites of ticks (Acari: Ixodidae) on domestic dogs in southeastern Oklahoma and northwestern Arkansas, USA. *Journal of Medical Entomology* **19**, 293–295.

2 Sucharit S and Rongsiyam Y (1990) *Rhipicephalus sanguinus Latrielle*, the causative agent of foreign body in the ear: distribution on the body of the dog. *Journal of the Medical Association of Thailand* **63**, 535–536.

3 Searle A, Jensen CJ and Atwell RB (1995) Results of a trial of fipronil as a adulticide on ticks (*Ixodes holocyclus*) naturally attached to animals in the Brisbane area. *Australian Veterinary Practice* **25**, 157–158.

4 Folz SD, Ash KA, Conder GA and Rector DL (1986) Amitraz: a tick and flea repellent and tick detachment drug. *Journal of Veterinary Pharmacology and Therapeutics* **9**, 150–156.

5 Hunter JS, Keister DM and Jeannin P (1996) A comparison of the tick control efficacy of Frontline Spray against the American dog tick and brown dog tick. *Proceedings of the 41st Annual Meeting of the American Association of Veterinary Parasitologists*, Louisville, 1996, p. 51.

6 Goldschmidt MH and Shofer FS (1992) Cutaneous papilloma. In *Skin Tumors of the Dog and Cat.* (eds MH Goldschmidt and FS Shofer) Pergammon Press, New York, pp. 11–15.

7 Bevier DE and Goldschmidt MH (1981) Skin tumors in the dog. Part I: Epithelial tumors and tumor-like lesions. *Compendium on Continuing Education* **3**, 389–400.

8 Moore PF and Schrenzel MD (1991) Canine cutaneous histiocytoma represents a Langerhans cell proliferative disorder based on an immunophenotypic analysis. *Proceedings of the American College of Veterinary Pathology* **42**, 119.

9 Goldschmidt MH and Bevier DE (1981) Skin tumors in the dog. Part III: Lymphohystiocytic and melanocytic tumors. *Compendium on Continuing Education* **3**, 588–594.

10 Goldschmidt MH and Shofer FS (1992) Canine cutaneous histiocytoma. In *Skin Tumors of the Dog and Cat.* (eds MH Goldschmidt and FS Shofer) Pergammon Press, New York, pp. 222–230.

11 Goldschmidt MH and Shofer FS (1992) Mast cell tumors. In *Skin Tumors of the Dog and Cat.* (eds MH Goldschmidt and FS Shofer) Pergammon Press, New York, pp. 231–251.

12 Tams TR and Macy DW (1981) Canine mast cell tumors. *Compendium on Continuing Education* **3**, 869–878.

13 Macy DW (1986) Canine and feline mast cell tumors: biologic behavior, diagnosis, and therapy. *Seminars in Veterinary Medicine and Surgery* **1**, 72–83.

14 Fadok VA (1987) Granulomatous dermatitis in dogs and cats. *Seminars in Veterinary Medicine and Surgery* **2**, 186–194.

DERMATOSES PRINCIPALLY AFFECTING THE CONCAVE ASPECT OF THE PINNA

1 Scott DW (1981) Observations on canine atopy. *Journal of the American Animal Hospital Association* **17**, 91–100.

2 Thomsen MK and Kristensen F (1986) Contact dermatitis in the dog. *Nordsik Veterinær Medicine* **38**, 129–147.

3 Olivry T, Prélaud P, Héripret D and Atlee BA (1990) Allergic contact dermatitis in the dog. *Veterinary Clinics of North America* **20**, 1443–1456.

DERMATOSES PRINCIPALLY CAUSING SYMMETRICAL PINNAL ALOPECIA

1 Kemppainen RJ and MacDonald JM (1993) Canine hypothyroidism. In *Current Veterinary Dermatology* (eds CE Griffin, KW Kwochka and JM MacDonald) WB Saunders, Philadelphia, pp. 265–272.

2 Miller WH jnr (1990) Follicular dysplasia in adult black and red Doberman Pinschers. *Veterinary Dermatology* **1**, 181–187.

3 Miller WH jnr (1990) Color dilute alopecia in Doberman Pinschers with blue and fawn coat colors: a study on the incidence and histopathology of this disorder. *Veterinary Dermatology* **1**, 113–122.

4 Beco L, Fontaine J, Gross TL and Charlier G (1996) Color dilute alopecia in seven Dachshunds: a clinical study and the hereditary, microscopical, and ultrastructural aspects of the disease. *Veterinary Dermatology* **7**, 91–97.

Chapter Five

Otitis Media, Otitis Interna

- Otitis media

- Otitis interna

- References

OTITIS MEDIA

KEY POINTS

- The term otitis media implies inflammation within the confines of the middle ear, usually bacterial in origin.
- Otitis media is common and often unrecognized
- In the vast majority of dogs with otitis media, clinical signs relate to the accompanying otitis externa.
- Neurologic signs accompanying otitis media are unusual.
- Systemic antibacterial therapy, in association with local drainage, is the medical treatment of choice.
- Surgical treatment may be necessary if the condition proves refractory to medical management.

ETIOLOGY

Otitis media is common and is almost invariably accompanied by otitis externa[1, 2, 3]. Furthermore, in the vast majority of cases the infection within the middle ear appears to result from extension of otitis externa, rather than from ascending infection via the auditory tube or as a result of hematogenous infection[1]. However, it may be that the role of the auditory tube in the etiology of canine otitis media has not been fully appreciated, since its normal physiologic role is critical to middle ear homeostasis, both microbiologic and environmental[4, 5]. Most cases of otitis media appear to be missed since in one study the duration of the condition, before diagnosis, was in excess of two years in over half the cases[3].

The microorganisms isolated from cases of otitis media are principally those associated with otitis externa, i.e. *Staphylococcus intermedius*, *Pseudomonas* spp., *Proteus* spp., *Escherichia coli*, and *Malassezia pachydermatis*[1, 2]. However, aerobic bacteria were isolated from nearly half the normal middle ears sampled in one study[6], suggesting a normal flora, presumably derived from pharyngeal flora ascending the auditory tube. The bacteria recovered were principally *E. coli*, staphylococci, and *Branhamella* spp., together with yeast[6].

Otitis media usually results as an extension of otitis externa through the tympanum, which may subsequently heal, even in the presence of otitis media. However, the bacteria recovered from behind an intact tympanum in cases of otitis media are not always the same species, or with the same antibacterial sensitivity, as those within the external ear canal[2]. Bacteria (especially *S. intermedius* and *Pseudomonas*

> The most common bacteria isolated from cases of otitis media are those associated with otitis externa.

spp.) and yeast were most commonly found in the external ear canal, whereas bacteria alone were more common in the middle ear. A greater variety of bacteria, including anaerobes, Group D streptococci, and *E. coli*, were found in the middle ear compared to the external ear canal[2].

Other causes, particularly of unilateral otitis media, include foreign bodies which have penetrated the tympanum, inflammatory polyps, and neoplasms such as fibromas and squamous cell carcinomas[1].

The pathologic changes within the infected middle ear were reported by Little *et al*[7]. All the cases in their study were accompanied by pathologic changes within the external ear canal, supporting the theory of an association between the two conditions. There was epidermal hyperplasia with a replacement of the normal stratified squamous epithelium by pseudo-stratified columnar type. The underlying dermis was infiltrated by a mixed inflammatory cell population and it took on the appearance of granulation tissue, occasionally with spicules of bone within it. Secretory cells and gland-like structures appeared within this inflamed granulation tissue. Most of the tympanic membranes were thickened.

Cholesteatomas

Cholesteatomas are slowly enlarging, cystic lesions within the middle ear cavity. They are lined by stratified squamous epithelium and keratin squames are shed into them. They are thought to arise when a pocket of the tympanic membrane contacts, and adheres to, inflamed mucosa within the middle ear[7]. Cholesteatomas are associated with chronic otitis externa, particularly if there is marked stenosis, or even total occlusion, of the external ear canal. In addition to otitis externa they may be associated with local pain, pain when eating, and head tilt[7]. Radiographically, cholesteatomas are associated with increased density within the middle ear cavity and disruption or a change in shape of the middle ear cavity. There is usually stenosis and calcification of the external ear canal[7].

CLINICAL SIGNS

The most common clinical signs associated with otitis media are those of otitis externa or, rarely, of otitis interna[1, 8, 9]. Pain may be a feature in some cases and animals may resent patting of the aural region or may exhibit frantic head shaking (**274**). Otitis externa is often present and animals commonly have a history of chronic or recurrent otitis externa[8]. Neurologic signs are unusual but include head tilt (**275**), ataxia, nystagmus,

> Otitis media is often confused with otitis interna and masked by otitis externa.

Horner's syndrome (**276**), or facial nerve paralysis (**277, 278**)[7, 9, 10]. Keratoconjunctivitis sicca may, rarely, result from otitis media, following damage to the parasympathetic innervation of the lachrymal gland[9].

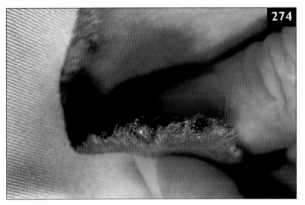

274 Pinnal trauma as a consequence of otitis media. This dog displayed incessant head shaking.

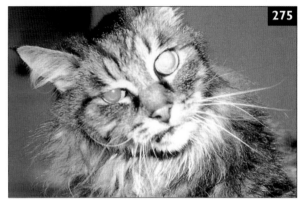

275 Dramatic head tilt to the right in a domestic longhaired cat with peripheral vestibular disease associated with otitis media.

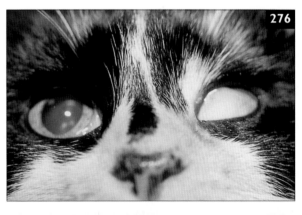

276 Horner's syndrome on the left-hand side. The markedly prolapsed third eyelid prevents examination of the pupil. This cat had a nasopharyngeal polyp which passed through the middle ear, then through the tympanic membrane into the external ear canal where it produced signs of an obstructive otitis externa.

277, 278 Horner's syndrome and facial nerve paralysis in a Staffordshire Bull Terrier. There is right-sided head tilt, a myotic right pupil, and facial paralysis resulting in drooping of the lips on the right-hand side of the face.

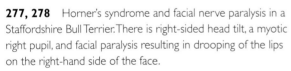

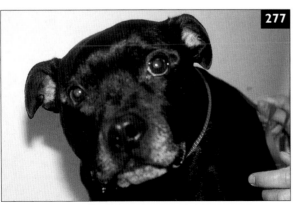

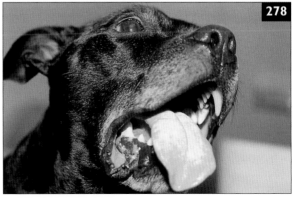

Otitis interna may occur following extension of infection into the inner ear via the oval window. Signs of otitis interna include[1, 8]: deafness, head tilt and circling toward the affected side; nystagmus with the fast component away from the affected side; and asymmetric ataxia.

MAJOR DIFFERENTIAL DIAGNOSES

Idiopathic canine and feline vestibular syndromes are the most common non-middle ear disorders associated with peripheral vestibular signs[10]. However, in contrast to otitis media these diseases usually show signs of gradual clinical improvement in 1–10 days[10].

DIAGNOSIS
Otoscopy

Otoscopy has good specificity but poor sensitivity[11]. Otitis media should be suspected in all cases of chronic otitis externa or in cases with recurrent episodes of otitis externa. The presence of a ruptured tympanic membrane is diagnostic (**279**). However, the presence of inflammation and exudate within the external ear canal makes meaningful examination of the tympanum difficult[11] (Chapter 2: Otoscopic appearance of the external ear canal and tympanum). Furthermore, the presence of an intact tympanum does not rule out otitis media since the defect in the tympanum often heals, even in the presence of ongoing otitis media[2]. These complications make definitive otoscopic diagnosis difficult.

Radiography and other imaging modalities

Radiographic techniques have good specificity but poor sensitivity, being able to delineate soft tissue, fluid, or bony changes within the middle ear in only about 70% of cases[10]. They are particularly useful in evaluation of bone involvement (e.g. petrous temporal bone) and in cases where neoplasia is suspected[12]. The open-mouth views are most useful[12], although in a series of cases in which otitis media persisted after bulla osteotomy the lateral oblique view was superior[12, 13]. The normal bullae have an identifiable air density within the tympanic cavity. Otitis media results in increased soft tissue density within the bullae (**280, 281**) and, if present, is a reliable indicator of disease within the middle ear[1, 12] (see Chapter 2: Radiographic features of the normal and abnormal ear). Positive contrast ear canalography may also be used to demonstrate otitis media[14].

Both CT and MRI have the potential to aid in the diagnosis of otitis media[15], although the clinician in practice will have difficulty accessing these techniques.

Tympanometry (impedance audiometry)

Tympanometry[11, 16] is non-invasive and has a high specificity and high sensitivity in detecting the presence of a ruptured tympanum. Unfortunately, in order to perform tympanometry in the dog it is necessary to adapt specialized equipment and it is unlikely to feature in the diagnostic armamentarium of any but the most specialized of clinics (see Chapter 2: Electrophysiologic procedures).

Culture and sensitivity following myringotomy

This technique, if performed carefully, has both good sensitivity and good specificity. However, it is necessary to rupture the tympanic membrane (myringotomy), if it is not already ruptured. Myringotomy is described in Chapter 2 (Other investigatory procedures).

279   Otoscopic view of a thickened and ruptured tympanic membrane.

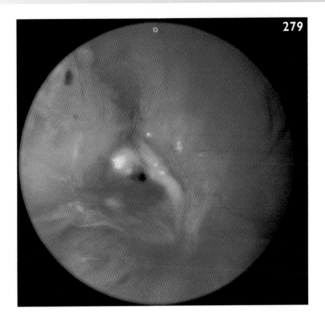

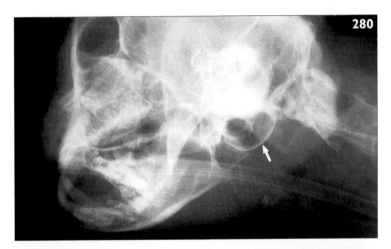

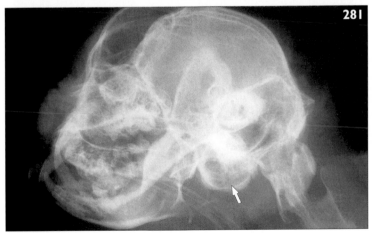

280, 281   Lateral oblique views of the tympanic bullae of a three-year-old Himalayan cat with left-sided otitis media associated with a nasopharyngeal polyp. Compare **280** (normal bulla on the right side, arrow) with **281** (soft tissue density within bulla on the left side, arrow).

MANAGEMENT

Given that most cases of otitis media are associated with otitis externa, the treatment of the former cannot be considered in isolation from the latter[1, 9, 10]. The approach to each case should be structured with this in mind and one authority[10] triaged animals into three groups:

Group 1

All new cases that have presented within the previous few days are treated with a cephalosporin or a fluoroquinolone antimicrobial agent at maximal doses for four weeks. Anti-inflammatory doses of prednisolone are given (1 mg/kg once daily for two weeks and then 1 mg/kg every other day for two weeks). If the tympanum is ruptured, a sample should be obtained from the middle ear for bacteriologic culture and sensitivity testing and treatment adjusted accordingly. Any apparent otitis externa is treated with ceruminolytics (if necessary) and dilute chlorhexidine (1:40) once daily, followed by gentle cleaning of the external ear canal. If indicated, clients can instil, twice daily, an appropriate non-oily (water-based) otic polypharmaceutic preparation. **NB:** Ensure that there is no aminoglycoside in the preparation if the tympanum is not intact.

Generally these animals show gradual improvement and the ataxia and head tilt resolves over 2–14 days. Resolution of nystagmus must not to be associated with successful treatment since the brain will compensate for aberrant input. Conversely, failure of nystagmus to resolve indicates treatment failure. Animals with otitis externa are subjected to dermatologic work up to establish whether there is an underlying cause that can be addressed. Careful attendance to these principles will minimize the number of animals which go forward to radical surgery.

Group 2

Cases which have not resolved within four weeks or so, or who presented originally having shown symptoms for a number of weeks, or those cases presenting with chronic or recurrent otitis externa, are subject to radiography (if not yet performed) and worked up for surgery. If available, CT or MRI would be indicated prior to surgery. Those with otitis externa are subject to total ear canal ablation and lateral bulla osteotomy. Those with no evidence of otitis externa are subject to ventral bulla osteotomy. The aim of treatment with these patients is to alleviate the otitis externa and to establish drainage of, and the opportunity for flushing of, the bulla. The bulla is flushed daily for 7–10 days and appropriate antibacterial therapy, based on bacterial culture and sensitivity, is instituted. The same glucocorticoid regime is used as described above, again designed to suppress inflammation within the bulla.

Group 3

Cases which fail to resolve after surgery are radiographed again and, if thought necessary (failure to demonstrate lesions with radiography), may be subjected to CT or MRI if not already performed. The bulla is curetted and a drain placed to facilitate daily flushing. Systemic antibacterial agents, based on culture and sensitivity testing, are prescribed for two months. Prednisolone, starting on the eighth day post-operatively, is given for one month as described above.

PROGNOSIS

If the inflammatory process is identified early, the cause identified, and effective treatment instituted, the prognosis for recovery is good. Minor residual vestibular deficits, such as head tilt or mild ataxia, may persist but the animal soon adapts to the 'new' head position. Neurologic signs associated with otitis media, such as facial nerve paralysis and Horner's syndrome, may persist and complications associated with these deficits can occur (see Chapter 7: Neurologic signs related to middle ear disease).

Some cases of otitis media (and, indeed, some cases of otitis interna) develop osteomyelitis of the osseous bulla and petrous temporal bone. Occasionally the infection ascends the vestibulocochlear and facial nerves to the brainstem, resulting in a brainstem abscess or meningitis associated with central vestibular signs[2]. Central vestibular infections can progress rapidly and cause death despite appropriate and aggressive treatment[2].

OTITIS INTERNA

KEY POINTS
- The true incidence of otitis interna is not known.
- There are no data relating to the normal microbial flora of the inner ear or, indeed, as to whether a microbial flora is present or not.
- Most cases of otitis interna are thought to result as an extension from otitis media.

INTRODUCTION
Otitis interna has been reported to account for half of the cases presenting with acute peripheral vestibular signs, at least in dogs[1]. However, the relative incidence of otitis interna versus otitis media may be somewhat less in reality. This may be a reflection of the severity of the clinical signs, which are much more dramatic in a case of vestibular dysfunction. Otitis media may be a chronic disease (possibly masked by chronic otitis externa) with less dramatic neurologic signs, such as facial nerve paralysis.

ETIOLOGY
There appears to be a strong association between otitis interna, otitis externa, and otitis media[1]. Thus, the most likely etiology of otitis interna is extension of otitis media[1,2], itself usually an extension of otitis externa (see Otitis media). Otitis media, and hence an associated otitis interna, may also result from hematogenous spread and ascending infection along the auditory tube[3]. Unfortunately, there are no reports describing the normal microbial flora of the inner ear, or even if one exists, either in health or in the presence of otitis interna. It would be reasonable to assume that similar pathogens affect the middle and the inner ear, although similar assumptions about the relationship between the microbial flora of the external ear and middle ear have been proven to be incorrect[4].

Inflammatory changes in the middle ear may cause a conductive hearing impairment, as only the transmission of sound waves through the tympanic bulla is affected; the hair cells within the cochlea are unaffected. However, some studies have described sensorineural deafness associated with otitis media[5]. If severe otitis media persists, combined conductive and sensorineural deafness may occur as fibrotic changes may develop in the inner ear.

CLINICAL SIGNS
The most commonly observed clinical signs of otitis interna include head tilt towards the affected side, spontaneous horizontal or rotatory nystagmus, and an asymmetric limb ataxia with preservation of strength[2]. In the acute stage the animal may be severely disorientated, circling and falling to the affected side. Sometimes, coordination and equilibrium are so affected that the animal may not be able to stand or walk. Vomiting or anorexia is commonly reported[2]. Acquired onset of deafness may be noted in some animals.

The clinical signs of otitis interna are very difficult to differentiate from those caused by other peripheral vestibular diseases such as idiopathic vestibular disease and neoplasia. Readers are referred to Chapter 7: (Neurologic signs related to inner ear disease) for a detailed discussion.

DIAGNOSIS
A thorough analysis of the case history will help to establish the presence of systemic diseases, hypersensitivities, defects in keratinization, or localized conditions (such as otodectic mange) which may underlie otitis externa and otitis media. A detailed description of the animal's behavior and clinical signs observed at home can sometimes provide evidence of middle or inner ear disease that is not always apparent on physical examination.

A careful physical examination should encompass the entire body in a systematic manner. Swelling, lumps, or pain may be found on careful palpation of the temporomandibular joints and around the base of the ears. Localized discharge may indicate a para-aural sinus. Signs of pruritus (alopecia, excoriation, hyperemia), a history of recurrent aural hematomata, or head shaking should alert the clinician to underlying dermatologic disease. The pharyngeal area should be examined for signs of inflammation or masses that may have spread to, or originated within, the middle ear via the auditory tube.

Given that otitis media may be clinically 'silent', or masked by chronic otitis externa, it could be inferred that otitis interna can be present in the absence of overt signs of otitis media.

A complete neurologic examination should document all parts of the nervous system, without bias, in order to distinguish peripheral versus central vestibular disease. This should report on mental status, behavior at home and in the examination room, head position, gait, and muscle strength. All the cranial nerves should be assessed individually. Proprioception, motor function, and spinal reflexes should be tested and evaluated. A more detailed neurologic examination of the ear is described in Chapter 2 (Neurologic examination of the ear).

Otic examination and visualization of the tympanic membrane, under sedation or general anesthesia, are the logical next steps (see Chapter 2: Otoscopic appearance of the external ear canal and tympanum). Myringotomy (see Chapter 2: Other investigatory procedures) and the subsequent submission of samples from the middle ear for bacterial culture and sensitivity are recommended in all cases of suspected otitis media/interna.

Imaging of the middle ear is best performed in a general practice setting by means of radiography (see Chapter 2: Radiographic features of the normal and abnormal ear), although recent studies have shown radiographs to be a poorly sensitive means of documentation of otitis media compared to CT or MRI[6, 7]. The inner ear is still poorly documented using the current means of imaging. MRI is the only means reported of imaging the peripheral vestibular system[7].

MANAGEMENT

The goal of treatment is to remove the underlying cause of otitis interna:

- Every effort should be made to identify if otitis media/externa is present. If otitis media or otitis externa is present, treat accordingly (see Otitis media; and Chapter 7: Medical management of ear disease).
- Consider referral for CT or MRI to rule out neoplasia.
- In the absence of any obvious pathology observed on advanced imaging, and once endocrine disease has been ruled out, it is reasonable to assume that either an idiopathic or an infectious cause is at the origin of the clinical signs. Long-term systemic antibacterial treatment is recommended, for a period of 6–8 weeks.

REFERENCES

OTITIS MEDIA

1 Neer TM (1982) Otitis media. *Compendium on Continuing Education* **4**, 410–417.

2 Cole LK, Kwochka KW, Kowalski JJ and Hillier A (1998) Microbial flora and antimicrobial susceptibility patterns of isolated pathogens from the horizontal ear canal and middle ear in dogs with otitis media. *Journal of the American Veterinary Medical Association* **212**, 534–538.

3 Little CJL, Lane JG and Pearson GR (1991) Inflammatory middle ear disease of the dog: the pathology of otitis media. *Veterinary Record* **128**, 293–296.

4 Bluestone CD and Doyle WJ (1988) Anatomy and physiology of the eustachian tube and middle ear related to otitis media. *Journal of Allergy and Clinical Immunology* **81**, 997–1003.

5 Bluestone CD (1983) Eustachian tube function: physiology, pathophysiology, and role of allergy in pathogenesis of otitis media. *Journal of Allergy and Clinical Immunology* **72**, 242–251.

6 Matsuda H, Tojo M, Fukui K, Imori T and Baba E (1984) The aerobic bacterial flora of the middle and external ears in normal dogs. *Journal of Small Animal Practice* **25**, 269–274.

7 Little CJL, Lane JG, Gibbs C and Pearson GR (1991) Inflammatory middle ear disease in the dog: the clinical and pathological features of cholesteatoma, a complication of otitis media. *Veterinary Record* **128**, 319–322.

8 Spreull JSA (1964) Treatment of otitis media. *Journal of Small Animal Practice* **5**, 107–152.

9 Bruyette DS and Lorenz MD (1993) Otitis externa and otitis media: diagnostic and medical aspects. *Seminars in Veterinary Medicine and Surgery (Small Animal)* **8**, 3–9.

10 Parker AJ and Chrisman CL (1995) How do I treat? Otitis media-interna in dogs and cats. *Progress in Veterinary Neurology* **6**, 139–141.

11 Little CJL and Lane JG (1989) An evaluation of tympanometry, otoscopy and palpation for assessment of the canine tympanic membrane. *Veterinary Record* **124**, 5–8.

12 Remedios AM, Fowler JD and Pharr JW (1991) A comparison of radiographic versus surgical diagnosis of otitis media. *Journal of the American Animal Hospital Association* **27**, 183–188.

13 Smeak DD, Crocker CB and Birchard SJ (1996) Treatment of otitis media that developed after total ear canal ablation and lateral bulla osteotomy in dogs: nine cases (1986–1994). *Journal of the American Veterinary Medical Association* **209**, 937–942.

14 Trower ND, Gregory SP, Renfrew H and Lamb CR (1998) Evaluation of the canine tympanic membrane by positive contrast ear canalography. *Veterinary Record* **123**, 78–81.

15 Dvir E, Kirberger RM and Terblanche AG (2000) Magnetic resonance imaging of otitis media in the dog. *Veterinary Radiology and Ultrasound* **41**, 46–49.

16 Penrod JP and Coulter DB (1980) The diagnostic use of impedance audiometry in the dog. *Journal of the American Animal Hospital Association* **16**, 941–948.

OTITIS INTERNA

1 Schunk KL and Averill DR (1983) Peripheral vestibular syndrome in the dog: a review of 83 cases. *Journal of the American Veterinary Medical Association* **182**, 1354–1357.

2 Shell L (1995) Otitis media and interna. In *Kirk's Current Veterinary Therapy XII.* (ed JD Bonagura) Philadelphia, WB Saunders, pp. 1128–1131.

3 Neer TM (1982) Otitis media. *Compendium on Continuing Education* **4**, 410–417.

4 Cole LK, Kwochka KW, Kowalski JJ and Hillier A (1988) Microbial flora and antimicrobial susceptibility patterns of isolated pathogens from the horizontal ear canal and middle ear in dogs with otitis media. *Journal of the American Veterinary Medicial Association* **212**, 534–538.

5 Morizono T (1990) Toxicity of ototopical drugs: animal modelling. *Annals of Otolaryngology, Rhinology and Laryngology* **99**, 42–45.

6 Love NE, Kramer RW, Spodnick GJ and Thrall DE (1995) Radiographic and computed tomographic evaluation of otitis media. *Veterinary Radiology and Ultrasound* **36**, 375–379.

7 Dayrell-Hart BL (1997) MR Imaging of the vestibular apparatus of the dog. *Proceeding of the 15th Annual Meeting of the American College of Veterinary Internal Medicine* 1997, Lake Buena Vista, pp. 606–607.

Chapter Six

Para-Aural Abscess

PARA-AURAL ABSCESSATION

KEY POINTS

- Para-aural abscessation results in chronic soft tissue swelling or discharge in the parotid area.
- The clinical signs result from leakage of purulent otic discharge into the surrounding tissues.
- Most commonly, para-aural abscessation follows otic surgery, particularly total ear canal ablation and bulla osteotomy.
- Otitis media is almost always present.
- Most cases require corrective surgery.

ETIOLOGY

Para-aural abscessation occurs when purulent discharge extends from the deeper parts of the external ear canal, or the middle ear cavity, to the surrounding soft tissues via a fistula or sinus. Ultimately there is soft tissue swelling and discharge, usually in the parotid area[1]. In addition there may be head tilt toward the affected side, pain on opening the mouth, and resentment of palpation in the region of the inflammation[2, 3]. Para-aural abscessation is more common in dogs than in cats[1], which is not surprising when the underlying causes are considered.

In a series of 17 dogs with para-aural abscess reported by Lane and Watkins[1], 50% of the cases had ongoing otitis externa, 50% had suffered previous otic surgery, and all the cases had otitis media. Between 3% and 5% of dogs undergoing total ear canal ablation and lateral or ventral bulla osteotomy may develop postoperative fistulation[4–8]. Most commonly this represents failure to remove all remnants of secretory tissue from the external ear canal, auditory meatus, or tympanic cavity. However, osteomyelitis of the ossicles, inadequate drainage of the middle ear (via the auditory tube), and iatrogenic parotid gland damage may also result in the syndrome[3, 4, 5, 8]. Cocker Spaniels, in particular, feature in reviews of postoperative para-aural abscessation[2, 3].

Neoplasia within the external ear canal may result in para-aural abscessation[1], although the neoplasm must occlude the external ear canal completely in order for this to happen. Traumatic separation of the auricular and annular cartilages results in blockage of the external ear canal and may result in para-aural abscessation[9]. Atresia of the external ear canal should be considered in the differential diagnosis of para-aural abscessation in young animals[1]. However, both of these conditions should be considered rare causes of para-aural abscessation.

DIAGNOSIS

The clinical signs of soft tissue pain, swelling, and sinus formation in the region of the parotid gland are highly suggestive of a para-aural abscess (**282, 283**). Foreign body penetration (either pharyngeal or percutaneous) and salivary gland pathology (iatrogenic at surgery or, rarely, necrosis or neoplasia) are the most likely differential diagnoses and both are rare causes of sinus formation on the lateral aspect of the head.

Exploration of the sinus with a probe will usually allow confirmation that the discharge is from the middle or external ear[1]. Otic examination (assuming that at least part of the external ear canal is present) will usually allow recognition of obstruction[1]. Radiography may be helpful in making a diagnosis and in allowing recognition of any associated soft tissue damage[1]. However, the sensitivity of the technique, with regard to demonstrating increased bulla opacity, is debatable[2, 3]. Changes were reported to be most obvious on lateral oblique views[3]. Contrast radiography (fistulograms) may also be helpful in documenting the association between sinus and bulla[2, 3].

MANAGEMENT

Surgical management of this condition is usually necessary. Systemic antibacterial treatment, based on culture and sensitivity, for 3–6 weeks may induce remission of the clinical signs in dogs which have had total ear canal ablation and bulla osteotomy, although recurrence after cessation of therapy is common[3].

The objectives of surgery are to relieve or remove the obstruction within the canal and to eliminate any suppurative foci within the external and middle ears[1]. In many cases this will at the least mandate resection of the vertical canal. However, total ear canal ablation with concurrent bulla osteotomy is probably the treatment of choice in spontaneous cases[1]. In cases resulting from previous bulla surgery, re-exploration is mandatory.

When sinus formation occurs as a sequela to total canal ablation and bulla osteotomy, it is essential that a thorough search is made for epithelial remnants and infected foci. A second, lateral approach to the bulla is complicated by scar tissue and loss of surgical landmarks, and it carries a risk of iatrogenic damage to the facial nerve[7]. Ventral bulla osteotomy avoids this, allows for a cleaner, more rapid dissection, and has therefore been recommended on this basis[3]. Furthermore, it allows easier visualization of the tympanic cavity[10, 11]. The ventral route allows ready access to the dorsal areas of the tympanic cavity. The most common location of the epithelial remnants is the dorsal rim of the osseous portion of the external ear canal or the caudolateral aspect of the tympanic cavity[3]. However, in another study[2], 40% of cases (ten dogs in total) had remnants of horizontal ear canal attached to the osseous external acoustic meatus. There is little prospect of exposing this area with a ventral approach.

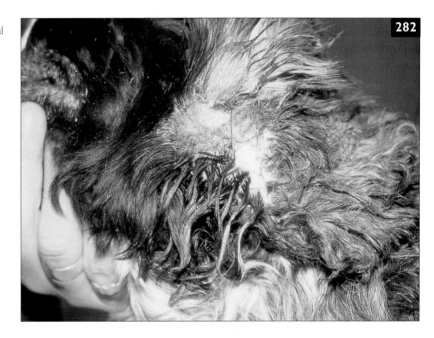

282 Cocker Spaniel with a para-aural abscess. Note the area of matted hair below the pinna.

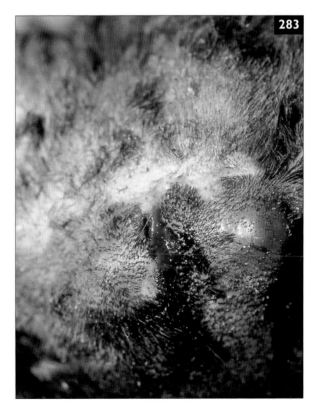

283 Close up of area after clipping. Note the serosanguinous discharge from the sinus and the tense, swollen areas of incipient sinus formation.

REFERENCES

1 Lane JG and Watkins PE (1986) Para-aural abscess in the dog and cat. *Journal of Small Animal Practice* **27**, 521–531.

2 Holt D, Brockman DJ, Sylvestre AM and Sadanaga KK (1996) Lateral exploration of fistulas developing after total ear canal ablations: 10 cases (1989–1993). *Journal of the American Animal Hospital Association* **32**, 527–530.

3 Smeak DD, Crocker CB and Birchard SJ (1996) Treatment of recurrent otitis media that developed after total ear canal ablation and lateral bulla osteotomy in dogs: nine cases (1986–1994). *Journal of the American Veterinary Medical Association* **209**, 937–942.

4 Smeak DD and de Hoff WD (1986) Total ear canal ablation: clinical results in the dog and cat. *Veterinary Surgery* **15**, 161–170.

5 Mason LK, Harvey CE and Orsher RJ (1988) Total ear canal ablation combined with lateral bulla osteotomy for end-stage otitis in dogs: results in 30 dogs. *Veterinary Surgery* **17**, 263–268.

6 Sharp NJH (1990) Chronic otitis externa and otitis media treated by total ear canal ablation and ventral bulla osteotomy in thirteen dogs. *Veterinary Surgery* **19**, 162–166.

7 Matthiesen DT and Scavelli T (1990) Total ear canal ablation and lateral bulla osteotomy in 38 dogs. *Journal of the American Animal Hospital Association* **26**, 257–267.

8 Beckman SL, Henry WB and Cechner P (1990) Total ear canal ablation combining bulla osteotomy and curretage in dogs with chronic otitis externa and media. *Journal of the American Veterinary Medical Association* **196**, 84–90.

9 McCarthy PE, Hosgood G and Pechman RD (1995) Traumatic ear canal separations and para-aural abscessation in three dogs. *Journal of the American Animal Hospital Association* **3**, 419–424.

10 Boothe HW (1998) Ventral bulla osteotomy: dog and cat. In *Current Techniques in Small Animal Surgery*. 4th edn. (ed MJ Bojrab) Williams and Wilkins, Baltimore, pp. 109–112.

11 Seim HB III (1993) Middle ear. In *Textbook of Small Animal Surgery*. 2nd edn. (ed D Slatter) WB Saunders, Philadelphia, pp. 1568–1576.

Chapter Seven

Medical Management of Ear Disease

APPROACH TO THE DIAGNOSIS OF OTITIS EXTERNA

INTRODUCTION

The approach to a case of otitis externa is no different to that of any disease. A look at the signalment will allow the clinician to consider breed, age, and sex predisposition to otitis externa. A case history may be sufficient to allow a working diagnosis of a foreign body to be made. In other cases it may be apparent that the dog has suffered occasional bouts of bilateral otitis externa before and, in these cases, a more detailed approach is necessary.

Consideration of the history and signalment will allow the clinician to make a provisional differential diagnosis, which will be further amended once the physical examination has been performed. At this point, pertinent laboratory tests are performed and a working diagnosis made. Treatment can be supplied and the response noted.

CONCEPT OF PRIMARY CAUSE, PREDISPOSING FACTORS, AND PERPETUATING CHANGE

August[1] proposed that the approach to otitis externa should be considered in a new light. He proposed a triad of factors: primary, predisposing, and perpetuating. Based on this concept it is helpful to approach otitis externa in a similar fashion and each case should be considered in the following, non-exclusive classification:

- Is there a primary cause? Primary causes are capable of causing otitis externa in their own right and include ectoparasites such as *Otodectes cynotis* and *Otobius megnini*, foreign bodies, otic neoplasia and inflammatory polyps, and the immune-mediated disorders such as drug eruption, allergic contact dermatitis, and the pemphigus group diseases.
- Are there any predisposing factors? Predisposing factors make otitis externa more likely by changing the internal environment in such a fashion that humidity within the ear canal rises, surface maceration occurs, and microbial proliferation follows. Predisposing factors include:
  - Anatomic factors such as the amount of soft tissue within the confines of the auricular cartilage and the presence of hair follicles, particularly compound hair follicles, within the external ear canal, e.g. stenotic ear canals (Shar Peis) or hair within the ear canal (Cocker Spaniels).
  - The effects of pathologic changes which occur as a result of previous episodes of otitis externa.
  - Underlying disease such as defects in keratinization, atopy, dietary intolerance, and food allergy.
  - Otitis media, an underrecognised factor in recurrent otitis externa.
  - Water within the external ear canal, which may precipitate acute gram-negative infection or *Malassezia pachydermatis* otitis externa.
  - The external environment may also be pertinent since humidity and high temperature are known to be correlated with an increased incidence of ear disease.
- Are there perpetuating factors? Perpetuating factors occur as a consequence of otitis externa. They tend to aggravate the otitis and further induce pathologic changes within the lining of the external ear canal. Perpetuating factors include:
  - Microbial infection with organisms such as *Staphylococcus intermedius*, *M. pachydermatis*, and gram-negative bacilli such as *Pseudomonas* spp.
  - Pathologic responses to otitis externa such as epidermal hyperplasia, which tends to cause luminal stenosis, and ceruminous gland hyperplasia, which results in a change in cerumen.
  - Otitis media, which may occur as a consequence of otitis externa.
  - Inappropriate medication which may irritate the external and middle ear or increase humidity within the external ear canal.

> Clinicians should attempt to identify and treat the primary causes of ear disease, diagnose and treat any predisposing factors, and try and prevent the onset of perpetuating factors.

SIGNALMENT

Breed

Some breeds, for example Cocker Spaniels and Persian cats, are predisposed to defects in keratinization, which may be associated with a ceruminous otitis externa. Breeds of dog recognized as particularly prone to otitis externa include Springer Spaniels, Miniature Poodles, Shar Peis, and German Shepherd Dogs. Dogs with pendulous pinnae are not necessarily predisposed to otitis externa but they may be susceptible to a rapidly progressive infection, should otitis externa develop. Breeds with excessive hair within the external ear canals, such as Poodles, may be predisposed to accumulations of cerumen and debris, which may provoke otitis externa. Yorkshire Terriers are predisposed to bilateral pinnal alopecia and hyperpigmentation. Longhaired breeds of cats and show cats are commonly affected by dermatophytosis. White haired cats and dogs are predisposed to actinic radiation damage to the pinnae.

Age

Young animals are often affected with *O. cynotis*, but this may not be associated with pruritus, particularly in kittens. In cats the peak incidence of otitis externa is between one and two years of age, presumably reflecting exposure to, and hypersensitivity to, *O. cynotis*. In older cats bilateral otitis externa is almost always associated with *O. cynotis* infection whereas unilateral otitis externa may reflect cat bite abscess or obstructive otitis secondary to polyps or neoplasia. Young animals are predisposed to dermatophytosis.

In dogs, young animals (and very old animals) are underrepresented in studies of the incidence of otitis externa. The peak incidence of otitis externa occurs in dogs between three and six years of age. Otic foreign bodies are unusual in young animals. Underlying disease, such as a defect in keratinization, atopy, or a dietary intolerance, may cause uni- or bilateral otitis externa and may occur in young animals, particularly in predisposed breeds.

Sex

There is no sex predisposition to otitis externa.

HISTORY

The key aims of history taking are:
- To make a definitive diagnosis, thus allowing specific treatment.
- To identify whether or not there is any evidence of underlying disease which may be predisposing the animal to otitis externa.

The history should encompass all aspects of the dog's management and lifestyle in an attempt to identify the cause of the otitis externa.

Management and lifestyle
- Diet: to identify deficiencies such as zinc and essential fatty acids.
- Water intake: any polyuria/polydipsia?
- Housing: kenneled or indoors?
- Exposure to sunlight: actinic radiation damage.
- Exercise: swimming predisposes to ear disease.
- Work: (working dogs predisposed to foreign bodies?).
- Grooming requirements: clipper burn on the pinnae, failure to pluck the ear canals, irritation following plucking, contagion at clipping parlor?
- Presence of other animals (*Otodectes cynotis*, *Sarcoptes scabiei*, dermatophytosis).
- Hunting cat (*Spilopsyllus cuniculi*, feline poxvirus infection, ticks).

Evidence of underlying disease
- Recurrent episodes of ear disease should raise the suspicion of an underlying disease, particularly if bilateral.
- Facial, otic, and pedal pruritus suggest atopy.
- Erythema in the ear, facial, neck, and truncal folds, and perhaps crust, scale, and erythema on the pinnae and trunk, suggest a defect in keratinization.
- A seasonal pattern is most likely to reflect atopy or seasonal exposure to ectoparasites such as mosquitoes, flies, harvest mites (*Neotrombicula* spp.), and rabbit fleas (*S. cuniculi*).
- Dietary intolerance is often associated with otitis externa.
- Allergic contact dermatitis may affect the concave, ventral aspect of the pinnae.
- Endocrinopathies may be associated with a ceruminous otitis externa.
- Sudden onset of severe, ulcerative bilateral otitis, perhaps in association with other skin disease, or systemic signs should raise the suspicion of drug eruption or immune-mediated disease.

Failure to consider the possibility of underlying disease, and addressing it, may result in permanent changes to the external ear canal, these changes themselves predisposing the dog to recurrent episodes of otitis externa.

Medications

Topical application of otic medication may induce an irritant or allergic contact dermatitis. The clinical sign which might suggest this is continued otitis in the face of repeated application of a medication. Neomycin is the most often cited agent in this regard, although propylene glycol also may be irritant.

PHYSICAL EXAMINATION

Having established the immediate and past history, the dog should be given a full clinical examination. In particular, evidence of internal disease and endocrinopathies should be sought. Thus, lymph nodes and testes should be palpated, the oral cavity examined, the chest auscultated, the abdomen palpated, and the perineum checked. Only after this general physical examination should the dermatologic assessment take place.

Pinnal scratch reflex

In some pruritic canine dermatoses, rubbing the distal edge of the pinna between finger and thumb nail induces a scratch reflex from the ipsilateral hindlimb. This positive scratch reflex is most commonly associated with scabies, although it is not pathognomonic. Pediculosis, *M. pachydermatis* dermatitis, and atopy also may result in positive scratch reflexes.

OTIC EXAMINATION

Gross examination of the pinnae

- Peripheral crust and scale may suggest scabies, pediculosis, a defect in keratinization, zinc deficiency, endocrinopathy, or fly bite or mosquito hypersensitivity.
- Erythema on the convex aspect, particularly distal, suggests actinic radiation damage.
- Erythema on the concave aspect suggests atopy or allergic contact dermatitis.
- Alopecia may be due to pruritus (scabies, pediculosis, hypersensitivity) or dermatophytosis.
- Alopecia and hyperpigmentation may reflect an endocrinopathy.
- Curling of the pinnae in the cat is almost pathognomonic for relapsing polychondritis.
- Vesicles, pustules, and crust may be due to superficial pyoderma, pemphigus foliaceus, or zinc deficiency.
- Punched out ulcerations on the convex aspect may be due to feline cowpox.
- Punched out ulcerations on the concave aspect may reflect vasculitis.

Gross examination of the external ear canal

- Calcification of the otic cartilage, which can be palpated, suggests the presence of chronic otitis externa.
- Malodor of the external ear canal may be associated with *M. pachydermatis* infection, gram-negative bacterial infection, devitalized tissues, or neoplasia.
- The amount of hair around the entrance to and within the external ear canal should be assessed. The clinician may need to remove this hair in order to complete an auroscopic examination.
- The areas hidden within the cartilage folds at the entrance to the ear canal should be examined for ectoparasites, particularly ticks and trombiculid mites.
- Erythema is often associated with swelling of the soft tissues of the external ear canal and stenosis of the lumen. In some cases the stenosis is so severe that it is impossible to insert the cone of an otoscope into the canal. Erythema of the vertical canal, in combination with a normal, or nearly normal, horizontal canal is very suggestive of atopy.
- Ulceration of the otic epithelium is usually associated with gram-negative bacterial infection but it may be a sign of immune-mediated disease.
- The nature, color, and odor of any discharge should be noted. However, whether any conclusions as to the causal organism, based on the physical nature of the discharge, are valid is debatable. Cytologic examination of the discharge is much more reliable in this regard.

Physical examination. The external ear should not be considered in isolation from either the skin or the internal mileau.

Otoscopic examination of the external ear canal

Many animals will allow otoscopic examination of the external ear canals with only gentle manual restraint being necessary. However, in cases of otitis externa the swelling and inflammation of the epithelial tissues make the process uncomfortable and usually some form of chemical restraint is necessary.

The external ear canal should be assessed for foreign bodies and ectoparasites, hair, accumulations of cerumen, erythema, stenosis, ulceration, and polyps or neoplasia. The tympanum should be examined for color, distension, and integrity.

Cytologic examination of cerumen and otic exudate

Cytologic and microscopic examination of otic discharge is much more meaningful than attempting to classify the etiology of the otitis on the basis of the physical characteristics of any discharge. Samples may be collected with cotton swabs. One swab should be applied to, and gently rolled in, a small pool of liquid paraffin (or other mineral oil) on a clean glass slide. A cover slip is applied and the slide examined for ectoparasites. Another swab is rolled onto a clean glass slide which is then air dried, or briefly heat fixed, and stained with a modified Wright's stain such as Diff-Quik. Further samples may be stained with Gram's stain if desired.

Microscopic examination of these samples will allow identification of ectoparasites, inflammatory cells, nucleated keratinocytes, cocci, bacilli, and yeast. This information is very useful when the clinician is formulating a treatment plan.

Other diagnostic aids
Bacterial culture and sensitivity testing

In most cases examination of cytologic samples will provide all the information necessary for effective treatment to be instituted. Microbial culture and sensitivity testing of samples from the external ear canal is, however, useful in certain cases:

- In cases of recurrent, or refractory, otitis externa.
- If ulceration of the epithelial lining of the external ear canal is present.
- If gram-negative infection is suspected.
- If otitis media is suspected (when samples from the middle ear will also be necessary).

Radiography and other imaging modalities

Radiography is used to delineate otitis media. Radiographic investigation (or CT or MRI) is indicated if the tympanum is abnormal, distended, or torn, or if the clinical signs suggest the presence of otitis media.

Biopsy

Otic tumors or polyps are usually subject to excision biopsy. Punch biopsy and excision biopsy of the epithelial lining of the deeper portions of the external ear canal is difficult, although pinch biopsy samples can be obtained using endoscope forceps.

ACUTE OTITIS EXTERNA

KEY POINTS

- Pay great attention to the first onset of otitis externa; it may be the best chance to identify the cause and treat it before chronic changes ensue.
- Owners usually fail to distinguish between pinnal pruritus and otitis externa.
- Bilateral otitis usually reflects an underlying disease.
- Remember that otitis media is commonly present, or may be induced by, otitis externa. Check the status of the tympanum before prescribing treatment.
- Do not rely on a quick otoscopic examination. History, physical examination, otoscopy, and otic cytology are required for a minimum database.
- Do not provide broad-spectrum, polypharmaceutical otic medications without a minimum database.
- Make a re-examination appointment; do not allow the owner to make therapeutic decisions.

HISTORY AND CLINICAL SIGNS

Most cases of acute otitis externa are presented because of pruritus or head shaking. There may be minimal discharge (**284**) or, in some cases, profuse exudate and malodor (**285**). Ulceration of the vertical canal (**286**) and concave aspects of the pinnae (**287**) may be a feature, particularly of cases where there is gram-negative infection. Infection with gram-negative bacteria usually produces a painful ear canal and dogs may be very subdued in these cases. Pyrexia, lymphadenopathy, and signs of systemic illness, however, are rare.

The dog's response to otic pruritus may result in pyotraumatic dermatitis ('hot spot', 'wet eczema') on the lateral aspect of the head (**288**). Aural hematoma formation (**289**) may also be noted in association with otitis externa, although current thoughts are that there may be no direct relationship between these conditions[1].

Cats may exhibit very severe self-trauma in the periaural region in some instances and clinicians should be careful to rule out ear disease before considering dietary intolerance (food allergy), which is a major cause of facial trauma in cats[2].

Acute otitis externa is a common complaint and the first task facing the clinician is to answer two questions:

- Is the condition really acute or has it been slowly developing?
- Is there a reason to suspect underlying disease?

True acute otitis externa is, in reality, not that common. In one study of 515 dogs with otitis externa[3] only 17% presented with acute suppurative otitis. Otic foreign bodies and acute gram-negative infection,

following swimming or grooming, are the most likely causes in dogs[3]. *Malassezia pachydermatis*, *Pseudomonas* spp. (and other gram-negative bacteria) were most often isolated from these ears[3]. Otic foreign bodies are rare in cats and gram-negative infections in the feline external ear canal are almost unknown[4].

Most cases of otitis externa which are presented as acute have usually been present for some time before clinical signs are noted by the owner. Although many of these will have some degree of abnormality consequent upon the duration of ear disease, it is usually possible to discern a primary cause of the otitis externa. A useful diagnostic clue can be gleaned from discovering the temporal relationship between otic discomfort and the presence of a discharge[5].

Pruritus prior to a discharge is most commonly seen in acute otitis externa such as that caused by a foreign body, which is nearly always unilateral, although both ear canals should be inspected. In dogs, otodectic mange may be associated with pruritus before significant erythema or discharge is apparent, but more usually there is a crumbly, brown discharge within the ear canal. Otitis externa due to

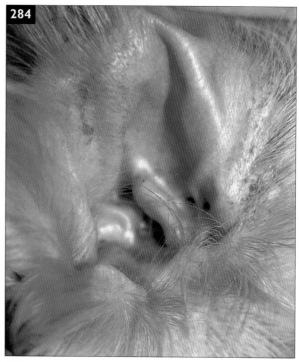

284 Acute otitis externa associated with a grass awn foreign body. There is minimal discharge and only a little erythema. The most dramatic clinical sign was peracute otic pruritus.

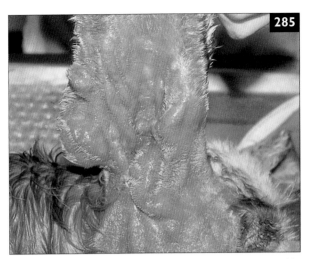

285   Acute otitis externa in a Cocker Spaniel associated with malodor, otic pain, and otic discharge. Acute gram-negative bacterial otitis externa associated with a defect in keratinization.

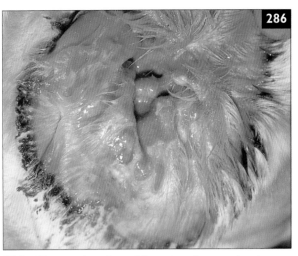

286   Discrete ulcerations of the external ear canal and immediately adjacent skin of a Labrador Retriever. Gram-negative bacterial otitis externa associated with swimming.

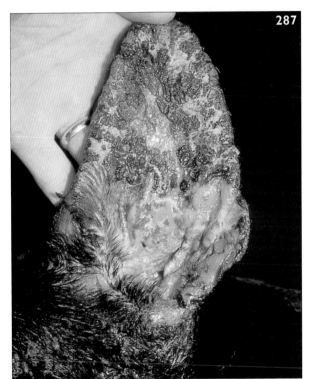

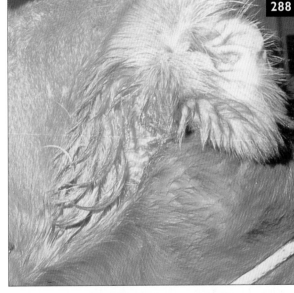

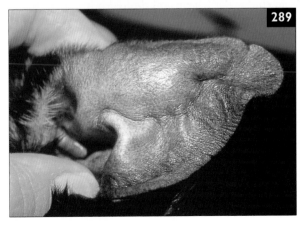

287   Acute otitis externa in a Doberman Pinscher with ulceration and crusting affecting the concave aspects of the pinna. Gram-negative bacterial otitis externa associated with swimming.

288   Pyotraumatic dermatitis ('hot spot') on the lateral aspect of the head of a dog associated with otic pruritus.

289   Aural hematoma associated with otitis externa.

hypersensitivity is nearly always bilateral. Atopy may cause otic pruritus in the absence of a discharge, although there will usually be detectable erythema on the concave aspect of the pinna and in the vertical canal. Dietary intolerance, although rare, may cause similar signs.

Discharge prior to pruritus is most commonly seen in cases where there is underlying disease, particularly a defect in keratinization. In many of these cases there is a ceruminous discharge apparent even before otic inflammation occurs, and in some cases there may be significant otic pathology at the time of presentation. Similarly, ceruminous otitis externa may be seen in cases of endocrinopathy, particularly gonadal endocrine disease, which is often associated with seborrhea. *Otodectes cynotis* infection in cats is frequently accompanied by significant dark brown, crumbly discharge in the absence of pruritus. Cats are frequently presented for an otic discharge and associated malodor secondary to an inflammatory polyp or otic neoplasm.

Cats may traumatize the area surrounding the ear in an attempt to alleviate the irritation, and crusting excoriations in the immediate surrounding area of the ear may be noted.

INVESTIGATIONS

Once a history has been elicited the clinician is in a position to rank the differential diagnoses (*Table 13*). The animal must then be given a clinical examination to ascertain whether the otitis is part of a more generalized problem or if it is an isolated event, and for the cause to be identified.

Otic examination
Pinnae
The pinnae should be checked for the presence of a pinnal scratch reflex (not pathognomonic for scabies but very suggestive) and the presence of papules, pustules, crust, scale, or alopecia, which may indicate that the owner has misinterpreted pinnal pruritus as ear disease. Erythema and early lichenification of the proximal, concave aspect of the pinnae is common in atopy and may be an early pointer to the presence of the disease.

Vertical ear canal
The upper aspect of the external ear canal is examined initially with the naked eye. The diameter of the canal is assessed and the color and nature of the epithelium noted, as is the presence or absence of hair or discharge.

The external ear canal should be wide and free from obstruction. In medium-sized and large dogs it is possible to see a considerable distance into the normal ear canal. The presence of hair in the upper portion of the external ear canal may inhibit examination but if the hair is gently plucked, a good view is usually possible. Inflammatory polyps and verrucose thickening of the epithelium may occlude the external ear canal and the polyps themselves may be obscured by discharge.

The color and nature of the otic epithelium should be assessed. The normal epithelium is a smooth, clean pink surface gently undulating over the underlying cartilage. Erythema and lichenification are early signs of chronic change. Ulceration is not common, but when it is present it is more usually associated with gram-negative infection than with immune-mediated disease.

The presence of hair within the external ear canal is normal, although the density of hair follicles and the ratio of simple follicles to compound follicles varies. Most dogs have sparsely distributed, typically simple hair follicles whereas some breeds, notably Cocker Spaniels, have compound follicles throughout the whole length of the external ear canal[6]. Excessive hair will tend to stabilize cerumen and scale and allow local accumulation to occur, thus aggravating any tendency to ceruminous otitis externa.

The vertical portion of the external ear canal can also be palpated as it passes ventrally under the skin to meet the horizontal canal. Any stenosis of the ear canal, consequent upon hyperplastic changes in the epithelium, will reduce its pliability and may evoke pain. Calcification of the external ear canal also may be detected by palpation.

Presence and nature of the discharge
Otic discharge may vary from minimal to profuse. Although there may be some correlation between the physical nature of the discharge and the major microbial pathogens, it is unwise to rely on this as a guide to treatment. In some animals with a keratinization defect (Cocker Spaniels, for example) there may be a profuse discharge which harbors no pathogens and only a scant growth of commensal organisms. Perhaps the most widely accepted relationship is that between *O. cynotis* and a dark brown, dryish, crumbly discharge.

Vertical ear canal. Gross examination of the affected ear canal, and the nature of the animal's reaction to examination and palpation, will indicate if sedation and cleaning are necessary before meaningful examination can be achieved.

On balance it is best simply to note the physical nature of the discharge and to rely on cytologic examination to establish any etiologic relationship between discharge and causal agent.

Otoscopic examination
Vertical canal

Otoscopic examination of the vertical canal should not be neglected on the grounds that a visual examination is possible without the use of an otoscope. The magnification provided by the lens allows for easier identification of otodectic mites, although failure to visualize mites should not be taken as a reliable finding: cytologic examination of otic discharge is much more reliable.

A close examination of the epithelial lining is possible and its condition, as well as the presence and nature of any cerumen or discharge, should be noted. The location and degree of luminal stenosis can also be assessed otoscopically. This may allow a presumptive diagnosis of an inflammatory polyp, mural granuloma, or neoplasm occluding the lumen. In cases of mural hyperplasia associated with allergic skin disease, particularly atopy, the luminal stenosis may be markedly reduced following application of topical glucocorticoids. Serial otoscopic examination will allow the clinician to monitor the response to treatment.

Table 13: Important points to establish when taking a history, and the type of information which they elicit. Answers to these question should allow the clinician to rank a differential diagnosis and prioritize investigatory tests.

Signalment
- Breed. Certain breeds are predisposed to otitis externa, defects in keratinization, atopy, and immune-mediated disease. Cats are predisposed to inflammatory polyps.
- Age. *Otodectes cynotis* and atopy occurs in young animals.
- Sex. Female gonadal endocrinopathies; females are predisposed to immune-mediated disease. Young males dogs may be predisposed to otic foreign bodies.

Background
- Where and when obtained? *O. cynotis* is more common in rescue cats; scabies is more common in puppies from puppy farms.
- Other animals in the household? *O. cynotis*, scabies, and dermatophytosis are all contagious and potentially zoonotic.

Diet and water intake
- Polyuria/polydipsia is a common pointer to systemic disease; nutritional deficiency may be identified; necessary information for formulating a restricted diet if the clinician suspects dietary intolerance.

Management and lifestyle
- Confined or allowed out? Ectoparasites are usually acquired from other animals or from the environment.
- Exercises over rough ground or not? *Neotrombicula* spp. infestations, ticks, and otic foreign bodies are more common in this environment than on parkland, for example.
- Regular contact with other animals? Ectoparasites and dermatophytosis are contagious.
- Regular swimmer? Gram-negative infections.
- Does the cat hunt? Feline cow pox, salmonellosis, and possibly rickettsial diseases may be acquired by contact with, or devouring of, affected prey.
- Recent grooming, ear canals plucked? Traumatic damage to the external ear canal.

Previous history of ear disease
- Has the animal had ear disease before? Consider contagious diseases, underlying disease, and predisposing causes. Remember that otitis media may present as recurrent otitis externa. When, which ear, and how often? Any evidence of a seasonal pattern? Occasional relapse might suggest a predisposing cause, whereas frequent relapse might be more typical of an underlying disease.
- What was used to treat it? *Malassezia pachydermatis* and *O. cynotis* will not respond to antibacterial agents; neomycin, in particular, is a sensitizing agent.
- What was the response? Good response with relapse suggests predisposing cause or underlying disease. Failure to respond suggests a failure to prescribe correct treatment, infection with a resistant microbe, or allergic contact sensitivity to one of the agents in the otic preparation. Also, the clinician should consider otic disease which might be refractory to topical treatments such as polyps and neoplasia, food allergy, or hypersensitivity.

Pointers to other disease
- Seasonality. Atopy or seasonal ectoparasites such as *Neotrombicula* spp., or *Spilopsyllus cuniculi*.
- Pruritus elsewhere or evidence of scale, crust, or alopecia. Atopy, ectoparasite infestation, defect in keratinization, food allergy or intolerance, immune-mediated or autoimmune disease.

Horizontal ear canal and tympanum

In most cases of mild to moderate otitis externa it is possible to visualize the distal portion of the horizontal ear canal, at least in medium and large sized, tractable patients. Small dogs, cats, and animals with swollen ears may greatly resent the procedure and in these cases sedation will be necessary. The otoscopic examination should permit the clinician to assess whether epithelial changes, discharge, and luminal stenosis are similar in both the vertical and horizontal portions of the canal. In addition to examining and noting the physical nature of the epithelium, the clinician may be able to visualize the tympanum. However, since it is not possible adequately to assess the patency of the tympanum in most cases, specific tests may be necessary to establish the presence of a damaged tympanum and otitis media (see Chapter 5: Otitis media, otitis interna). The simplest test is described by Griffin[5]. A soft rubber feeding tube is gently passed through the cone of the otoscope and pushed toward the tympanum. If the tympanum is intact the tip of the tube will remain in sight, via the otoscope. If the tip passes out of sight, presumably through a ruptured tympanum into the middle ear, otitis media is presumed. Griffin pointed out that this technique is difficult if there is marked proliferation in the horizontal canal.

Cytologic examination

Microscopic examination of cytologic preparations taken from the external ear canal form a key part of the diagnostic work up, since it is from examination of these samples that treatment will be prescribed. The presence, or absence, of otodectic mites may be difficult to assess if the clinician relies on otoscopic examination alone. Furthermore, the shape, (yeast, coccus, bacillus) and gram-staining status of any microbes can be assessed.

The clinician may decide that further diagnostic information is not needed and prescribe treatment based on otoscopic and cytologic evaluation alone. However, the presence of bacilli, particularly gram-negative bacilli, mandates culture and sensitivity testing. In the meantime, treatment can be commenced on an empirical basis, pending laboratory results.

Microbial culture and sensitivity

Under most circumstances clinicians prescribe otic antimicrobials for acute otitis externa on an empirical basis, usually as part of a polypharmaceutical product. Certainly, there is little value in performing culture and sensitivity testing without first examining an otic cytologic preparation. Evidence is needed that any organisms recovered from the external ear canal on

> The importance of cytologic evaluation of otic discharge cannot be overstated.

culture are acting as pathogens and are not simply part of the normal otic flora. The presence of an inflammatory infiltrate (neutrophils, macrophages, perhaps in association with cocci and/or gram-negative bacilli) is a prerequisite. The value of otic cytology in this situation is that it also allows the clinician a more extensive database on which to make an empirical prescription pending culture and sensitivity testing.

Culture and sensitivity testing is mandatory in cases of otitis media. Furthermore, care must be taken to ensure that the microbial sample taken from the middle ear is not contaminated while passing through the external ear canal (see Chapter 5: Otitis media, otitis interna). Samples from the external ear canal should also be submitted for culture and sensitivity testing since there is every probability that a different spectrum of microbes, with a different antimicrobial pattern, is present on either side of the tympanum.

MANAGEMENT

- Identify any primary or underlying causes of ear disease such as ectoparasites, foreign bodies, or systemic disease. These must be treated, or managed, if the otitis externa is to be cured or controlled.
- Identify any predisposing or perpetuating factors which will potentiate the ear disease or induce relapse. These include microbial infections, epithelial and glandular hypertrophy, luminal stenosis, and compound hair follicles within the deeper portions of the external ear canal. These must be managed if relapsing ear disease is to be prevented.
- Identify if otitis media is present. This must receive priority in the treatment plan.
- Clean and dry the external ear canal.
- Instill and dispense an appropriate otic medication. This will either be an acaricide or a combination of an antimicrobial and glucocorticoid designed to reduce the infection and inhibit inflammation. Both of these actions will tend to reduce the onset of hyperplasia within the glandular and epithelial components of the external ear canal.
- Re-examine the dog. Do not let the owner decide that the dog is in remission and suspend treatment without a proper examination. The interval between examinations will vary according to the identified cause. Thus, four or five days is appropriate in the case of a foreign body, ten days in the case of microbial infection, and two weeks if *O. cynotis* is present.

GRAM-NEGATIVE OTITIS EXTERNA

KEY POINTS

- Gram-negative otitis externa is usually suppurative and painful.
- Bathing, grooming, and foreign bodies are the most common conditions associated with acute gram-negative otitis externa.
- Bacterial culture and sensitivity testing is mandatory as multiple-resistant strains may be recovered.
- 2% or 2.5% acetic acid may be used for treatment on an empirical basis pending laboratory results.

HISTORY AND CLINICAL SIGNS

Most cases of gram-negative otitis externa are acute in onset, unilateral, painful rather than pruritic, suppurative, and ulcerated[1]. The most common causes in one survey of 550 dogs with otitis externa were otic foreign body, grooming, and bathing, rather than underlying disease[2]. This finding was supported in another large study (of 752 dogs with otitis externa) in which underlying disease was not a feature of gram-negative otitis in dogs[1].

Otic inflammation, an increase in humidity, and a rise in pH within the external ear canal appear to be necessary for *Pseudomonas* spp. to establish[3]; inflammation *per se* is not sufficient in the normal external ear canal. However, predisposing factors such as hirsute ear canals, narrow ear canals, and pendulous pinnae may make the external ear canal more susceptible to gram-negative infection. Hence, Cocker Spaniels (**290**) are predisposed[4, 5]. Gram-negative infections of the external ear canal appear to be more common in tropical climates[5], possibly because of increased temperature and increased humidity in the environment affecting, or potentiating, alteration in the otic microclimate.

Acute gram-negative suppurative otitis (**291**) is most often associated with *Pseudomonas* spp. infection, although it may commonly be associated with other gram-negative bacteria[2] and *Malassezia pachydermatis*. *Staphylococcus intermedius* was not isolated in any of the 65 cases of *Pseudomonas* spp. otitis externa in one study[2].

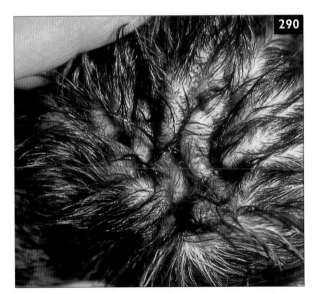

290 Cocker Spaniel with chronic otitis externa secondary to a defect in keratinization. There is a gram-negative bacterial infection.

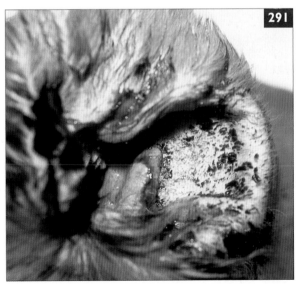

291 Suppurative otitis externa associated with gram-negative bacterial infection.

Because of the severity of the clinical signs these cases rarely become chronic before being presented to the veterinarian, therefore ulceration (**292, 293**) rather than hyperplasia is the most common finding on gross and otoscopic examination[1, 2]. However, in some cases there is extension into the middle ear[2].

DIAGNOSTIC APPROACH

Because gram-negative otitis externa is often a very painful condition, affected animals may greatly resent any attempt at investigation, and sedation, or even general anesthesia, will be necessary. If cytologic examination (**294**) suggests that bacilli, particularly gram-negative bacilli, are associated with otitis externa, samples should be submitted for bacteriological culture and sensitivity testing for two reasons: (1) *Pseudomonas* spp. may be resistant to many antibacterial agents, including gyrase inhibitors. (2) Otitis media may be present, necessitating long-term, systemic antibacterial therapy. The ear canal should be flushed and a careful examination made for an otic foreign body. The clinician should bear in mind that these ear canals may be ulcerated and that application of alcohol-containing cleansers and drying agents may cause pain. An attempt should be made to assess the integrity of the tympanum since many agents, which might be expected empirically to be useful against *Pseudomonas* spp., are ototoxic if they reach the middle ear. Examples of potentially ototoxic agents include gentamycin, neomycin, propylene glycol, acetic acid, and chlorhexidine[6]. Although underlying disease is not a common feature of acute gram-negative otitis externa, it should be borne in mind in animals which suffer recurrent episodes of otitis externa. Hypersensitivity, defects in keratinization, and endocrinopathy should be ruled out before idiopathic disease is diagnosed.

MANAGEMENT

- Ensure adequate restraint.
- Submit samples for bacteriological culture and sensitivity.
- Clean and dry the external ear canal.
- Pending laboratory results, apply a 2–5% solution of acetic acid to the external ear canal, twice daily. If the tympanum is ruptured, consider enrofloxacin diluted 1:6 in saline, instilled directly into the external ear canal.

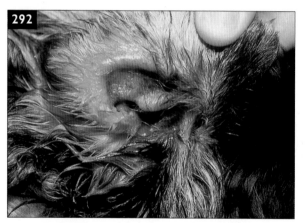

292 Suppurative, ulcerative otitis externa associated with gram-negative bacterial infection.

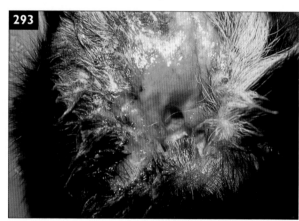

293 Acute, erosive gram-negative otitis externa.

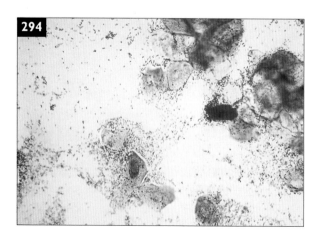

294 Cytologic preparation from a Cocker Spaniel with acute gram-negative bacterial otitis externa. Note the nucleated squames and masses of bacilli.

- When bacteriological results are to hand, institute specific treatment.
- If concurrent gram-negative otitis media is diagnosed, prescribe a systemic fluoroquinolone such as enrofloxacin (5–7.5 mg/kg q12h or 20 mg/kg q24h) in addition.

If multiple resistant *Pseudomonas* spp. is recovered, consider one, or several, of the following options:

Silver sulfadiazine

1% silver sulfadiazine cream applied daily for ten days is effective but, being rather viscous in nature, it is hard to apply to the depths of the external ear canal[7]. However, dilutions of the cream with water, to a concentration as low as 1/100, will exceed the minimal inhibitory concentration (MIC) of *P. aeruginosa* and be fluid enough to penetrate the depths of the ear canal[8]. A 0.1% solution may be prepared by mixing 1.5 ml silver sulfadiazine cream into 13.5 ml water or saline[9]. This may be instilled into the ear canal twice daily.

Acetic acid

Application of aqueous solutions of acetic acid (2–5%) to the external ear canal is effective at inducing a sufficiently low pH that *Pseudomonas* spp. cannot survive[10]. The 5% solution may be irritating and should only be used with caution in the presence of a ruptured tympanum[6, 11]. Anecdotal reports suggest that the 2% or 2.5% solution may be safe to use in the presence of a ruptured tympanum[11, 12].

Fluoroquinolone antibacterial agents

Antibacterial agents such as enrofloxacin, marbofloxacin and ciprofloxacin are highly effective against gram-negative bacteria such as *P. aeruginosa* and *Proteus* spp.[13, 14]. A specific otic preparation containing marbofloxacin, clotrimazole and dexamethazone is available in some countries. There is evidence (manufacturer's internal data) that adjunctive treatment with systemic administration may enhance the 'time to cure interval'. In those countries where a specific otic preparation is not available then systemic administration of fluoroquinolones may be augmented by local administration of diluted solutions of these agents into the external ear canal. Recommended oral doses are 20 mg/kg once daily for enrofloxacin[9, 15] and 2 mg/kg once daily for marbofloxacin. Caution should be used when treating skeletally immature dogs with systemic fluoroquinolones as damage to articular cartilage may ensue. Care should be taken to ensure that the external ear canal is cleaned and thoroughly dried before instilling topical enrofloxacin, since it is inactivated in an acidic environment[9, 16]. A dilution of the injectable solution (20 mg/ml) at the rate of 1:6 in water or isotonic saline has been recommended as being efficacious when instilled directly into the external ear canal[9].

Other antibacterial agents

Imipenem and carbenicillin are both active against *P. aeruginosa*, although imipenem has met with resistance problems because of its widespread use in the human field[17]. Topically applied ticarcillin, in conjunction with prednisolone (1–2 mg/kg p/o q12h) and an acetic acid-based topical otic cleanser, has been reported to be effective[18]. If the tympanum is ruptured, the ticarcillin is administered three times daily intravenously until healing is observed[18]. The topical solution is made by mixing a 6g vial of ticarcillin powder with 12 ml of sterile water[9]. This may be divided into 2 ml aliquots and frozen, where it will remain stable for up to three months. The vials are thawed and mixed with 40 ml saline, each again being divided into aliquots, this time of about 10 ml. These are given to the client to freeze at home. When required they are thawed for use, the surplus being kept in the refrigerator for up to seven days[9].

Potentiating the effect of topical antibacterial agents with EDTA-tris

Ethylene-diamine tetra-acetic acid (EDTA) binds divalent cations, enhances membrane permeability, and alters ribosome stability[19]. *P. aeruginosa* and *S. intermedius*, which are resistant to enrofloxacin and cephalexin (respectively), may be rendered sensitive by pretreatment of the external ear canal with EDTA-tris[20]. *In vitro* studies with *Pseudomonas* spp. isolated from cases of canine otitis have also demonstrated the bactericidal potential of EDTA-tris[21]. EDTA-tris is prepared in the following ways:

- By adding 6.05 g EDTA (disodium) and 12 g tromethamine (Trizma base) to distilled water, sufficient to make 1 liter. The pH is adjusted to pH8 with HCl and the solution autoclaved for 15 minutes to ensure sterility[11].
- By adding 24.2 g tromethamine and 4.8 g EDTA (disodium) to 3,900 ml distilled water. Adjust the pH to pH8 using white vinegar (5% acetic acid). Autoclave to ensure sterility[9].

The ear canal is treated with 2.5 ml of the EDTA-tris solution ten minutes prior to application of antibacterial solution (such as gentamycin, cephalexin, or a gyrase inhibitor), twice daily for 7–10 days. In some countries, EDTA-tris is available commercially in an otic preparation. This has rapidly become the treatment of choice for gram-negative otitis.

CHRONIC, OR RECURRENT, OTITIS EXTERNA IN DOGS

KEY POINTS

- Most cases of chronic otitis externa are bilateral.
- Defects in keratinization, hypersensitivities, and otitis media are the most common causes of chronic, or recurrent, otitis externa.
- Less common causes include allergic contact dermatitis and multiresistant microorganisms.
- Chronic otitis externa is usually either ceruminous or erythematous and hyperplastic.
- Surgery will be necessary unless chronic pathologic change can be prevented or reversed.

HISTORY AND SIGNALMENT

From a practical point of view, recurrent otitis externa and chronic otitis externa present similar problems. Indeed, given that relapsing otitis externa will eventually result in chronic disease, the former could be viewed as an early stage of the latter. Both conditions have the potential for inducing irreversible, pathologic changes within the external ear canal, and in both instances the clinician is required to institute a diagnostic work up in order to identify the underlying or predisposing cause(s).

Many breeds are predisposed to chronic otitis externa and clinicians should 'flag' even the first episode as a possible harbinger of future problems. Thus, Cocker Spaniels are not only predisposed from an anatomic point of view but also from the frequency with which defects in keratinization and ceruminous otitis externa occur. Similarly, atopic West Highland White Terriers are predisposed. Larger breeds (Basset Hounds with seborrhea and Labrador Retrievers with atopy, for example) appear to have some resistance to the onset of chronic pathologic changes, perhaps because the external ear canals are much wider and the local microclimate less subject to change. On the other hand, German Shepherd Dogs are notorious for developing chronic obstructive otitis externa, even though they have wide external ear canals and erect pinnae.

> In a surprising number of cases owners are unaware of the changes taking place within the ear, and they are surprised when the degree of change, and its significance, is pointed out.

PHYSICAL EXAMINATION

Some animals will severely traumatize the area around the pinnae and erythema, alopecia, and crusting may be detected. Similarly, dogs with chronic otitis externa will develop hyperpigmentation and lichenification in the periaural region (**295**).

Affected dogs should be given a thorough examination in an attempt to identify whether the otitis is associated with dermatologic lesions. The type of change within the external ear canal may give a pointer to the pattern of dermatologic lesion to look for, although clinicians should not be too dogmatic about this as cross-over occurs.

In a dog with ceruminous otitis (**296–298**) the clinician should search for evidence of defects in keratinization and endocrinopathies.

295 Hyperpigmentation around the base of the pinna and the opening to the external ear canal in this terrier with chronic otitis externa.

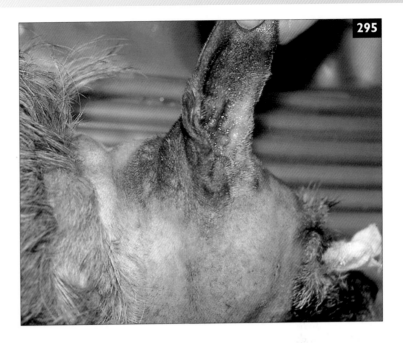

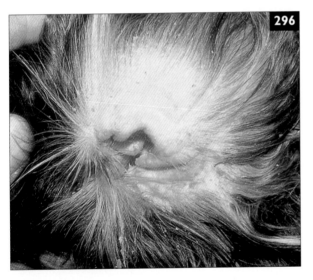

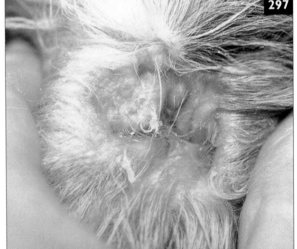

296 Moderate ceruminous otitis externa in a Cavalier King Charles Spaniel. Note the greasy scale adhering to the surrounding hair.

297 Moderate ceruminous otitis externa in a German Shepherd Dog with a Sertoli cell tumor.

298 Severe hyperplasia and chronic ceruminous otitis externa.

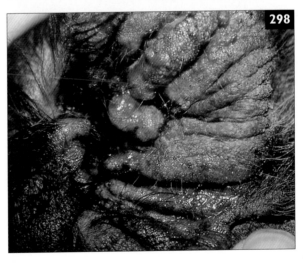

Accumulations of greasy scale around the nipples (**299**), comedones, follicular casts on hair shafts (**300**), and erythema, perhaps with greasy scale, in the ventral neck folds, axillae, and groins suggest a defect in keratinization. There may be scale, crust (**301**), and even alopecia on the dorsal trunk. There may be secondary pyoderma and *Malassezia pachydermatis* infection.

In a dog with erythematous hyperplastic changes (**302–304**) characteristic of hypersensitivity, the clinician should look for similar changes on the concave aspect of the pinnae (**305**), in the dorsal and plantar interdigitae (**306**), on the flexor aspect of the carpus (**307**), and on the extensor aspect of the tarsus. In addition, the coat may be rather harsh and dry and be accompanied by a fine scale. There may be a secondary superficial pyoderma and *M. pachydermatis* infection.

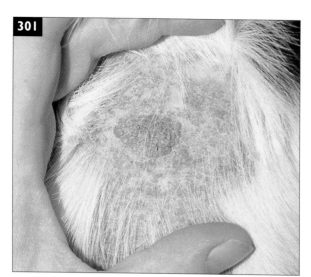

299 Greasy scale adhering around the nipples. Note also the comedones.

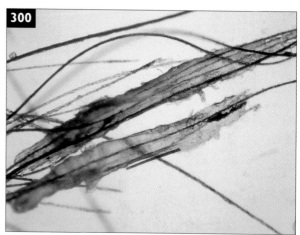

300 Follicular casts adhering to hair shafts. Follicular casts reflect abnormal follicular keratinization.

301 Erythema, alopecia, and patches of crust in a Cocker Spaniel with a defect in keratinization.

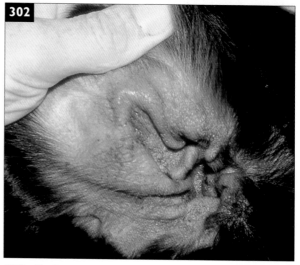

302 Erythematous, hyperplastic otitis externa in a Rottweiler.

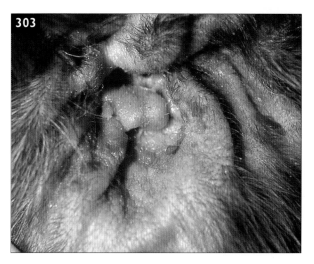

303 Erythematous, hyperplastic otitis externa.

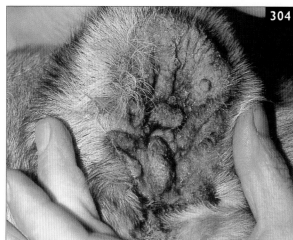

304 Erythematous, hyperplastic otitis has continued in this German Shepherd Dog with atopy, even though the dog has been subject to lateral wall resection.

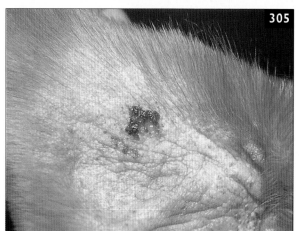

305 Erythematous, hyperplastic changes on the concave aspect of the pinna in a dog with atopy.

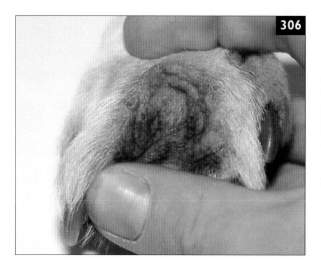

306 Hyperpigmentation following chronic inflammation in the interdigital areas of a Labrador Retriever with atopy.

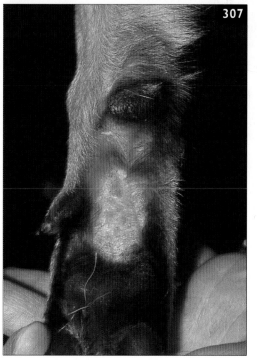

307 Discrete patch of erythema and alopecia immediately distal to the accessory carpal pad on the plantar aspect of the distal limb of a German Shepherd Dog with atopy.

Otic examination and other investigations

Most cases of chronic or recurrent otitis externa manifest some degree of hyperplasia of the epithelial lining of the external ear canal (**308**). Although this may be not be readily apparent on gross examination, it will be visible on histopathologic examination of biopsy samples. The epithelial lining may appear grossly normal or may have a cobblestone-like pattern (**309**) if glandular and epithelial hyperplasia is present. In some cases the canal may be stenosed by proliferative epithelial changes (**310**), which are often localized or polyploid in the cat. Epithelial hyperplasia and accumulation of cerumen may result in complete obstruction of the horizontal canal. The deeper portion of the horizontal ear canal and tympanum is completely hidden from view and protected from topical treatment – 'false middle ear'.

Attempting to classify the changes within the ear canal, as ceruminous or erythematous hyperplastic, is helpful from a management point of view. However, the basic elements of the otic examination should still be carried out. Given that many of these animals will have a degree of stenosis within the canal and that all are at risk for concurrent otitis media, the investigation should probably be performed under sedation so that radiography of the bullae, assessment of the tympanum and, possibly, myringotomy can be performed.

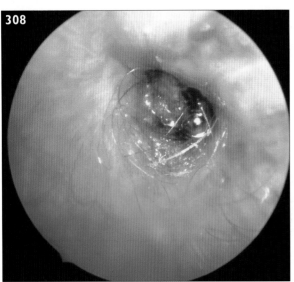

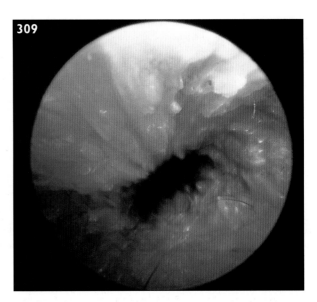

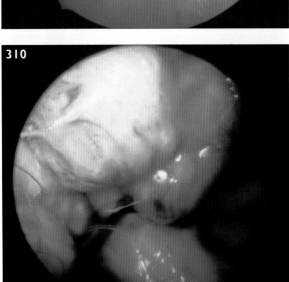

308 Otoscopic picture of the external ear canal of an atopic dog. Note the erythema and early hyperplasia.

309 Otoscopic picture of more advanced hyperplastic changes in an external ear canal; the 'cobblestone' pattern is clearly visible.

310 Otoscopic view of an external ear canal almost completely obstructed by hyperplastic epithelium.

Otoscopic examination may reveal large quantities of ceruminous discharge in some cases (**311, 312**); in other ears there may be minimal discharge. Air-dried smears should be examined unstained and after staining with Diff-Quik (**313–315**). Yeast and bacteria may be identified (**315**), in addition to cellular elements and variably proteinaceous exudate. Air-dried smears should be examined before and after staining.

It cannot be stressed too much that the quantity, physical nature, and color of otic exudate cannot be reliably correlated with any particular microbial infection.

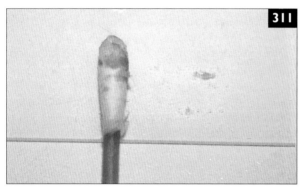

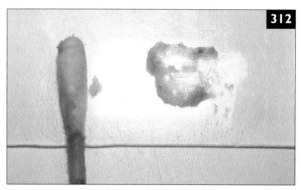

311, 312 Photographs of air-dried cerumen from normal (**311**) and ceruminous-type (**312**) ear canals demonstrating the breadth of appearance of the sample.

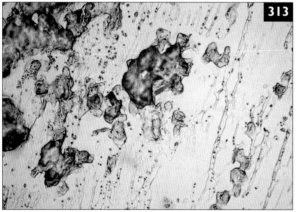

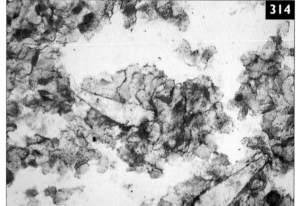

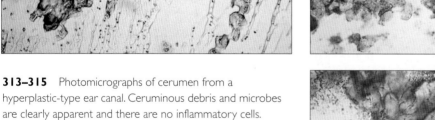

313–315 Photomicrographs of cerumen from a hyperplastic-type ear canal. Ceruminous debris and microbes are clearly apparent and there are no inflammatory cells.

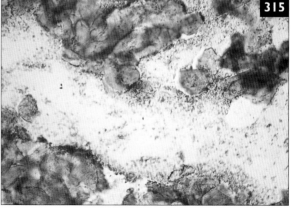

All cases of chronic otitis externa should have bacterial culture and sensitivity performed on samples from both ears, and from both sides of the tympanic membrane if otitis media is present.

Not all exudate contains pathogenic microorganisms. Microscopic examination of otic exudate only allows identification of the relative number and physical classification of organisms; yeast, coccus, bacillus, gram positive, or gram negative, for example. The presence of a neutrophilic infiltrate may suggest an infectious process, or at least that inflammation is present. Absence of such an inflammatory infiltrate might strongly suggest that any microorganisms are non-pathogenic and that any discharge relates to ceruminous gland hyperactivity (which can be prodigious) and epithelial hyperproliferation, rather than to infection. Histopathologic examination of biopsy samples may be useful in identifying the degree of fibrosis present (316, 317). Topical glucocorticoids may be useful in suppressing mural edema and hyperplasia, provided fibrosis is minimal.

MANAGEMENT
Otitis externa associated with hypersensitivity
Most commonly the hypersensitivity will be atopy, although dietary intolerance and food allergy may be associated with chronic otitis externa. Erythematous, hyperplastic otitis externa is usually associated with hypersensitivity and in many cases there is minimal microbial multiplication, at least in the early stages. As with atopic dermatitis, the microbial proliferation is usually staphylococcal and malassezial in nature, rather than gram negative:

- Identify and institute treatment for the underlying disease.
- Control secondary malassezial and bacterial multiplication.
- Assess the status of the tympanum and ascertain whether otitis media is present. If so, treat it.
- Apply topical otic glucocorticoids to suppress inflammation, reduce epithelial hyperproliferation, and minimize fibrosis.
- Maintain remission with regular application of otic cleansers, antimicrobial ointments, and occasional otic glucocorticoid preparations,
- Consider ablation of the external ear canal if these measures fail to prevent progressive pathologic changes.

Application of topical glucocorticoids to these ear canals (and to the concave aspect of the pinnae) can produce a spectacular reduction in the degree of inflammation and otic stenosis which is present, often obviating the requirement for surgery. However, regular use of potent glucocorticoids, even in otic preparations, can induce iatrogenic hyperadrenocorticism[1]. Therefore, although a potent fluorinated steroid may initially be indicated, the clinician should switch to a minimally potent agent such as prednisolone, prednisone, or hydrocortisone for maintenance.

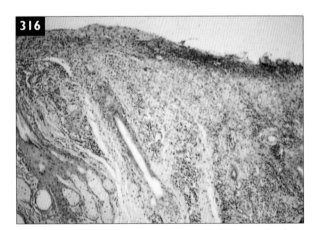
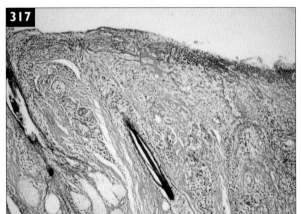

316, 317 Photomicrographs of histopathologic samples from a case of chronic otitis externa. Epidermal hyperplasia, an inflammatory infiltrate, and dermal edema (**316**). The same section but stained to highlight fibrosis (**317**). This degree of fibrosis is not amenable to topical glucocorticoids; surgery rather than medicine is indicated.

Otitis externa associated with a defect in keratinization

Ceruminous otitis externa is not always complicated by infection, but chronic cases usually are. In particular there is a tendency for gram-negative bacteria to proliferate early in the course of the disease and this must be identified and treated. Furthermore, there may be concurrent otitis media and this must be ruled in or ruled out before long-term measures are instituted:

- Consider surgical ablation at an earlier rather than a later stage, and be sure to warn the owner that surgery may well be necessary at some point.
- Keep the external ear canal and the surrounding area as clean as possible. Pluck hair regularly out of the external ear canal, and keep the concave aspect of the proximal pinna and surrounding area clipped short. Local shampooing may be helpful in keeping greasy scale to a minimum; use a degreasing, keratolytic, or keratoplastic product such as benzyl peroxide or one of the tar/sulfur/salicylic acid combination products.
- Regular use of an acetic acid based aqueous cleanser (2.5% or 5% concentration) will help to keep the otic pH acid and suppress gram-negative overgrowth. Commercial products may be used, as may equal quantities of white vinegar and water, or alcohol[2, 3].
- Regular use of ear cleansers which loosen cerumen and inhibit microbial growth may help to prevent accumulation of such debris and prevent relapse into overt otitis externa.
- Occasional, sometimes more frequent, use of cleansers such as carbamide peroxide and dioctyl sodium sulfosuccinate will help to flush out accumulations of ceruminous debris, although a drying agent, such as one based on isopropyl alcohol, should be used after these products[2].
- Otic polypharmaceutical preparations with combinations of glucocorticoids and antimicrobial agents, based on bacterial culture and sensitivity, may be indicated if the measures outlined above fail to prevent otitis externa developing.
- Consider ablation of the external ear canal if these steps fail to prevent progressive pathologic changes.

Otitis externa associated with otitis media

Although otitis media usually results as an extension of otitis externa through the tympanum[4], it may itself be a cause of recurrent otitis externa. Diagnosis may be difficult since the tympanic defects may heal, in spite of the presence of infection within the middle ear. Furthermore, bacteria recovered from cases of otitis media, behind an intact tympanum, are not always the same species, or with the same antibacterial susceptibility, as those within the external ear canal[5].

Otitis externa associated with allergic contact dermatitis

Allergic contact dermatitis to environmental allergens (for example carpet or grass) may affect the medial aspect of the pinna but is unlikely to cause otitis externa. However, reactions to otic medications have been reported, most commonly to neomycin and propylene glycol. Whether the reaction to propylene glycol is a true allergic reaction and not simply an irritant dermatitis is not clear. However, this is immaterial from a practical point of view. What the clinician and client will note is that the otitis is aggravated by the treatment.

Otitis externa associated with resistant microorganism

In a survey of the bacterial flora associated with otitis externa in dogs and cats[6], 15% of the staphylococci were resistant to more than three antibacterial agents. However, none were resistant to all the commonly used antibacterial agents. Furthermore, in a review of cases in which otic surgery had failed[7], resistant bacterial infection was not considered a significant factor. Multiple-resistant, gram-positive otitis externa is, it appears, a recognized problem in veterinary medicine.

If otitis media is suspected, it must be treated aggressively. Management of otitis media is detailed in Chapter 5 (Otitis media, otitis interna).

In practice the most difficult organism to treat is *Pseudomonas aeruginosa*, which may only be sensitive to parenteral agents *in vivo*. Approaches to gram-negative infection are detailed earlier in this chapter (Gram-negative otitis externa).

CHRONIC, OR RECURRENT, OTITIS EXTERNA IN CATS

KEY POINTS

- Recurrent otitis externa is rare in cats.
- As in dogs, the initial challenge to the clinician is to identify whether the otitis is recurring because of a disease within the ear or is a manifestation of systemic disease.
- Systemic causes of otitis externa are unusual in cats and most cases result from *Otodectes cynotis* infection, yeast infection, or polyps or neoplasia. Otodemodicosis may be found.
- Hypersensitivities such as atopy and dietary intolerance are rare.
- Indications for surgery, other than for polyps and neoplasia, are very rare.

ETIOLOGY

Otodectes cynotis infection

Many cats develop a local hypersensitivity to *O. cynotis*[1] and exhibit otitis externa characterized by variable erythema, variable pruritus, and a crumbly black brown discharge (**318**). Some animals may exhibit local self-trauma (**319**) whereas others may harbor huge numbers of mites within the external ear canal and show no obvious sign of discomfort. These are easily recognized and treated. Animals exhibiting intense self-trauma with little obvious pathology are more difficult to diagnose, as are those with only one or two mites in the external ear canal: the mites are sufficient in number to cause disease but very hard to see. Problems with diagnosis may also occur in multicat households, where control may be difficult and low numbers of mites are endemic.

Combined environmental, otic, and topical (or systemic) acaricidal treatment should be carried out in these cases. Ivermectin is particularly useful as it will eliminate mites within the ear canal and any ectopic mites on the body surface. It is important that all animals in the household are treated, whether dogs or cats[2]. *Demodex gatoi* has been reported to cause chronic ceruminous otitis externa in cats.

Malassezia pachydermatis or *M. sympodialis* infection

The status of yeast within the feline external ear canal is probably analogous to the status of *M. pachydermatis* in the canine, i.e. it is an opportunist pathogen[3]. Bond *et*

Microscopic examination of stained cytologic preparations is mandatory.

Microscopic examination of collected cerumen may be a more reliable method of detecting *O. cynotis* than otoscopic examination.

al.[4] reported the recovery of *M. pachydermatis* and *M. sympodialis* from the feline external ear canal and also stated that aural yeast infection may be associated with otic pruritus. Feline malassezial otitis externa may be associated with minimal pathologic changes, raising the suspicion of hypersensitivity rather than infectious disease. Many otic polypharmaceutical preparations contain only acaricides, antibacterial agents, and topically acting glucocorticoids, and these will not be effective in eliminating yeast infection. Non-response to treatment with such medications compounds the error of assuming hypersensitivity when in fact there is an infectious disease.

Treatment with an otic preparation containing an antifungal is curative, although reinfection may occur. This may reflect abnormal otic expression of adhesion molecules, or a systemic aberration that is not clinically expressed and hence difficult to diagnose.

Polyps and otic neoplasia

Most inflammatory polyps arise from the epithelium of the middle ear or auditory tube[5]. Inflammatory polyps arising from the epithelium of the auditory tube or middle ear may occur in cats as young as three months of age[6]. If they grow laterally through the tympanum and into the external ear canal (**320**), they may be associated with otic discharge, inflammation, head shaking, and Horner's syndrome.

Otic neoplasia in the cat is usually malignant, typically adenocarcinomas or squamous cell carcinomas[7, 8]. Animals often present with malodor and otic pruritus (**321**).

Hypersensitivity

Atopy

Although atopy is a very common cause of otitis externa in dogs, it appears to be much less so in cats, perhaps due to differences in anatomy, such as a relatively wide canal, lack of hair within the canal, and an upright pinna[9]. There may also be differences in the cerumen which make microbial overgrowth less likely, even in the face of chronic inflammation. Intradermal skin testing is more difficult to perform in the cat compared to dogs and many clinicians will make a provisional diagnosis of atopy on the basis of ruling out all other potential diagnoses.

Dietary intolerance

Dietary intolerance (food allergy) is rare in the cat. However, pinnal erythema and otitis externa may be associated with intolerance to dietary components[10]. Perhaps more commonly there is facial and head pruritus with the pinnae and periaural areas being affected (**322**) rather than the external ear canals[10, 11, 12]. The most common allergens in proven cases of feline dietary intolerance are beef, milk, and fish[13]. Diagnosis is based on a resolution of the clinical signs while an exclusion diet is fed. A period of 3–16 weeks may elapse before complete recovery is noted.

Allergic contact dermatitis

Allergic contact dermatitis is extraordinarily rare in cats. However, allergic contact dermatitis to topical neomycin is recognized by some clinicians. Certainly, the diagnosis should be considered in all cases of refractory otitis externa.

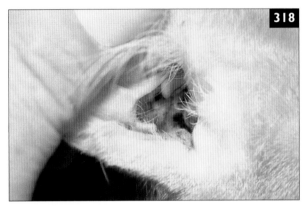

318 *Otodectes cynotis* infestation in a cat. Note the discharge within the ear canal.

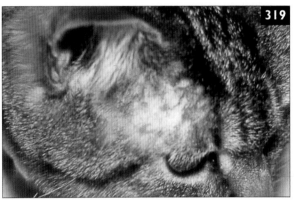

319 Self-excoriation as a consequence of otic pruritus.

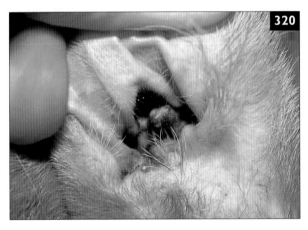

320 Pigmented polyp apparent at the entrance to the external ear canal.

321 Hemorrhagic tumor in the external ear canal.

322 Severe self-trauma to the head and neck in a case of food allergy.

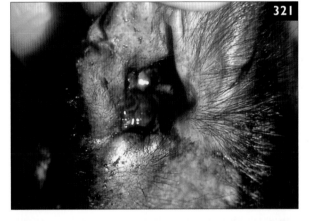

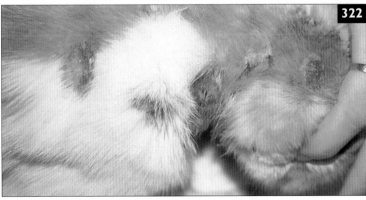

NEUROLOGIC SIGNS RELATED TO MIDDLE EAR DISEASE

KEY POINTS

- The neurologic structures crossing the middle ear include the facial nerve and the sympathetic supply to the eye and eyelids.
- Middle ear disease can result in ipsilateral facial nerve dysfunction, Horner's syndrome, and conductive deafness.
- Causes of middle ear disease principally include infection, neoplasia, trauma and, in cats, polyps.
- Conductive deafness associated with middle ear disease carries a better prognosis than sensorineural deafness.

INTRODUCTION AND NEUROANATOMY

The middle ear consists of an air-filled tympanic cavity connected to the nasopharynx via the auditory tube, and closed to the outside by the tympanic membrane. In the dog the tympanic cavity has a small dorsal epitympanic recess and a large ventral tympanic bulla. The middle portion of the tympanic cavity contains the three auditory ossicles and their two associated muscles[1] (see Chapter 1: Gross and microscopic anatomy of the ear: structure and function). In the cat the middle ear cavity is divided into two parts by a bony septum, incomplete dorsally. These two compartments lie dorsolaterally and ventromedially, the latter being larger than, and extending caudally to, the former. The larger compartment corresponds to the fundic portion of the tympanic bulla in the dog. The tympanic membrane forms the major portion of the lateral wall of the smaller compartment, which also contains the bony part of the auditory tube[2].

Facial nerve

The facial nerve (cranial nerve [CN] VII) is a mixed nerve, providing motor innervation for all of the superficial muscles of the head, face, and external ear (mimetic muscles) as well as the caudal belly of the digastricus muscle, the stylohyoid muscle, the platysma of the neck, and the stapedius muscle in the middle ear. It also contains preganglionic parasympathetic fibers, as well as afferent sensory neurons coming from the taste buds of the rostral two-thirds of the tongue and other visceral receptors in the soft palate, nasopharynx, and nasal cavity via the chorda tympani. The parasympathetic fibers synapse in ganglia that send postganglionic fibers to the lacrimal gland; the glands of the nasal mucosa (via the major petrosal nerve); the dorsal buccal, mandibular, and sublingual salivary glands; and the buccal and lingual mucosa. The somatic efferent fibers of the facial nerve have their cell body located in the motor nucleus of the facial nerve in the brainstem. The intermediate nerve constitutes the sensory and preganglionic root of the facial nerve. Its cell bodies are located in the parasympathetic nucleus of the facial nerve, situated dorsally and cranially to the motor nucleus in the brainstem. The sensory nerve fibers have their cell bodies in the geniculate ganglion[3].

The central course of CN VII is beyond the scope of this book. However, for an understanding of neuropathies that can be associated with middle ear disease, a good appreciation of the course of the facial nerve in relation to the tympanic bulla is important.

The intermediate nerve and motor fibers join just distal to their emergence from the brainstem. The facial nerve leaves the cranial cavity via the internal acoustic meatus, together with the vestibular and cochlear nerves. Within the meatus the cochlear nerve diverges and the vestibular nerve divides into a superior and an inferior portion. The superior part remains in contact with the facial nerve as they traverse the dorsal part of the internal acoustic meatus and enter the facial canal together[3] (**323, 324**).

After pursuing a sigmoid course throughout the temporal bone, the facial nerve emerges at the stylomastoid foramen situated dorsally and laterally to the tympanic bulla (**325**).

The initial 3 mm (0.1 in) of the facial canal, starting at the internal acoustic meatus, is straight. The canal makes its first turn on arriving at the thin medial wall of the fossa m. tensor tympani. At this turn, or genu, of the facial canal there is an indistinct enlargement of the sensory geniculate ganglion of the facial nerve. In the concavity of this bend is the rostral half of the vestibule. As the canal straightens after the first turn, and before the second turn begins, it opens into the cavity of the middle ear lateral to the vestibular window. This is where the facial nerve is exposed to diseases affecting the middle ear. The direction of the second bend of the canal is the reverse of that of the first, so that the whole passage is S-shaped but does not lie in one plane[4]. The facial nerve then exits the skull via the stylomastoid foramen to be distributed in branches (the auriculopalpebral, dorsal, and ventral buccal nerves) to the muscles of the ears, cheek, lips, and nose[5].

323   Ventral aspect of the skull of a dog with the bulla removed. The acoustic meatus (1), the internal aspect of the stylomastoid foramen (2), the jugular foramen (3), the promontory (4), and the facial canal (dotted line) are visible.

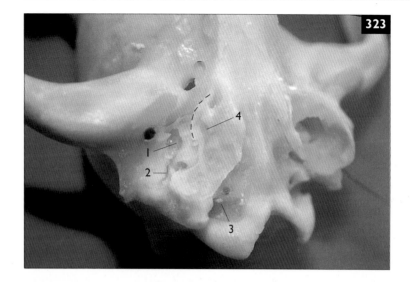

324   Dorsal view of the skull of a dog with the calvarium removed. The internal acoustic meatus (1) and the jugular foramen (2) are visible.

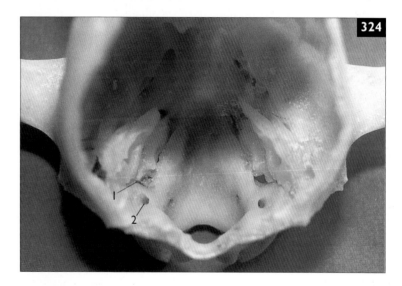

325   Lateral view of the caudal part of the skull of a dog. The stylomastoid foramen (1) is clearly visible immediately caudal to the external acoustic meatus (2).

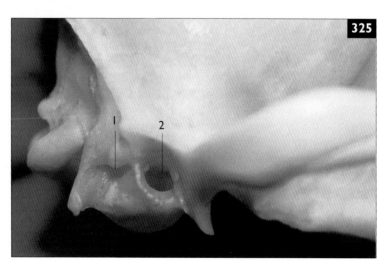

Sympathetic innervation of the eye

In order to understand the reasons for the occurrence of Horner's syndrome with middle ear disease, and its accurate diagnosis, it is important to have a basic understanding of the anatomy of the autonomic nervous system. This system is concerned with the motor innervation of smooth muscles, cardiac muscles, and glands, as well as fat. It is further subdivided into sympathetic and parasympathetic parts, which are 'three-neurons' systems. Both parts of the autonomic nervous system are under the influence of higher centers located in the midbrain, pons, medulla and, most importantly, the hypothalamus. The first neuron of the chain descends from the hypothalamus through the brainstem and the spinal cord in the tecto-tegmento-spinal tract. It synapses in the gray matter of the thoracic and lumbar segments with the second neuron of the chain, the preganglionic neuron, which has its cell body in the gray matter of the central nervous system (brainstem and spinal cord). Its axon leaves the central nervous system via a cranial or spinal nerve and synapses in a peripheral ganglion with the third neuron (postganglionic neuron) which terminates in the structure to be innervated. In the sympathetic system, also called the thoracolumbar system, the cell bodies of the preganglionic neuron are located in the intermediate horn of the gray matter in the spinal cord, from the first thoracic to the fifth lumbar spinal segments. With a few exceptions, the neurotransmitter released at the presynaptic end of the postganglionic axon is norepinephrine[6, 7].

The sympathetic innervation of the eye responds to stimulation eliciting excitement, fear, or anger. The cell bodies of the preganglionic neurons destined to innervate the pupil are located in the first three or four thoracic spinal segments. The axons pass through the ventral gray horn and adjacent white matter into the ventral roots and the proximal portion of the spinal nerve corresponding to these segments. Before the spinal nerve branches, these preganglionic axons leave it via the segmental ramus communicans, which joins the thoracic sympathetic trunk inside the thorax ventrolateral to the vertebral column and close to the surface of the cranial lung lobe[8]. The axons usually progress cranially without synapse in a trunk ganglion. They pass through the cervicothoracic (stellate) and middle cervical ganglia and course cranially in the cervical sympathetic trunk, which is part of the vagosympathetic trunk. Medial to the origin of the digastricus muscle and ventromedial to the tympanic bulla, the cervical sympathetic trunk separates from the vagus nerve and terminates in the cranial cervical ganglion. At this level the preganglionic axons synapse with the third neuron. The axons for ocular innervation course rostrally through the tympano-occipital fissure with the internal carotid artery and pass between the tympanic bulla and the petrosal bone into the middle ear cavity, closely associated with the ventral surface of the petrosal bone (**326**).

The axons continue rostrally between the petrosal bone and the basisphenoid to join the ventral surface of the trigeminal ganglion and the ophthalmic branch of the trigeminal nerve in the cavernous sinus. This ophthalmic nerve enters the periorbita through the orbital fissure. The postganglionic axons are distributed by way of the ophthalmic nerve branches to the smooth muscles of the periorbita, the eyelids, including the third eyelid, and the iris muscles, particularly the dilator of the pupil. The normal tone of the smooth muscles of the periorbita and eyelids keeps the eyeball protruded and the eyelids retracted. The sympathetic tone also keeps the pupil partially dilated in normal conditions and aids dilation during periods of stress, fear, pain, and darkness[6, 9] (**327**).

Although it is important to remember that the sympathetic innervation of the eye is counterbalanced by parasympathetic innervation, a detailed description of the latter system is beyond the scope of this book, but it can be found in anatomy and neuroanatomy texts[1, 6, 10] (**328**).

MIDDLE EAR DISEASE: CAUSES AND CONSEQUENCES

The main causes of middle ear disease include neoplasia, infection, polyps, and trauma. A detailed discussion of polyps and otitis media can be found in Chapter 3 (Nasopharyngeal and middle ear polyps) and Chapter 5 (Otitis media, otitis interna), respectively. Neoplasms involving the middle ear include adenocarcinoma of the tympanic bulla[11], squamous cell carcinoma[12], and fibrosarcoma[11] (see Chapter 3: Otic neoplasia). Traumatic causes of middle ear disease are mostly due to road traffic accidents.

The main neurologic consequences of middle ear disease are conductive deafness, facial nerve paralysis, and Horner's syndrome.

Conductive deafness

Conductive deafness occurs when there is a failure of proper transmission of sound vibration to the inner ear and auditory nervous system[13]. Therefore, this type of hearing impairment results from problems in the external or middle ear, such as external ear occlusion (in extreme cases of chronic otitis externa), rigidity or rupture of the tympanic membrane, damage to the ossicular chain, and fluid or soft tissue accumulation within the tympanic bulla. The most common cause of conductive deafness is chronic otitis externa or otitis media, sometimes in association with cholesteatoma[14]. However, while severe hearing loss can be present in dogs affected by severe otitis, few become totally deaf[15]. Cleaning of the external ear has been reported to be a potential cause of

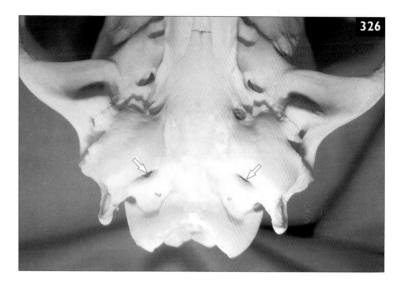

326 Ventral view of the skull of a dog with the tympano-occipito fissures marked (arrows).

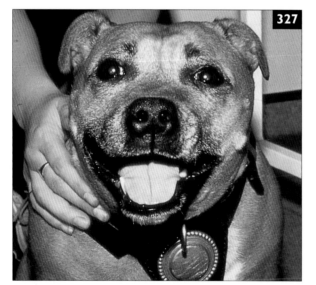

327 Staffordshire Bull Terrier with left-sided facial nerve paralysis exhibiting asymmetry of the lip commisures.

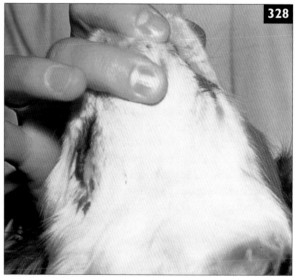

328 Cavalier King Charles Spaniel exhibiting asymmetry of the lip commisures as a result of right-sided facial nerve paralysis.

> It is important that conductive deafness is differentiated from sensorineural deafness, particularly when an animal is considered as a candidate for an auditory prosthesis, as the prognosis is rather different.

deafness. Although damage to bony ossicles is a rare cause of deafness[16], it can occur after overzealous flushing and curettage of the tympanic bulla. Nonetheless, gentle cleaning of the ear canal tends to improve the hearing function of dogs, which indicates the profound effect of physical obstruction of the external ear canal by debris[15].

Treatment

Ear cleaning. As suggested by Eger and Lindsay[15], ear cleaning (see Chapter 9: Cleaning the external ear canal) can improve the hearing function of dogs, as long as it does not cause more damage (rupture of the tympanic membrane, disruption of the ossicle chain, ototoxicity).

Surgical options. Surgical management of external and middle ear disease is described in Chapter 11 (Surgical resection, aural ablation, and bulla osteotomy). Studies by McAnulty *et al.*[17] demon-strated that ventral tympanic bulla osteotomy does not have any deleterious effect on hearing, as measured by brainstem auditory evoked potential (BAEP), in a majority of treated dogs. However, total ear canal ablation with lateral tympanic bulla osteotomy causes irreversible hearing loss unless the tympanic membrane and ossicles are retained, which tends to be a cause of postoperative complications[18].

Hearing aids. Hearing aids for veterinary patients have been developed. They are similar to a miniature public address system, containing a miniaturized microphone and a battery-powered amplifier and speaker housed in a suitable container. The amplified sound is introduced into the ear by various means that have evolved with experience of tolerance in dogs. The latest model, described by Marshall[19], is mounted in a case worn on the collar of the dog. The amplified sound is fed into the ear via a flexible plastic tube, which is held in the ear by acoustic foam. Success depends largely on the training provided by the dog's owner, as well as the owner's patience in conditioning the dog to wear the instrument.

More recently, the surgical placement of a bone-anchored hearing aid (BAHA) was described in a dog with bilateral chronic otitis which had been treated by bilateral total ear canal ablation and lateral bulla osteotomy[20]. (**NB:** The inner ear must function normally, with a hearing threshold below 45 dB [as assessed by bone-conducted BAER].) The BAHA implant allows the by-pass of the resected or redundant ear canals and tympanic bullae and permits stimulation of the cochlea by bone-conducted sound through the skull. With the BAHA in place, BAER testing shows a good hearing threshold at 30 dB (sound pressure level [SPL]) while without the BAHA no BAER line is reproducible even at 70 dB (SPL).

The principal consideration is whether amplifying devices are indicated in the ageing canine. Indeed, studies suggest that presbycusis is due to a degeneration of neurons[21] which would not support the use of a sound amplifier if the sound cannot be perceived at the receiving end. This was the perceived opinion early in human research. However, experience accumulated over 20 years contradicts this early impression. Indeed, it is stated that the great majority of people who wear and benefit from hearing aids have sensorineural loss. Similar experience is reported in veterinary patients. Nevertheless, it remains important to understand that amplification cannot help totally deaf animals[19].

Prognosis

The prognosis associated with conductive deafness is essentially based on the underlying cause. An objective evaluation of the hearing level with BAEP is indicated (see Chapter 2: Electrophysiologic procedures). Further investigation of the cause of deafness should yield a definitive diagnosis and a treatment plan. As mentioned above, surgical treatment may or may not help with recovery of the hearing ability. It is also important to remember that the hearing impairment can be worsened by inappropriate or aggressive medical treatment (see Chapter 8: Ototoxicity and other side-effects of otic medications).

Facial nerve paralysis
Clinical signs
The cardinal signs of facial nerve paralysis include ear and lip droop, asymmetrical commissures of the lips, widened palpebral fissure, ipsilateral sialosis, and collection of food on the paralyzed side of the mouth (**327, 328**, see page 187). Cranial nerve reflexes and responses requiring facial nerve function (palpebral and corneal reflexes, menace response) are decreased or absent[22]. If the parasympathetic fibers conveyed in the facial nerve are affected, this can lead to reduced tear production and result in keratoconjunctivitis sicca[23] (**329**).

Hemifacial spasm, which is a constant contraction of all the facial muscles on one side of the head, has been observed in dogs. On the affected side the nose is pulled caudally and the lips may feel hypertonic. The palpebral fissure is smaller due to partial closure of the eyelids, and the ear is slightly elevated. In most dogs some slight movement can be elicited in the eyelids and sometimes in the ear and nose. The facial muscles on the opposite side function normally. This syndrome has been attributed mainly to hyperirritability of the facial nerve caused by otitis media, although it can occur spontaneously or follow total facial nerve paralysis[6].

Neuroanatomic localization and associated neurologic signs

The facial nerve can be affected, like all cranial nerves, at the level of its nucleus in the brainstem, or anywhere along its axon, within the skull, during its exit of the skull, and outside of the skull. Neurologic signs associated with facial nerve paralysis often allow a more precise localization of the problem:

- If the lesion is located within the brainstem, neurologic signs affecting adjacent structures will be observed simultaneously causing, for instance, ipsilateral conscious proprioception deficits with upper motor neuron (UMN) signs. Other cranial nerves, such as CNs V, VI, and VIII, may be affected as well.
- If the facial nerve is affected along its passage through the petrosal bone, the vestibulocochlear nerve is most likely to be affected and this will cause concomitant ipsilateral signs of peripheral vestibular disease and deafness.
- If the facial nerve is affected after it emerges from the stylomastoid foramen, the parasympathetic fibers in the major petrosal nerve will be spared[23] and paralysis of the facial muscles will not be accompanied by the dry eye and nasal mucosa that are often associated with total facial neuropathy.

Differential diagnosis

Facial nerve paralysis can occur without any lesion in the middle ear. The clinician presented with a case of facial nerve paralysis should consider carefully all possible differential diagnoses and localizations of the problem before narrowing investigations to the middle ear.

Metabolic facial nerve paralysis has been reported to be associated with hypothyroidism, often in conjunction with neuropathies involving other cranial nerves or even peripheral appendicular nerves. The exact pathogenesis of hypothyroid neuropathy is still poorly understood and results of thyroid hormone replacement in affected animals have been variable[16, 24].

Neoplastic causes of facial nerve paralysis include pituitary tumor[6] and insulinoma, which is often associated with a subclinical peripheral neuropathy[25]. Fibrosarcoma and squamous cell carcinoma of the tympanic bulla in cats can cause facial nerve paralysis, amongst other cranial nerve involvement[26].

Idiopathic facial nerve paralysis is reported in both dogs and cats. In a retrospective study it was judged to be the cause of 74.7% of cases in dogs and 25% of cases in cats[5]. The onset is usually sudden and the course variable[6]. The condition is usually unilateral but can be bilateral. Idiopathic facial nerve paralysis has been reported mainly in mature dogs and cats. Some breeds, such as Cocker Spaniels, Welsh Corgis, Boxers, English Setters, and domestic longhaired cats, are more predisposed[5, 27].

Inflammatory causes of facial nerve paralysis include polyradiculoneuritis, such as Coonhound paralysis in the USA[16], and brachial plexus neuritis[6]. Granulomatous meningoencephalomyelitis can involve the facial nerve nucleus, amongst other structures of the central nervous system[28].

Infectious causes of facial nerve paralysis are mainly localized to the middle ear and are the most common cause for this cranial nerve deficit. In cases of otitis media, concomitant signs of ipsilateral peripheral vestibular disease are most common[26].

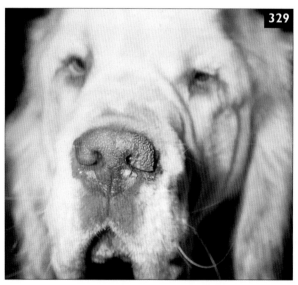

329 Clumber Spaniel with left-sided facial nerve paralysis. Note the ipsilateral (left) neurogenic dry nose and dry eye. (Illustration courtesy J Sansom.)

Trauma, such as fracture of the petrosal or basioccipital bone, can also be a cause of facial nerve paralysis. In this case it is mostly associated with signs of ipsilateral peripheral vestibular disease[6]. Surgical trauma subsequent to middle ear surgery is also one of the most commonly reported causes of facial nerve paralysis.

Investigation

Aural examination and radiographs of the skull and tympanic bullae help rule out obvious signs of trauma and otitis media. However, radiography is not a very sensitive means of investigating otitis media and advanced imaging techniques such as CT or MRI should be pursued. Electromyography will confirm the presence of denervation if the clinical signs have been present for five days or more. However, this will not identify the cause of the neuropathy. In all cases of confirmed facial nerve paralysis, tear production should be assessed by Schirmer tear testing and fluorescein staining should be performed to rule out exposure keratitis. Both tests should be monitored on a monthly or two-monthly basis[22].

Treatment

Treatment of facial nerve paralysis is based on the underlying cause and aims at avoiding the occurrence of exposure keratitis or keratoconjunctivitis sicca. Artificial tears should be applied in confirmed dry eyes and animals should be kept out of draughts and dusty environments. If motor function does not return within three months post diagnosis, a temporary or permanent tarsorrhaphy can be performed to prevent traumatic keratitis.

Prognosis

Recovery of facial muscle function is guarded. It can take weeks or months and, more often than not, the paralysis is permanent.

Horner's syndrome

Clinical signs

The classic features of Horner's syndrome are well recognized (**330–332**):
- Anisocoria with ipsilateral miosis.
- Ptosis of the upper eyelid.
- Narrowing of the palpebral fissure.
- Enophthalmos.
- Protrusion of the third eyelid.

The affected pupil is not pinpoint but is definitely smaller than the normal pupil. It is best assessed in the dark, as the affected pupil cannot dilate beyond the size of the pupil created by the resting iris sphincter muscle.

Therefore, dark adaptation accentuates the anisocoria, with the normal pupil dilating widely and the affected pupil being incompletely dilated[9]. The size of the pupils in the dark is best evaluated by eliciting a tapetal reflex during distant direct ophthalmoscopic examination, the ophthalmoscope being held at arms length from the animal (**333, 334**).

Theoretically, ptosis is caused by loss of sympathetic innervation of the smooth muscle of the upper eyelid; however, some experts believe that ptosis may occur secondarily to the enophthalmos[9].

Narrowing of the palpebral fissure is caused by a combination of ptosis of the upper eyelid, enophthalmos, and elevation of the lower eyelid[9].

Enophthalmos is the result of lack of sympathetic supply to the musculus orbitalis of the periorbital sheath, which pushes the globe forward. The retractor bulbi is left without antagonism, which allows further retraction of the globe[9].

Protrusion of the third eyelid is not always present in Horner's syndrome but it is the most consistent sign after miosis. Protrusion of the third eyelid is mainly caused by denervation but it is also accentuated by the enophthalmos[9].

Other changes occasionally reported with long-term Horner's syndrome include peripheral vasodilation causing locally increased skin temperature and hyperemia, best observed in the ipsilateral ear and nasal mucosa[6, 28, 32]. This phenomenon is reported to be the cause of a change in coat color in affected Siamese cats[9, 29, 30]. It has also been noted that the affected iris of the cat changes color three-and-a-half years after cervical ganglionectomy[31].

Neuroanatomic localization and associated neurologic signs

As with any neurologic disorder, it is important to localize the lesion before establishing a list of differential diagnoses specific to the neuroanatomic location.

Brainstem. Damage to the hypothalamus or tecto-tegmental-spinal tract in the brainstem can result in 1st order Horner's syndrome. As these structures are placed fairly deeply in the parenchyma, they are unlikely to be the only ones affected, and most of the time they are associated with rather severe neurologic signs affecting the long tracts and adjacent brainstem nuclei such as the cranial nerves or the vegetative respiratory and cardiovascular centers. The deficits observed can include dyspnea, arrhythmia, altered mental status, and proprioceptive deficits affecting the ipsilateral thoracic and pelvic limbs, at least in theory. In practice most cases present with tetraparesis and tetraplegia. The segmental spinal reflexes are normal to increased in both the thoracic and the pelvic limbs, indicating an UMN lesion.

Spinal cord. The 1st sympathetic neuron of the chain travels in the tecto-tegmento-spinal tract in the white matter of the spinal cord until it synapses with the 2nd neuron at the level of spinal segments T1, T2, and T3. Lesions affecting the tecto-tegmento-spinal tract in the spinal cord are unlikely to be discreet enough to cause a Horner's syndrome as the sole clinical sign. Long tracts are likely to be affected as well, causing proprioceptive deficits in the ipsilateral thoracic and pelvic limbs.

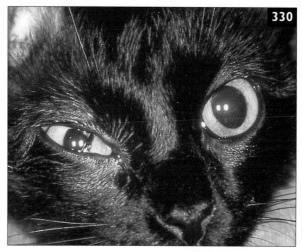

330   Domestic shorthaired cat with right-sided Horner's syndrome. There is myosis, a protruded third eyelid, and a drooped upper eyelid. Compare with the normal left eye.

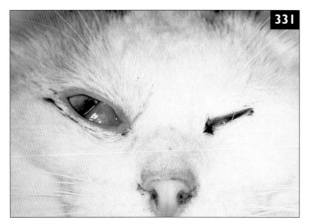 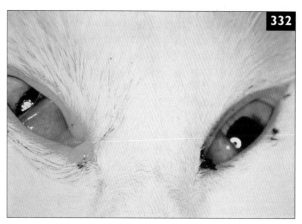

331, 332   Domestic shorthaired cat with right-sided Horner's syndrome and right-sided facial nerve paralysis. Note the prolapsed third eyelid, myotic pupil, and asymmetric eyelid aperture, as well as the absence of a blink reflex in the affected eye in **331**.

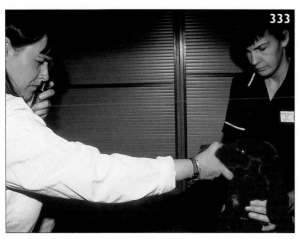 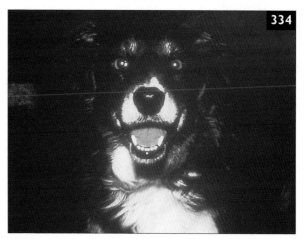

333, 334   Evaluation of the tapetal reflex performed during distant direct ophthalmoscopic examination in a darkened room (**333**). In **334** the tapetal reflex is easily seen. Note the anisocoria.

The segmental spinal reflexes vary with the localization of the lesion along the cervico-thoracic spine:

- Between C1 and C5 spinal segments the reflexes indicate an UMN lesion in both the thoracic and the pelvic limbs.
- Between C6 and T3 spinal segments the reflexes are decreased to absent in the thoracic limb, indicating a lower motor neuron (LMN) lesion whilst they indicate an UMN lesion in the pelvic limb. With a lesion at this level of the spinal cord, it is possible to observe ipsilateral deficits of the cutaneous trunci (panniculus) reflex, as its efferent (motor) arm, the lateral thoracic nerve, emerges from spinal segments C8–T1.
- A lesion to the tecto-tegmento-spinal tract between C1 and C8 causes a 1st order Horner's syndrome, whilst lesions located between T1 and T3 spinal segments affect the cell body of the 2nd neuron in the chain and cause a 2nd order Horner's syndrome.

Lesions located in the central nervous system causing Horner's syndrome are rarely discreet enough to cause neurologic deficits limited to the ipsilateral side, and it is not unusual to observe neurologic deficits in all four limbs.

Ventral roots of T1, T2, T3, and proximal spinal nerves. Lesions to the ventral roots cause a 2nd order Horner's syndrome associated with LMN signs to the ipsilateral thoracic limb and possibly cutaneous trunci deficits, but they should not affect the ipsilateral pelvic limb. LMN injuries are the most common cause of Horner's syndrome in animals[33].

Sympathetic trunk. Damage to the 2nd neuron of the chain in the sympathetic trunk before it synapses with the postganglionic neuron can occur at the level of the cranial mediastinum, the thoracic inlet, or in the neck where it courses with the carotid artery, the vagus nerve, and the recurrent laryngeal nerve. Signs associated with a 2nd order Horner's syndrome at this level include laryngeal and esophageal dysfunction. Lesions in the mediastinum do not tend to produce other neurologic deficits but may cause dyspnea.

Middle ear. Diseases of the middle ear may be the most common cause of Horner's syndrome[9]. Clinical signs associated with middle ear disease can be associated or not with signs of otitis externa and/or otitis interna (see Chapter 5: Otitis media, otitis interna). Facial nerve paralysis is another sign often observed with Horner's syndrome due to a lesion localized to the middle ear, as well as ipsilateral vestibular disease if the problem extends to the inner ear (**335, 336**).

Cavernous sinus. The cavernous sinus is a paired venous sinus that lies on each side of the floor in the middle cranial fossa and runs from the orbital fissure to the petro-occipital canal. Lesions located at the level of the cavernous sinus are rare. They can affect the sympathetic innervation of the pupil and produce a Horner's syndrome as part of a clinical syndrome. However, the majority of cases reported presented mainly with deficits of the parasympathetic innervation of the eye, as well as involvement of CNs III, IV, VI, and the ophthalmic and maxillary branches of CN V. The most common signs are ophthalmoparesis or ophthalmoplegia, mydriasis and absent pupillary light reflex, ptosis, decreased corneal sensation, and decreased retractor occuli reflex. In one

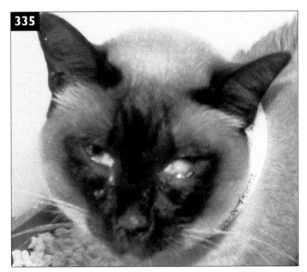
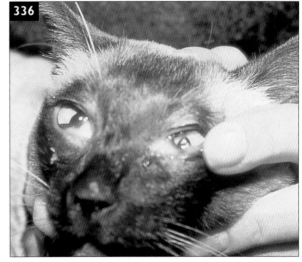

335, 336 Siamese cat with retropharyngeal lymphoma extending to the middle ear and causing bilateral Horner's syndrome and left-sided facial paralysis. Note the absence of a blink reflex in the left eye.

series of 12 cases, only one had signs of partial Horner's syndrome[33].

Retrobulbar area. Retrobulbar lesions can cause Horner's syndrome. In these cases it is often associated with other clinical signs due to compression or damage to the surrounding structures, i.e. exophthalmos, retrobulbar compression of the optic nerve causing abnormal pupillary light response, and visual deficits and ophthalmoplegia/ophthalmoparesis.

Pharmacologic localization

Often, the neuroanatomic localization of the cause of the Horner's syndrome cannot be determined by physical examination alone. Therefore, attempts to determine whether the lesion is pre- or postganglionic can be helpful[9]. Although the classically described cocaine and epinephrine tests are used by some clinicians, they rarely produce a clear localization of the lesion site[34].

Pharmacologic testing theoretically allows the classification of Horner's syndrome into three categories[23]:
- A 1st order Horner's syndrome where the 1st neuron of the chain is affected.
- A 2nd order Horner's syndrome where the 2nd neuron of the chain is affected (preganglionic).
- A 3rd order Horner's syndrome where the postganglionic neuron, the 3rd in the chain, is affected.

During pharmacologic testing, both the normal and the abnormal eye should be tested for comparison and each eye should receive the same amount of drug[9]. Under normal circumstances the following sequence of events accounts for stimulation of the iris dilator:
- Sympathetic nerve impulses are transmitted to the ends of postganglionic nerve fibers, at which time norepinephrine is released.
- Norepinephrine rapidly crosses the neuromucular junction, and the iris dilates.

In Horner's syndrome, when these nerve fibers are non-functional or are destroyed, the iris does not dilate and the unopposed iris sphincter maintains the pupil in a contracted miotic status. The released norepinephrine can undergo several fates:
- It may be removed by capillary circulation.
- It can be destroyed enzymatically.
- It can undergo re-uptake by the nerve from which it was released.

0.001% epinephrine. Diffusion and re-uptake are probably the most significant routes for inactivation of norepinephrine after its release[35]. Topically applied 0.001% epinephrine is subject to the same route of inactivation as endogenously released norepinephrine. If a low concentration is applied exogenously, some will diffuse into the circulation and the rest will be taken up into the nerve endings.

Therefore, in the normal eye there will not be sufficient concentration of epinephrine to cause dilation. However, in the eye with a postganglionic Horner's syndrome the sympathetic nerve is no longer intact. Thus, one route of inactivation of the epinephrine, namely uptake into the nerve endings, has been lost[35]. According to Canon's law of denervation supersensitivity, weak concentrations of epinephrine may then be strong enough to cause rapid dilation of the affected pupil[36]. The cat and dog have some degree of supersensitivity with a preganglionic lesion, although it is only 10% of that seen after postganglionic denervation[35]. However, results of testing with epinephrine have proved to be inaccurate and some authors recommend the use of 10% phenylephrine, which penetrates the cornea more effectively[8, 35].

10% phenylephrine. Ten percent phenylephrine is a direct-acting sympathomimetic drug. It should be used at least 24 hours after a positive hydroxyamphetamine test (i.e. incomplete to no mydriasis)[34]. After denervation the iris dilator muscle becomes hypersensitive to catecholamines. Hypersensitivity is greater in postganglionic denervation than in preganglionic denervation[37]. Therefore, if the lesion is postganglionic, mydriasis and retraction of the protruded 3rd eyelid occur in the affected eye within 5–20 minutes after instillation of 10 % phenylephrine[10, 34]. In the case of a 2nd order Horner's syndrome the abnormal pupil dilates in about 45 minutes, and in the normal eye, or 1st order Horner's syndrome, mydriasis occurs between 60 and 90 minutes[10].

1% hydroxyamphetamine. One percent hydroxyamphetamine is an indirect-acting sympathomimetic which acts by causing endogenous norepinephrine release from adrenergic nerve endings. Therefore, it can help distinguish between pre- and postganglionic lesions. When the lesion is central or preganglionic, mydriasis results after 1% hydroxyamphetamine is placed in a Horner's-affected pupil, just as in the control eye.

In these lesions the nerve endings of the postganglionic neurons are unimpaired and therefore they liberate their endogenous norepinephrine stores. Since this drug is dose dependent, a sufficient quantity needs to be administered equally to each eye to achieve mydriasis of the control eye to assure valid testing. A greater number of drops are required in dark irides. The test may require one hour to complete and requires multiple instillations. When the lesion is postganglionic, the norepinephrine stores contained in the adrenergic nerve terminals are reduced or absent, depending on the duration of the lesion and the location of the damage from the nerve endings. This type of Horner's pupil dilates incompletely or not at all, depending on the state of the nerve terminals[9, 34] (*Table 14*).

5% or 6% cocaine. Five percent[34] or 6%[37] cocaine potentiates or produces adrenergic effects by blocking the transport of catecholamines back into the sympathetic postganglionic fibres[35]. While cocaine is valuable in confirming Horner's syndrome, it is considered unreliable in predicting the site of a lesion in cats and dogs[38].

Differential diagnosis

Although all the clinical signs constituting Horner's syndrome are rarely present simultaneously for any other reason, the above mentioned clinical signs taken individually can be caused by a variety of specific disorders. It is important to keep these options in mind when investigating the origin of Horner's syndrome. For instance, the differential diagnosis for miosis includes anterior uveitis, corneal ulceration with secondary miosis, causes of synechia, and spastic pupil syndrome in cats[8, 9]. Anisocoria can also occur following cranial trauma.

The differential diagnosis for enophthalmos and protrusion of the third eyelid includes microphthalmia, phthysis bulbi, dehydration, chronic orbital inflammation, or loss of orbital fat due to excessive weight loss[39]. Protrusion of the third eyelid can also be associated with tetanus or Haw's syndrome in the cat[40]. The main clinical signs of Haw's syndrome are chronic diarrhea and depression and they are usually self-limiting[41]. However, systemic disorders such as dehydration, weight loss, and tetanus usually affect both eyes symmetrically. Blepharospasm due to primary ocular disease can mimic narrowing of the palpebral fissure.

There are many causes of Horner's syndrome, but it is essential that, as in any other neurologic disease, the causes are assessed in the context of the likelihood of their occurrence at the identified neuroanatomic localization.

Congenital Horner's syndrome has been reported in a Basset Hound, which showed clinical signs from the time its eyes opened[42].

Neoplastic processes can affect the sympathetic pathway anywhere along its way from the hypothalamus to the muscle dilator of the pupil. Many types of tumor have been described in cats and dogs. They include intramedullary or extradural lymphoma compressing the thoracic spinal cord, leiomyosarcoma[29]

or thymoma in the anterior mediastinum, thyroid adenocarcinoma[40], salivary gland adenocarcinoma[43], and metastatic carcinoma involving the maxillary and palatine bones or the regional lymph nodes[29, 41, 44]. Other less common neoplastic causes of Horner's syndrome include myelomonocytic neoplasia of peripheral nerves, especially the trigeminal nerve in dogs[45], and retrobulbar squamous cell carcinoma in the cat[46].

Iatrogenic causes of Horner's syndrome are mainly due to trauma during middle ear surgery or cleaning of the external ear canal[32]. It is also reported as a common complication of neck surgery for cervical spinal cord compression[38], thyroid[47] and parathyroid gland excision[48], as well as surgical correction of osteochondritis dissecans in the shoulder[49]. Horner's syndrome can occur following placement of intrathoracic drains[50] or aortic catheterization[51].

Idiopathic Horner's syndrome is diagnosed in over 50% of canine cases[32] and over 40% of feline cases[38, 52]. It has been reported as a breed predisposition in the Golden Retriever[53].

Infection localized to the middle ear is one of the main causes of Horner's syndrome in cats and dogs[52]. *Toxoplasma gondii* was reported to cause Horner's syndrome, amongst many other clinical signs, in one dog[54].

Inflammatory causes of Horner's syndrome are unusual. In these cases signs of sympathetic involvement tend to be associated with other signs of neurologic disease. Idiopathic pyogranulomatous meningoencephalomyelitis in Pointers is one of the causes reported.[55] Trigeminal neuritis causing bilateral paralysis of the muscles of mastication and a dropped jaw can also cause Horner's syndrome, presumably from involvement of the postganglionic sympathetic axons coursing in the ophthalmic branch[6].

Traumatic causes of Horner's syndrome include chronic intervertebral disk protrusion consistent with lower cervical spondylomyelopathy. This latter etiology was reported at the level of C6–C7 in a Doberman Pinscher[29]. Some authors have reported that spinal cord lesions cranial to C6 severe enough to cause Horner's syndrome usually cause respiratory failure, leading to death[56]. Other frequently reported traumatic causes include rib fracture, high rise falls, stake and choke chain injuries, bite wounds, and jugular puncture[29, 40]. Road traffic accidents (RTAs) are the most common cause of Horner's syndrome. An RTA resulting in avulsion of the brachial plexus can include the spinal nerve roots T1, T2, and T3 and cause an associated ipsilateral preganglionic Horner's syndrome. Postganglionic Horner's syndrome caused by trauma can be brought on by fracture or hemorrhage in the middle ear.

Cardiovascular causes of Horner's syndrome are mainly represented by fibrocartilaginous emboli in the cervical spinal cord. In these cases the associated neurologic signs are characterized by sudden onset, non-progressive, non-painful ipsilateral hemiplegia[57].

Diagnosis

Investigation of Horner's syndrome should always start with a precise localization in mind. However, despite the above mentioned theory of pharmacologic localization, it is not always possible to localize Horner's syndrome very precisely. The next step, therefore, involves exploring all localizations and all differential diagnoses in context with the set of clinical signs observed.

Investigative procedures should commence with routine hematology, a complete serum biochemistry profile, and serum titers for toxoplasmosis, FeLV/FIV

in cats, and *Neospora caninum* in dogs. Imaging procedures should include radiographs of the thorax, the cervical and thoracic spine, and the tympanic bullae, and orbital ultrasonography. More advanced imaging of the skull and orbit, or even of the neck and thorax, can be pursued with MRI or CT, associated with CSF sampling and analysis.

Prognosis

The prognosis for recovery from Horner's syndrome is mainly associated with the underlying disease. If the cause of the problem is transient, pre- and post-ganglionic innervation will re-establish itself. Preganglionic lesions may require as long as six months to re-establish; postganglionic lesions carry a better prognosis[29, 40, 58]. Resolution time is shortest for animals with traumatic causes and longest for those with Horner's syndrome of iatrogenic or idiopathic origin[32].

Table 14: Localization of the lesion in Horner's syndrome using pharmacologic agents. (Modified from Neer 1984[9], Theisen et al. 1996[33], and Gum 1991[37])

Neuron involved	Location of lesion	Localization of clinical signs	Pharmacologic test
Central (1st order) tecto-tegmento-spinal tract	Hypothalamus	Temperament change, polyuria/polydipsia, polyphagia, hypersexuality.	1% hydroxyamphetamine: normal mydriasis in both eyes. 10% phenylephrine: minimal dilation of both pupils.
	Brainstem	Ipsilateral UMN hemiparesis/hemiplegia, cranial nerve deficits (CN IV-VII), dyspnea, cardiac arrhythmias, altered mentation.	6% cocaine: impaired mydriasis of affected pupil; full mydriasis of normal pupil.
	Cervical spinal cord	Ipsilateral UMN hemiparesis/hemiplegia.	
Pre-ganglionic (2nd order)	Thoracic spinal cord (T1–T3)	Ipsilateral UMN deficits to pelvic limb and LMN deficit to thoracic limb.	1% hydroxyamphetamine: normal mydriasis. 10% phenylephrine: minimal to no dilation of both pupils.
	Ventral roots (T1–T3)	Ipsilateral brachial plexopathy, LMN deficits to thoracic limb, ipsilateral cutaneous trunci reflexe deficit.	6% cocaine: no dilation of affected pupil, full mydriasis of normal pupil.
	Cranial thoracic sympathetic trunk	Possible dyspnea.	
	Cervical (vago) sympathetic trunk	Laceration, sinuses (foreign bodies), swelling (abscess, tumor), pain (trauma), laryngeal hemiparesis/hemiplegia.	
Post-ganglionic (3rd order)	Middle ear	Ipsilateral peripheral vestibular signs, facial nerve paralysis.	1% hydroxyamphetamine: incomplete to no mydriasis of affected pupil, full mydriasis of normal pupil.
	Cavernous sinus	Ipsilateral cranial nerve deficits (III, IV, VI, ophthalmic and maxillary branches of V).	10% phenylephrine: mydriasis of affected pupil, minimal dilation of normal pupil.
	Retrobulbar	Ipsilateral cranial nerve deficits (II, III, IV, VI).	6% cocaine: no dilation of affected pupil, full mydriasis of normal pupil.

UMN = upper motor neuron   LMN = lower motor neuron

NEUROLOGIC SIGNS RELATED TO INNER EAR DISEASE

KEY POINTS
- The inner ear consists of one peripheral receptor for the sense of hearing and one for the organ of balance, the peripheral vestibular apparatus.
- The vestibular system is the primary sensory system responsible for maintaining an animal's balance or its normal orientation relative to the gravitational field of the Earth.
- Signs of inner ear disease include sensorineural deafness and peripheral vestibular disease, ataxia, head tilt, nystagmus, positional strabismus and, sometimes, nausea.
- Peripheral vestibular disease must be differentiated from central vestibular disease.

INTRODUCTION
The vestibular system has two main functions:
- To maintain the visual image by stabilizing the eyes in space during head movements.
- To stabilize the position of the head in space, thus ensuring that the position of the body is stable[1].

Clinically, signs of vestibular disease have been classified either as peripheral or central in order to help localization of the neurologic lesion and to aid in the ranking of a list of differential diagnoses. The anatomic structures concerned include peripheral receptors connected to central receptors.

RECEPTORS OF THE VESTIBULAR SYSTEM
Peripheral receptors
The peripheral vestibular system consists of the membranous semicircular canals, the utricle, and the saccule as well as the vestibular ganglion and the vestibular portion of CN VIII. It develops in conjunction with the receptor for the auditory system. Together they are the components of the inner ear and their anatomic structure has been detailed in Chapter 1 (Gross and microscopic anatomy of the ear: structure and function). Receptors located in the semicircular canals are responsive to angular (rotational) acceleration (or deceleration), while receptors located in the utricle and the saccule are responsive to linear acceleration (or deceleration) and gravity[1].

Vestibulo-cochlear nerve (CN VIII) – vestibular branch
The vestibular nerve is composed of bipolar neurons, with the cell bodies located in the vestibular ganglion.

The axons course through the internal acoustic meatus into the cranial cavity and enter the rostral medulla at the cerebello-medullary angle. Most of these axons terminate in the vestibular nuclei in the rostral medulla. A portion of them enter the cerebellum to terminate in the fastigial nucleus and the flocculonodular lobe[2].

Vestibular nuclei
Although a detailed description of the components of the central vestibular system is beyond the scope of this book, it is important to acquire at least a superficial knowledge of its anatomy and connections. This will allow a better understanding of the difference between clinical signs of peripheral disease as opposed to central vestibular disease.

There are four vestibular nuclei on either side of the medulla, adjacent to the wall of the fourth ventricle in the brainstem. They are grouped into rostral, medial, lateral, and caudal vestibular nuclei. There are numerous projections from the vestibular nuclei into the spinal cord (descending) and the brainstem (ascending):
- Descending pathways remain essentially ipsilateral in the spinal cord. They are responsible for the maintenance of posture and locomotion and are generally responsible for control over the antigravity muscles of the neck and limbs as well as the coordination of movements of the limbs and trunk with movements of the head[1, 3].
- Ascending pathways can be ispsilateral or contralateral. One of them, the medial-longitudinal fasciculus, establishes a connection between the vestibular nuclei and the nuclei of CNs III, IV, and VI, which are responsible for movements of the eyes. This connection provides coordinated, conjugated eye movements associated with changes in the position of the head. Other ascending pathways are directed towards the vomiting center in the reticular formation, which is the pathway underlying motion sickness[1, 3].

Other projections of the vestibular nuclei are directed towards the cerebellum. Through these pathways the vestibular system functions to coordinate the eye, trunk, and limbs with movements of the head. It maintains equilibrium during active and passive movement and when the head is at rest[3].

SIGNS OF VESTIBULAR DISEASE
Ataxia and abnormal posture
As a general rule, signs of vestibular dysfunction are those of loss of balance without loss of muscle strength. As the vestibular system is involved in coordination of movements of the limbs, neck, and trunk with those of the head, the gait observed can be described as ataxic (from the Greek *ataxia* = disorder: *a* = privative; *taxis* = order). Vision helps to compensate for the vestibular system deficit. Therefore, blindfolding an animal with suspected vestibular disease may accentuate the clinical signs. In most cases the disturbance is unilateral, although sometimes both sides may be affected simultaneously[3].

Nystagmus
Nystagmus is one of the described signs of disturbed vestibular function. Physiologic (or vestibular) nystagmus is a normal reflex which helps to maintain visual fixation on stationary points as the body or head rotates. It is usually elicited in both eyes simultaneously with any rapid head movements. Nystagmus is defined as an involuntary rhythmic eyeball oscillation. The movements can occur in any plane, and they can be either equal (pendular) or show a quick and slow phase (jerk). Physiologic nystagmus can be observed in the horizontal or in the vertical plane. Rapid dorsoventral flexion and extension of the animal's head and neck elicits a vertical nystagmus. Side-to-side movements of the head elicit a horizontal nystagmus. The quick phase of the nystagmus is in the direction of the rotation. The labyrinth initiates the slow component whereas the fast component is a function of a brainstem center.

Physiologic nystagmus can also be induced by fast rotation of the whole animal, and this is called postrotational nystagmus. During rotation the quick phase of the nystagmus is in the direction of the rotation. However, once the rotation stops, nystagmus continues to be elicited by movements of the viscous endolymph in the membranous labyrinth. The direction of the endolymph flow is now opposite to the direction of the rotation and the fast phase of the nystagmus becomes opposite to the direction of the rotation.

The individual labyrinths can be tested separately by the caloric test. Irrigation of the external ear canals with ice-cold water sets up currents in the endolymph, stimulating a caloric nystagmus directed to the side opposite to the one being stimulated. However, this test is unreliable and rarely used in the daily neurologic examination of the vestibular system.

If nystagmus occurs when the head is stationary and there is no rotation or movement of the surroundings, it is abnormal and is called spontaneous or resting nystagmus. Spontaneous nystagmus is therefore observed in the posture assumed by the animal and is due to an abnormal input from the vestibular system to the neurons innervating the extraocular muscles. Positional nystagmus is stimulated by changing the orientation of the head. Positional nystagmus may be 'direction-fixed' or 'direction-changing', which means that the direction of the fast phase can change when the head position is altered. More importantly, it can show:
- Latency, i.e. take 10–15 seconds to appear once a new head position is assumed.
- Adaptation, i.e. persist for only a short period after appearing.
- Fatigability, i.e. not reappear after repeated stimulation[4].

Abnormal nystagmus can be horizontal, vertical, or rotatory (i.e. around the axis of the eye). Pendular nystagmus is usually associated with congenital visual deficits and is not of vestibular origin. Both eyeballs are usually affected simultaneously and in the same direction. It has been described in Siamese cats and Belgian Sheepdogs and is reported to be due to a lack of development of the optic chiasm (optic nerve fibers continue into the ipsilateral optic tract without decussation). It has also been attributed to an abnormal sensory input to the system that controls eye movements, or even to an excessive contralateral projection of optic nerve axons in albino cats[3].

It has become customary to describe a nystagmus by the direction of its fast phase, although the slow phase (or drift) is actually the abnormal one when associated with vestibular disease[1, 3].

Strabismus

In normal individuals, when the head is extended dorsally (tonic neck reaction), the eyeballs should remain in the center of the palpebral fissure. This often fails to occur on the side of the vestibular disturbance and results in a dropped or ventrally deviated eyeball (ventral positional strabismus). Occasionally, in vestibular disease, an eye may be deviated ventrally or ventrolaterally without extension of the head, only to be corrected by moving the head or attracting the patient's gaze in a different direction. This is called vestibular strabismus (**337**). It is not due to a paralysis of a cranial nerve, as eye movements are otherwise normal.

Nausea and vomiting

These may be associated with any vestibular disorder but they are more commonly observed in cases of peripheral vestibular disease[2].

LOCALIZATION OF VESTIBULAR DISEASE (SEE *TABLE 15*)

Unilateral peripheral disease

Animals with unilateral peripheral vestibular dysfunction display a head tilt towards the side of the lesion (**338**) and/or spontaneous nystagmus and/or asymmetrical ataxia, with preservation of muscle strength (**339**).

The ataxia is characterized by leaning, drifting, rolling, or falling towards the affected side, and the animal may walk along a wall for additional support. It is common for an affected animal to fall over when shaking its head. The animal may circle in tight circles toward the side of the lesion, and there may be a curvature of the trunk with the concavity directed toward the affected side.

In cases of unilateral peripheral vestibular disease the nystagmus observed is spontaneous, either in a horizontal or a rotary direction. The direction (or fast phase) is always away from the affected side and does not tend to change with the head position. The direction of rotatory nystagmus is defined by the change in the 12 o'clock position of the limbus during the fast phase. Exceptionally, a direction-changing positional nystagmus is observed, which also shows latency, adaptation, and fatigability[4]. The postrotational nystagmus is depressed when the patient is rotated in a direction opposite to the side of a peripheral receptor lesion. The caloric nystagmus will not be observed when the affected side is tested[3].

Ventral positional or vestibular strabismus can be observed in the eye on the affected side. Nausea and vomiting are not infrequent and tend to resolve as the animal adapts to its new head position.

Bilateral peripheral disease

In these cases the ataxia and loss of balance are symmetrical, often resulting in a complete inability to stand, at least in the early days of the problem. The animal is crouched, close to the ground, with its limbs spread apart. Affected animals tend to be reluctant to move at all and if they walk, they stagger or fall to either side. Wide head sway is frequently observed. These patients do not tend to exhibit any nystagmus or strabismus.

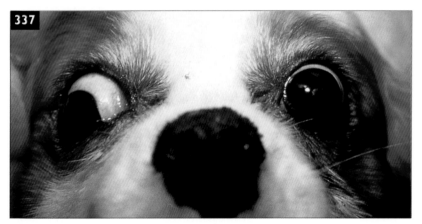

337   Cavalier King Charles Spaniel exhibiting positional ventral strabismus in the right eye due to vestibular disease associated with otitis media. (Illustration courtesy J Penderis.)

Table 15: Comparative neurologic signs of vestibular disease (after Schunk 1990[2]).

Clinical signs	Peripheral vestibular disease	Central vestibular disease
Head tilt	Yes, towards the affected side	Yes, towards the affected side
Nystagmus		
– direction	May vary with head position	May vary with head position
– horizontal	Yes	Yes
– rotary	Yes	Yes
– vertical	No	Yes
Strabismus	Yes	Yes
Ataxia (ipsilateral)	Yes	Yes
Proprioceptive deficits	No	Yes (ipsilateral hemiparesis)
Facial nerve paralysis	Possibly (with otitis media)	Possibly (+/- CNs V, VI, IX, X)
Horner's syndrome	Possibly (with otitis media)	No
Nausea	Yes, often	Sometimes
Mental status	Normal	May be affected

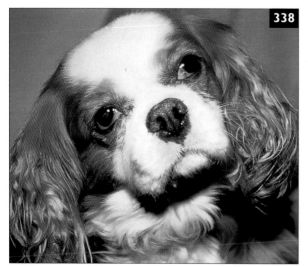

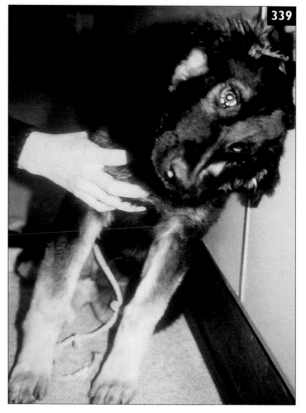

338 Cavalier King Charles Spaniel with right-sided peripheral vestibular disease. Note the head tilt and facial nerve paralysis. (Illustration courtesy J Penderis.)

339 Dog with unilateral vestibular disease exhibiting head tilt and ataxia. The dog is leaning against the wall for support. (Illustration courtesy P Cuddon.)

Central vestibular disease

Although detailed knowledge of the clinical signs associated with central vestibular disease are beyond the scope of this book, it is important to be able to recognize these signs as they allow differentiation of central versus peripheral disease. The neurologic signs that the animal will exhibit, in addition to the normal signs of the vestibular disease, reflect the principal neuroanatomic structures located in the brainstem near the vestibular nuclei.

The most commonly observed signs are due to disruption of long tracts from the cerebral cortex/brainstem to the spinal cord/peripheral nerves and back, passing by the vestibular nuclei. Other connections of the vestibular nuclei (e.g. with the cerebellum) can also be disturbed. Therefore, proprioceptive deficits will be reported in the ipsilateral limbs with normal to increased spinal reflexes (UMN paresis), cerebellar ataxia, or even other cranial nerve disturbances such as facial nerve paralysis. Note that facial nerve paralysis may also be associated with peripheral vestibular disease secondary to otitis media.

Nystagmus is present most of the time. It may be positional or spontaneous and it may be horizontal, rotatory, or vertical. The fast phase is away from the affected side but the direction may change with changes in the head position. The caloric test may elicit nystagmus in an inappropriate direction or dissociated (disconjugate) nystagmus, which suggests a lesion in the vestibular nuclei or the medial longitudinal fasciculus[1].

Positional strabismus can be observed in the ipsilateral eye.

Paradoxical vestibular syndrome

With unilateral peripheral vestibular disease, the head tilt is always towards the side of the lesion. The same applies for central vestibular disease except when the lesion is located at the cerebello-pontine angle or involves more precisely the caudal cerebellar peduncle. In these cases the head tilt and vestibular ataxia are directed towards the side opposite to that of the lesion. The nystagmus will be directed toward the opposite side as well. Cerebellar dysmetria and proprioception deficits will be observed on the affected side and will allow localization of the problem.

CAUSES OF PERIPHERAL VESTIBULAR DISEASE

As in all other aspects of neurologic diseases, it is of utmost importance to localize the disease and establish a list of differential diagnoses before proceeding to any kind of investigative procedures, as these can vary dramatically with the localization of the problem.

The most common way to avoid forgetting possible causes of vestibular diseases is to use the colloquial acronymic mnemonic 'DAMNIT' (D = degenerative diseases; A = abnormalities; M = metabolic diseases; N = neoplasia and nutritional; I = infectious, inflammatory, idiopathic; T = trauma and toxic substances). Cardio-vascular causes should not be forgotten, although they do not tend to play a significant role in dysfunction of the peripheral vestibular system in small animals.

Degenerative diseases

Degenerative peripheral vestibular diseases are mainly due to ototoxicity (see Chapter 8: Ototoxity and other side-effects of otic medication).

Abnormalities (usually congenital diseases)

Congenital peripheral vestibular disease has been described in several breeds of dogs and cats. It has been reported in German Shepherd Dogs[5], Doberman Pinschers[6, 7], English Cocker Spaniels[8], Tibetan Terriers[9], Labrador Retrievers[10], and Siamese and Burmese cats[3]. A congenital bilateral peripheral vestibular syndrome has been reported in Beagle and Akita puppies. Deafness has been associated only with the syndrome described in Beagles and Doberman Pinschers[7].

In most cases signs of peripheral vestibular disease may be noted from birth to four months of age. In German Shepherd Dogs and Siamese cats, abnormal nystagmus was not a common feature, although physiologic nystagmus could not be elicited. The clinical signs were reported to have regressed by 2–4 months of age and although normal function may have occurred, recurrences within a few months of recovery were not infrequent[3]. Signs of unilateral and bilateral peripheral vestibular disease were reported in the two litters of Doberman Pinschers reported by Forbes et al.[6]. They were associated with complete functional deafness and the prognosis was uncertain. The final histopathologic diagnosis was lymphocytic labyrinthitis of unknown origin. The involvement of the same bitch in both litters suggested a possible hereditary component[6]. Deafness was also a component of the syndrome in the litter of Dobermanns described by Wilkes and Palmer[7], and in these cases the prognosis for recovery was good.

Pedigree analysis showed that the condition was likely to be transmitted by an autosomal recessive gene[7].

In general, congenital vestibular disease is associated with a guarded to good prognosis. There is no treatment, and even if return to normal head position and gait is not always the case, affected animals tend to maintain a satisfactory quality of life as long as they can ambulate and feed adequately. The prognosis for the deafness associated with the vestibular syndrome is usually hopeless, as the degenerative changes observed in the cochlea are irreversible.

Metabolic diseases

Hypothyroidism is reported to cause peripheral vestibular disease in a number of dogs, associated or not associated with other signs of peripheral neuropathy or neuromuscular disease[11, 12]. In their study, Jaggy *et al.*[11] reported that of 29 dogs diagnosed with neurologic signs associated with hypothyroidism, nine presented for investigation of vestibular syndrome. The signs of vestibular disease were mostly associated with involvement of other cranial nerves (such as the facial nerve). They were first noticed ten days to four weeks before presentation, with a variable rapidity of onset. The clinical signs of vestibular disease appeared refractory to supplementation with levothyroxine (20 µg/kg p/o q12h), despite subsequent improvement of the other clinical signs of hypothyroidism within two months of treatment. One dog was followed up at three and four months. Its postmedication serum levothyroxine levels were found to be low and a month after the oral dose was doubled, all neurologic signs had resolved[11]. These reports should encourage the practitioner to investigate thyroid function in all cases of suspected vestibular disease.

Very little is known about the pathophysiology of peripheral neuropathy and hypothyroidism. Thyroxin is involved in cellular metabolism, influencing energy production via the activity of the ATP-dependent Na^+/K^+ pump. Therefore, a lack of thyroxin could be altering the pump-dependent axonal transport, leading to axonal degeneration and peripheral neuropathy[11].

Thyroid function is investigated by measuring resting serum total T4 and endogenous canine TSH concentrations. Treatment consists of a starting dose of levothyroxine of 20µg/kg p/o q24h for one week then q12h. The treatment is usually monitored 6–8 weeks later with a premedication and a 4–6 hours postmedication serum T4 assay. The normal resting T4 values are 16–45 nmol/l, whilst normal canine

TSH values are 0–6.0 ng/l. Ideally, the premedication T4 level should be in the upper half of the normal values. The therapeutic T4 levels 4–6 hours post-medication should be well above the upper normal limit. If that is not the case, the oral dose of levothyroxine should be increased by 5 µg/kg q12h and the same monitoring should be repeated six weeks later.

Neoplastic disease
Primary tumors

Primary tumors such as peripheral nerve sheath tumors (Schwannoma, neurofibroma, and neurofibrosarcoma) originating from the vesti-bulocochlear nerve are rare. If they do occur, they are slowly progressive and present with the usual signs of peripheral vestibular syndrome. The signs may progress to those of central vestibular disease if the neoplasm invades the posterior fossa and compresses the brainstem. The prognosis is often poor as surgical resection is difficult in this area. There are no published reports of cases treated with radiotherapy.

Secondary tumors

Secondary tumors arising from structures adjacent to the labyrinth may destroy or compress the inner ear and cause signs of peripheral vestibular disease. They include fibrosarcoma, chondrosarcoma, osteo-sarcoma, ceruminous adenoma, adenosquamous carcinoma[13], adenocarcinoma[14], and squamous cell carcinoma[15].

Polyps

Polyps can be defined as 'benign tumors', although they are described as inflammatory in most reports[16, 17]. Affected cats are generally less than two years of age. Polyps can arise from the nasopharyngeal area or the middle ear. They tend to cause mainly signs of middle ear and upper respiratory tract disease. Occasionally polyps can extend against the vestibular window and cause disruption of the vestibular system. The neurologic signs associated with middle ear disease have been discussed earlier (see Neurologic signs related to middle ear disease). The management of polyps in cats is discussed in detail in Chapter 3 (Nasopharyngeal and middle ear polyps).

Idiopathic diseases
Feline idiopathic vestibular syndrome

This is a disease of unknown cause. In the USA it tends to be seasonal, occurring mostly between early summer and early autumn (June to September). The clinical signs are those of peripheral vestibular disease. They include head tilt, ataxia, rolling, rotatory, or horizontal nystagmus, and occasional vomiting. They do not involve any other cranial nerve. The disease has no sex predilection and the age varies between one year and ten years, with a median of four years[18]. The signs are acute to peracute in onset, frequently developing in one hour or less, and they are usually unilateral. Affected animals tend to stabilize within 24 hours and the nystagmus disappears over several days. The ataxia resolves gradually, but may persist for up to 3–6 weeks. Exhaustive diagnostic work up is unremarkable, making idiopathic feline vestibular syndrome a diagnosis of exclusion. Except for supportive care in anorexic or vomiting cases, there is no treatment that will alter the course of the disease and the prognosis is generally excellent[19]. Most cats experience only one episode of idiopathic vestibular syndrome[18].

Canine idiopathic vestibular syndrome
This disease is recognized in older dogs, and it is also sometimes called 'old dog vestibular disease'. It is characterized by acute onset of head tilt, asymmetric ataxia, and nystagmus. The signs are very similar to those described for the feline idiopathic syndrome. The diagnosis, as in feline idiopathic vestibular syndrome, is one of exclusion. The syndrome is usually self-limiting within 72 hours, although some of the signs can persist for several days to weeks. No specific therapy is available[20]. It is rare for dogs to suffer more than one episode of this disease.

Infectious diseases
Infectious causes of otitis interna usually relate to associated otitis media. (See Chapter 5: Otitis media, otitis interna for further details.)

Inflammatory diseases
Unilateral or bilateral signs of peripheral vestibular disease have been observed with facial nerve paresis or paralysis in mature dogs without evidence of otitis media[3]. A few patients affected by this combination of neuropathy or neuritis recovered spontaneously. However, the author describing these clinical signs[3] did not report the investigative procedures that led to the exclusion of otitis media. As described in the study by Cole et al.[21], otitis media can be subclinical and should not be ruled out unless myringotomy is performed and followed by culture and sensitivity of the local microflora.

Traumatic causes
Trauma to the inner ear and peripheral vestibular system in small dogs and cats can arise as a result of encounters with larger animals or because of head injury subsequent to a road traffic accident. Fractures of the petrous temporal bone or hemorrhage within the tympanic bullae are more frequently reported in larger dogs[22], but they can occur in small animals and these differentials should be investigated. In these cases the signs of peripheral vestibular disease may be masked by neurologic symptoms indicating involvement of the central nervous system or musculoskeletal system, and they can be associated with facial nerve paralysis or Horner's syndrome (see Neurologic signs related to middle ear disease).

Toxic diseases
A large variety of drugs cause ototoxicity, affecting vestibular function, hearing, or both. Most of these agents initially cause damage to the receptors, leading eventually to degeneration of the nerve. Toxicity can occur from either systemic or topical therapy[23]. Causes and clinical signs of ototoxicity are discussed in detail in Chapter 8 (Ototoxicity and other side-effects of otic medication).

SENSORINEURAL DEAFNESS
Physiology of hearing
The pinna and external ear canal act as a collector of sound and they are useful in sound localization[24]. Sound waves in the external ear canal cause vibrations of the tympanic membrane. These vibrations are then transmitted through the ossicles, the malleus, the incus, and the stapes to the oval window of the cochlea (**340**) (see Chapter 1: Gross and microscopic anatomy of the ear: structure and function; and Chapter 2: Neurologic examination of the ear). Vibrations of the tympanum may be as small as the diameter of a hydrogen molecule and they are transmitted with negligible distortion but with increased power by the ossicles. Damage to these structures can result in conductive deafness despite a normal cochlea.

Muscle tension in the tensor tympanii muscle and the stapedius muscle attached to the stapes allows the animal to reduce or enhance sensitivity[25]. Vibrations are then further transmitted from the oval window into the perilymph of the scala vestibuli. This canal joins the scala tympani at the apex of the cochlea so that the inward deflection of the oval window produced by the stapes results in an outward deflection of the round window. Within the cochlear duct, hair cell stereocilia of the organ of Corti are embedded in the tectorial membrane (see Chapter 1: Gross and microscopic anatomy of the ear: structure and function) so that shearing forces from sound waves propagated along the scala vestibuli produce bending of the stereocilia, thereby depolarizing their cells. From there, synaptic connections between hair cells and spiral ganglion neurons result in transmission of information through the cochlear branch of the vestibulocochlear nerve[26].

Auditory function is present when the ear canals open at the age of 12–14 days in dogs and five days in cats. However, behavioral response to loud noises can be detected before the canals open[27]. Reported hearing frequencies range from 45–67 kHz in dogs and 45–78 kHz in cats[28, 29]. Electrophysiologic studies of the sense of hearing suggest that the most sensitive level of hearing is reached by the age of 20 days in dogs[30] and 30 days in cats[31]. The hearing threshold of veterinary patients who cannot respond reliably to conventional hearing tests can be estimated by brainstem auditory evoked response (BAER), an objective electrophysiologic test. The technical aspects of this test are discussed in detail in Chapter 2 (Electrophysiologic procedures). Studies report various hearing thresholds in dogs of different sizes and in different experimental settings. These thresholds vary between –5 dB nHL (normal hearing level)[32] up to 40 dB nHL[30] in the dog. (0 dB nHL is the average threshold for disappearance of hearing behavior in a normal human population.)

When evaluating hearing it is important to remember that vibration through air and surfaces can also be felt via extracochlear mechanoreceptors. An animal may react to the vibrations of a door slammed rather than actually hear the sound produced. Vibrations can also be 'heard' by transmission through the skull to the inner ear and auditory system. This is the basis for bone-conducted stimulation in auditory testing (see Chapter 2: Electrophysiologic procedures)[33].

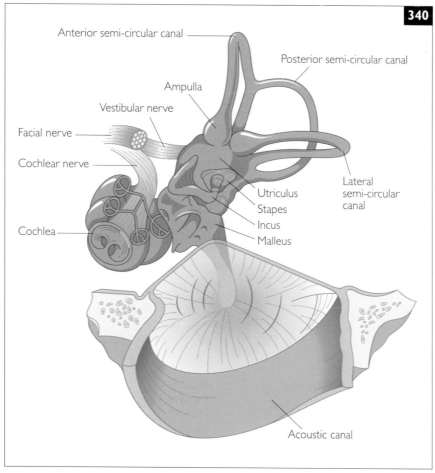

340 Schematic diagram showing the major relationships of the canine ear.

Classification of deafness

Peripheral deafness can be characterized by three pairs of descriptors:

- Inherited versus acquired.
- Congenital versus late-onset.
- Sensorineural versus conductive.

This results in eight classifications of deafness, but only three types are commonly seen in dogs and cats: inherited congenital sensorineural; acquired late-onset sensorineural; and acquired late-onset conductive. Inherited congenital sensorineural deafness is usually, but not always, associated with pigmentation genes responsible for white in the coat. Acquired late-onset sensorineural deafness is most often associated with ototoxicity or age (presbycusis), but it can also be associated with a breed predisposition or result from otitis interna, noise, and other causes. Acquired late-onset conductive deafness is associated with otitis media and is discussed earlier in this chapter (Neurologic signs related to middle ear disease). Acquired congenital deafness may result from malformation, intrauterine infections, or drug toxicity but these are uncommon[34].

Etiologies of deafness

Congenital sensorineural deafness

Prevalence. In 1896, Rawitz first described a case of canine congenital deafness in a white dog with blue eyes[35], and in 1898, Charles Darwin reported his observation of entirely white cats with blue eyes being generally deaf[36].

The incidence of congenital deafness in the canine and feline population is unknown but the occurrence of deafness may reach 30% in selected breeds, such as the Dalmatian; the incidence reported currently in the US is 8% bilateral deafness and 22% unilateral deafness[26].

Pathophysiology. Congenital deafness is a degenerative process that manifests itself at various ages. However, in an epidemiologic study of canine congenital deafness, 50% of the deaf animals were diagnosed before six months of age[37]. Although the degenerative process can start as early as one day after birth, congenitally affected dogs such as Dalmatians do not become deaf until 3–4 weeks after birth[34]. Inherited hearing dysfunction does not necessarily result in total deafness in all breeds affected. Although any breed of dog can be affected, a list of predisposed canine breeds has been established (*Table 16*) and is constantly growing. Reports of breed-associated congenital deafness in cats are not available but blue-eyed, white cats have a high incidence of deafness.

Genetics. Hereditary deafness associated with pigmentation abnormalities has been reported as a syndrome with a spectrum of features including piebaldism or partial albinism, deafness, heterochromia iridis (blue iris or irides attributable to absence of pigment), absence of retinal pigment, and absence of pigment in the cochlear stria vascularis[26, 38, 39].

In cats the syndrome results from a dominant autosomal gene W that is fully dominant with respect to the production of white fur and incompletely dominant in the production of a blue iris. However, gene W expresses incomplete penetrance with respect to deafness[40].

Table 16: List of breeds affected by congenital deafness[7, 8, 26, 34, 37, 44, 45, 50, 52–54].

Akita	Dachshund (Dappled)	Ibizan Hound	Saint Bernard
American Staffordshire Terrier	Dalmatian	Jack Russell Terrier	Schnauzer
Australian Blue Heeler	Doberman Pinscher	Kuvasz	Scottish Terrier
Australian Shepherd Dog	Dogo Argentino	Labrador Retriever	Sealyham Terrier
Beagle	English Bulldog	Maltese	Shetland Sheepdog
Bichon Frise	English Setter	Miniature Pinscher	Shropshire Terrier
Border Collie	Foxhound	Norwegian Dunkerhound	Siberian Husky
Boston Terrier	Fox Terrier	Old English Sheepdog	Springer Spaniel
Boxer	French Bulldog	Papillon	Walker American Foxhound
Bulldog	German Shepherd Dog	Pitbull Terrier	West Highland White Terrier
Bull Terrier	Great Dane	Pointer	White cats
Catahoula Leopard Dog	Great Pyrennees (Pyrenean	Poodle (Toy, Miniature)	
Cocker Spaniel	Mountain Dog)	Rhodesian Ridgeback	
Collie	Greyhound	Rottweiler	

Deafness in dogs is frequently associated with the presence of the merle or dapple (M) gene (e.g. Collie, Shetland Sheepdog, Harlequin Great Dane, Dappled Dachshund) and the piebald (S^P) or extreme piebald (S^w) gene (e.g. Bull Terrier, Great Pyrennees [Pyrenean Mountain Dog], Dalmatian) where large amounts of white are present in the fur.

The merle gene is dominant, and heterozygous dogs (Mm) show the 'merle' pattern (**341**). Homozygous individuals (MM) have a solid white coat and blue irises and they are often deaf and/or blind and sterile. Heterozygous merles can also be deaf, with the likelihood of deafness increasing with the amount of white in the coat.

Genetic transmission of deafness in dogs with the piebald and extreme piebald genes, such as the Dalmatian, is less clear. The gene responsible for deafness is neither dominant nor recessive and there is increasing suspicion that there is more than one gene involved in the transmission of this congenital disease. In the Dalmatian the underlying color of the coat is black (B) or liver (b, simple recessive). The extreme piebald gene (S^w) covers the color with white, and the dominant ticking gene (T) opens the spots through the white. In Dalmatians with a patch the gene S^w does not completely suppress the underlying coat colour; the S^w gene is only weakly expressed. Patched Dalmatians have been shown to have significantly lower deafness rates but patches are not allowed in the breed standard. Conversely, blue-eyed Dalmatians, where the normal brown iris pigment is suppressed, are significantly more likely to be deaf[41]. Dalmatians that are the offspring of one bilaterally hearing parent and one unilaterally deaf parent are twice as likely to be deaf (unilaterally or bilaterally) as dogs born from bilaterally normal parents[34, 42].

Histopathology. The histopathologic finding described in most breeds of dogs and cats with congenital sensorineural deafness is known as cochleosaccular-type of end organ degeneration. In Dalmatians degeneration begins in the middle coil of the cochlea, followed by the basal and then the apical coils[43]. The stria vascularis lining the outer wall of the cochlear duct is the major vascular area of the cochlea and this produces endolymph, which is necessary for the maintenance of cochlear hair cells. Sensorineural deafness may result from direct damage to hair cells by neuroepithelial degeneration or from hair cell loss secondary to strial degeneration[26].

In congenitally deaf animals this degenerative process includes collapse of the cochlear duct and the saccule, adhesion of the Reissner membrane to the basilar membrane, replacement of the hair cells in the organ of Corti by an irregular arrangement of cells, and presence of colloid bodies in the cochlear canal. The tectorial membrane has been reported to be swollen and tucked into the internal spiral sulcus and connective tissue can accumulate in the cochlear aqueduct[44]. The stria vascularis is atrophied throughout the cochlea and its blood supply is markedly less than normal. Secondary loss of spiral ganglion cells is also described at later stages. Melanin pigmentation is

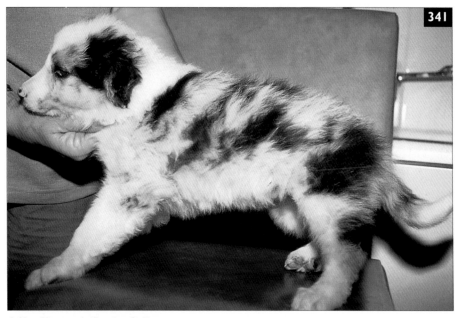

341 Blue merle Border Collie pup.

also diminished, which has to be considered in relation to the coat color of affected individuals. It is important to note that the temporal bone, middle ear, utricle, and semicircular canals were found to be normal[45, 46]. However, in congenitally deaf Dalmatians, anatomic alterations were observed in the temporal lobes of the cerebrum, the auditory pathways in the brainstem, and even in the acoustic nerve[47]. Although Ferrara *et al.*[47] suspected that these changes might be the primary cause of the deafness, they are most likely secondary to the lack of sensory input.

A few exceptions to the Dalmatian model of deafness exist. In Shropshire Terriers the deafness is due to a degeneration of the scala media[48], whereas a cochlear aplasia has been described in a Foxhound[49, 50]. In Doberman Pinschers the hearing impairment comes from direct loss of cochlear hair cells without any effects on the stria vascularis[51].

Acquired late-onset conductive deafness

Conductive deafness is most often secondary to chronic otitis externa and otitis media, where stenosis and eventual occlusion of the external ear canal or impaction from excess accumulation of cerumen occurs[34].

Acquired late-onset sensorineural deafness

Ototoxicity. Ototoxic agents may cause hearing loss or deafness by direct effects on cochlear or vestibular hair cells, or they may cause damage to the stria vascularis with secondary hair cell loss. Over 180 compounds and classes of compounds have been identified as ototoxic[34]. Otoxicity is discussed in Chapter 8 (Ototoxicity and other side-effects of otic medications).

Presbycusis. Presbycusis is the decline in hearing associated with various types of auditory system dysfunction that accompany ageing, and that cannot be accounted for by traumatic, genetic, or pathologic conditions[55]. Four types of presbycusis are described in man[56] and dogs:

- Sensory presbycusis, characterized by loss of hair cells and degeneration of the organ of Corti[2].
- Neural presbycusis, characterized by primary degeneration of neural elements, including the cells of the spiral ganglion and the fibers in the cochlear nerve[3, 57].
- Strial, or metabolic presbycusis, characterized by atrophy of the stria vascularis and a flat audiometric loss.
- Inner ear conductive or mechanical presbycusis, characterized by changes in the structure and mechanical properties of the basilar membrane[58].

Presbycusis is common in geriatric dogs[59]. Although it is a progressive phenomenon, owners often report sudden onset deafness. This is most likely due to the ability of the animal to compensate for hearing loss until nearly complete deafness occurs. Hearing aids have been successfully placed in dogs with residual hearing capabilities, but the ear plug is not always well tolerated by veterinary patients, particularly cats. The success of the hearing aid rests on the ability of the owner to train the dog to tolerate the presence of such a foreign body in the ear canal[34].

Noise. Noise-induced hearing loss or deafness can be temporary or permanent[60]. Temporary increases in hearing threshold occur after brief exposure to intense sounds (over 100 dB), with gradual recovery of function occurring over periods ranging from minutes to two weeks. Noise-induced hearing loss is thought to result from either disarrangement or breakage of hair cilia[61] but it can also result from damage to the tympanum or the ossicles. Continuous or repeated exposure to noise results in a progressive loss of hair cells and corresponding hearing threshold. Dogs regularly used to work with guns may develop noise-induced hearing loss[34].

Breed predisposition. Cavalier King Charles Spaniels are reported to develop an early onset hearing impairment. In one study, nine dogs were evaluated between the age of 14 and 93 months and found to have elevated hearing threshold as assessed by BAER[62]. This type of deafness could be classified as 'inherited late-onset conductive deafness'; the suspected genetic origin has not yet been demonstrated.

Infectious disease. Infectious otitis interna responsible for hearing loss is only a rare histopathologic diagnosis as affected animals maintain a satisfactory quality of life and their clinical signs seldom warrant euthanasia. However, an unusual case of sensorineural hearing loss due to *Prothoteca zopfii* is reported in the literature[63]. In the case described the agent was also causing blindness due to intraocular disease and postmortem examination revealed a polysystemic involvement.

Other causes. Hearing loss or deafness may also result from meningitis, anoxia, anesthesia, and trauma, or a combination of these causes[64].

Diagnosis of deafness

The diagnosis of deafness in veterinary patients is based initially on a high index of suspicion or astute observation by the owner or breeder. Indeed, since the ear canal does not open until a few days after birth, and deaf puppies and kittens often take cues from the response of their littermates, it is not uncommon for deafness to go unrecognized for several weeks. Bilaterally deaf puppies may display a more aggressive behavior, as they cannot hear the cries of pain when playing with their littermates. Deaf animals tend to sleep very deeply as they are unperturbed by auditory stimuli and do not wake up unless jostled. Bilateral deafness can be observed during a routine physical examination if the animal is blindfolded and vibrations are avoided during auditory stimuli. The minimum response expected is a Preyer's reflex (twitching of the ears in response to the sound). However, unilateral deafness is rarely picked up during routine physical examination as the normal ear compensates quite well for the dysfunctional ear. Extremely observant owners report that unilaterally deaf patients have difficulty orienting the origin of sounds, but this is an exception rather than the rule.

The only objective means of diagnosing deafness and establishing the degree of hearing loss is based on electrophysiologic evaluation of each ear by means of BAER. This may be one of a series of investigative procedures described in detail in Chapter 2 (Electrophysiologic procedures).

Prognosis and management of deafness

Despite progress made in the field of human deafness, very little has been done towards treating or assisting deaf veterinary patients. Canine hearing aids have been developed but their use remains anecdotal. They have been used mainly in animals which have retained some degree of hearing. They are known to be expensive and of short benefit to the treated animal. They work as amplifiers and therefore need the retained ability of the hearing apparatus to hear sounds, even at a very low level. Congenital deafness is an irreversible phenomenon, and as it tends to be complete in the affected ear in most cases, hearing aids would not be helpful.

Dogs and cats with unilateral congenital deafness make excellent pets, with owners often unable to detect any impairment. However, in order to prevent further spreading of the defect in the breed, owners should be discouraged from breeding from affected animals. Some animals may show difficulty localizing sounds or may not awaken to sounds if sleeping on the normal ear[34].

Animals with late-onset acquired deafness generally adapt well, but precautions must be observed to prevent vehicular injury or death and also bite injuries to humans, especially to children, when deaf dogs are startled[34]. Noise-induced hearing loss acquired slowly, over time, is unfortunately irreversible, as living for

years in a very noisy environment causes a gradual killing of hair cells. However, resting in a quiet environment (less than 70 dB) for three weeks can reverse impulsive noise-induced hearing loss as is observed in the case of dogs working with guns. The result of impulsive noise seems to be mainly a disarrangement of the cilia, which resolves with time and silence[61].

Animals bilaterally deaf from both congenital and acquired etiologies rely more on visual and odoriferous cues as well as on vibrations to cope with their disability. They can be trained to read their owner's body language and interpret cues such a flashing porch light or obedience-training shock collars set to the lowest shock level as a call back signal[34].

Despite the worry of their owners and those concerned with animal rights, the quality of life of deaf dogs and cats is not demonstrably diminished. These animals do not have any more diminished mental capabilities than their human counterparts. A dilemma often occurs when bilaterally deaf puppies are identified in a litter. The official position of the Dalmatian Club of America is that such animals should be euthanased, but this position is not universally accepted. This recommendation becomes even more difficult once the deaf animal has been placed in a home, as emotional attachment develops rapidly. Although it may not always be the case, congenitally deaf dogs are prone to untimely death by road traffic accident and they may develop anxious or aggressive personalities from continuously being startled. They are undoubtedly more difficult to rear and often end up in animal shelters because of their owner's inability to cope with the hearing impairment. When possible, cats should be confined to the house and dogs restricted to a fenced yard or to exercise only on the lead[34, 42].

Genetic counselling for breeders is delicate as the exact mode of inheritance is as yet undetermined. However, common sense dictates the elimination of affected individuals from breeding and systematically screening breeding stock and offspring, as the defect can be present in the litter from two healthy parents[34]. Screening schemes using BAER are currently organized at various veterinary centers in the UK and the USA in collaboration with the Dalmatian Club and other breed associations. It is important to remember that electrophysiologic testing (with BAER amongst other procedures) is the only objective means of evaluating the hearing status of veterinary patients (see Chapter 2: Electrophysiologic procedures).

REFERENCES

APPROACH TO THE DIAGNOSIS OF OTITIS EXTERNA

1 August JR (1988) Otitis externa: a disease of multifactorial etiology. *Veterinary Clinics of North America* **18**, 731–742.

ACUTE OTITIS EXTERNA

1 Joyce JA and Day MJ (1997) Immunopathogenesis of canine aural haematoma. *Journal of Small Animal Practice* **38**, 152–158.
2 White SD and Sequoia D (1989) Food hypersensitivity in cats: 14 cases (1982–1987). *Journal of the American Veterinary Medical Association* **194**, 692–695.
3 Kiss G, Radvanyi Sz and Szigeti G (1997) New combination for the therapy of canine otitis externa. I: Microbiology of otitis externa. *Journal of Small Animal Practice* **38**, 51–56.
4 Scott DW (1980) External ear disease. *Journal of the American Animal Hospital Association* **16**, 426–433.
5 Griffin CE (1993) Otitis externa and otitis media. In *Current Veterinary Dermatology*. (eds CE Griffin, KW Kwochka and JM MacDonald) Mosby, St Louis, pp. 244–262.
6 Stout Graham M, Kainer RA, Whalen LR and Macy DW (1990) Morphologic measurements of the external ear canal of dogs. *American Journal of Veterinary Research* **51**, 990–994.

GRAM-NEGATIVE OTITIS EXTERNA

1 Carlotti DN, Guaguere E, Denerolle P, Madin F, Collet JP and Leroy S (1995) A retrospective study of otitis externa in dogs. *Proceedings of the 11th Annual Meeting of the AAVD/ACVD*, Santa Fe, p. 84.
2 Kiss G, Radvanyi Sz and Szigeti G (1997) New combination for the therapy of canine otitis externa. I: Microbiology of otitis externa. *Journal of Small Animal Practice* **38**, 51–56.
3 Mathison PT, Simpson B, Heithamer T, McCurdy D and Fadok V (1995) Development of a canine model for *Pseudomonas* otitis externa. *Proceedings of the 11th Annual Meeting of the AAVD/ACVD*, Santa Fe, p. 21.
4 Fraser G (1961) Factors predisposing to canine external otitis. *Veterinary Record* **73**, 55–58.
5 Grono LR and Frost AJ (1969) Otitis externa in the dog. *Australian Veterinary Journal* **45**, 420–422.
6 Merchant SR (1994) Ototoxicity. In *Veterinary Clinics of North America*. (eds RAW Rosychuck and SR Merchant) **24**, 971–980.
7 Bogaard van den AEJM and Bohm ROB (1986) Silbersulfadiazincreme als therapie bei chronischen Pseudomonas infektionen des ausseren Gehorganges des hundes. *Prakt Tierarztl* **67**, 963–966.
8 Noxon JO, Kinyon JM and Murphy DP (1997) Minimum inhibitory concentration of silver sulfadiazine on *Pseudomonas aeruginosa* and *Staphylococcus intermedius* isolates from the ears of dogs with otitis externa. *Proceedings of the 13th Annual Meeting of the AAVD/ACVD*, Nashville, pp. 12–13.
9 Foster AP and DeBoer DJ (1998) The role of *Pseudomonas* in canine ear disease. *Compendium on Continuing Education* **20**, 909–919.
10 McKeever PJ (1996) Otitis externa. *Compendium on Continuing Education* **18**, 759–772.
11 Rosychuck RAW (1994) Management of otitis externa. In *Veterinary Clinics of North America*. (eds RAW Rosychuck and SR Merchant) **24**, 921–952.
12 Griffin CE (1993) Otitis externa. In *Current Veterinary Dermatology*. (eds CE Griffin, KW Kwochka and JM Macdonald) Mosby, St Louis, pp. 245–262.
13 Little CJL (1996) Medical treatment of otitis externa in the dog and cat. *In Practice* **18**, 66–71.
14 Waker RD, Stein GE, Hauptman JG and MacDonald KH (1992) Pharmacokinetic evaluation of enrofloxacin administered orally to healthy dogs. *American Journal of Veterinary Research* **12**, 2315–2319.
15 Rosin E, Fialkowski J and Kujak J (1996) Enroflaxacin and ciprofloxacin dosage in *Pseudomonas* infection in dogs. *Veterinary Surgery* **25**, 436–437.
16 McKellar QA (1996) Clinical relevance of the pharmacological properties of fluoroquinolones. *Proceedings of the 2nd International Veterinary Symposium on Fluoroquinolones*, pp. 14–21.
17 Salyer AA and Whitt DD (1994) *Pseudomonas aeruginosa*. In *Bacterial Pathogenesis: a Molecular Approach*. (eds AA Salyers and DD Whitt) ASM Press, Washington, pp. 260–270.
18 Nuttall TJ (1998) Use of ticarcillin in the management of canine otitis externa complicated by *Pseudomonas aeruginosa*. *Journal of Small Animal Practice* **39**, 165–168.
19 Yuan D and Shen V (1975) Stability of ribosomal and transfer ribonucleic acid in *Escherichia coli* B/V after treatment with ethylene-diamine tetra-acetic acid and rifampin. *Journal of Bacteriology* **122**, 425–432.
20 Farca AM, Piromalli G, Maffei F and Re G (1997) Potentiating effects of EDTA-tris on the activity of antibiotics against resistant bacteria associated with otitis, dermatitis and cystitis. *Journal of Small Animal Practice* **38**, 243–245.
21 Wooley RE and Jones MS (1983) Action of EDTA-tris and antimicrobial agent combinations on selected pathogenic bacteria. *Veterinary Microbiology* **8**, 271–280.

CHRONIC, OR RECURRENT, OTITIS EXTERNA IN DOGS

1 Moriello KA, Fehrer-Swaer SL, Meyer DJ and Feder B (1988) Adrenocortical suppression associated with topical otic administration of glucocorticoids in dogs. *Journal of the American Veterinary Medical Association* **193**, 329–331.
2 Griffin CE (1993) Otitis externa. In *Current Veterinary Dermatology*. (eds CE Griffin, KW Kwochka and JM Macdonald) Mosby, St Louis, pp. 245–262.
3 Chester DK (1988) Medical management of otitis externa. In *Veterinary Clinics of North America*. (ed JR August) **18**, 799–812.
4 Neer TM (1982) Otitis media. *Compendium on Continuing Education* **4**, 410–417.
5 Cole LK, Kwochka KW, Kowalski JJ and Hillier A (1998) Microbial flora and antimicrobial susceptibility patterns of isolated pathogens from the horizontal ear canal and middle ear in dogs with otitis media. *Journal of the American Veterinary Medical Association* **212**, 534–538.
6 Baba E, Fukata T and Saito M (1981) Incidence of otitis externa in dogs and cats in Japan. *Veterinary Record* **108**, 393–395.
7 Lane JG and Little CJL (1986) Surgery of the canine external auditory meatus: a review of failures. *Journal of Small Animal Practice* **27**, 247–254.

CHRONIC, OR RECURRENT, OTITIS EXTERNA IN CATS

1 Powell MB, Weisbroth SH, Roth L and Wilhelmsen C (1980) Reaginic hypersensitivity in *Otodectes cynotis* infestation of cats and mode of mite feeding. *American Journal of Veterinary Research* **6**, 877–881.

2 Scott DW and Horn RT (1987) Zoonotic dermatoses of dogs and cats. *Veterinary Clinics of North America* **17**, 117–144.

3 Mansfield PD, Boosinger TR and Attleburger MH (1990) Infectivity of *Malassezia pachydermatis* in the external ear canal of dogs. *Journal of the American Animal Hospital Association* **26**, 97–100.

4 Bond R, Anthony RM, Dodd M and Lloyd DH (1996) Isolation of *Malassezia sympodialis* from feline skin. *Journal of Medical and Veterinary Mycology* **34**, 145–147.

5 Katapkin AS, Matthieson DT, Noone NE et al. (1990) Results of surgery and long-term follow up in 31 cats with nasopharyngeal polyps. *Journal of the American Animal Hospital Association* **26**, 387–392.

6 Brownlie SE and Bedford PGC (1985) Nasopharyngeal polyp in a kitten. *Veterinary Record* **117**, 25–26.

7 van der Gaag I (1986) The pathology of the external ear canal in dogs and cats. *Veterinary Quarterly* **8**, 307–317.

8 London CA, Dubilzeig RR, Vail DM et al. (1996) Evaluation of dogs and cats with tumors of the ear canal: 145 cases (1978–1992). *Journal of the American Veterinary Medical Association* **208**, 1413–1418.

9 Scott DW (1980) Feline dermatology: a monograph. *Journal of the American Animal Hospital Association* **16**, 426–433.

10 Rosser EJ (1993) Food allergy in the cat: a prospective study of 13 cats. In *Advances in Veterinary Dermatology, Volume 2*. (eds PJ Ihrke, IS Mason and SD White) Pergammon Press, Oxford, pp. 33–39.

11 White SD and Sequoia D (1989) Food hypersensitivity in cats: 14 cases (1982–1987). *Journal of the American Veterinary Medical Association* **194**, 692–695.

12 Stogdale L, Bomzom L and van den Berg PB (1982) Food allergy in cats. *Journal of the American Animal Hospital Association* **18**, 188–194.

13 Wills JM and Harvey RG (1994) Diagnosis and management of food allergy and intolerance in dogs and cats. *Australian Veterinary Journal* **71**, 322–326.

NEUROLOGIC SIGNS RELATED TO MIDDLE EAR DISEASE

1 Evans HE (1993) The ear. In *Miller's Anatomy of the Dog*. (ed HE Evans) WB Saunders, Philadelphia, pp. 988–1008.

2 Little CJL and Lane JG (1986) The surgical anatomy of the feline bulla tympanica. *Journal of Small Animal Practice* **27**, 371–378.

3 Evans HE and Kitchell RL (1993) Cranial nerves and cutaneous innervation of the head. In *Miller's Anatomy of the Dog*. (ed HE Evans) WB Saunders, Philadelphia, pp. 953–987.

4 Evans HE (1993) The skeleton. In *Miller's Anatomy of the Dog*. (ed HE Evans) WB Saunders, Philadelphia, pp. 122–218.

5 Kern TJ and Hollis NE (1987) Facial neuropathy in dogs and cats: 95 cases (1975–1985). *Journal of the American Veterinary Medical Association* **191**, 1604–1609.

6 DeLahunta A (1983) *Veterinary Neuroanatomy and Clinical Neurology*. 2nd edn. WB Saunders, Philadelphia, pp. 115–129.

7 Stromberg MW (1993) The autonomic nervous system. In *Miller's Anatomy of the Dog*. (ed HE Evans) WB Saunders, Philadelphia, pp. 776–799.

8 Scagliotti RH (1980) Current concepts in veterinary neuro-ophthalmology. *Veterinary Clinics of North America: Small Animal Practice* **10**, 417–436.

9 Neer TM (1984) Horner's syndrome: anatomy, diagnosis, and causes. *Compendium on Continuing Education* **6**, 740–746.

10 Petersen-Jones SM (1995) Abnormalities of eyes and vision. In *Manual of Small Animal Neurology*. (ed SJ Wheeler) BSAVA, Cheltenham, pp. 125–142.

11 Busch DS, Noxon JO and Miller LD (1992) Laryngeal paralysis and peripheral vestibular disease in a cat. *Journal of the American Animal Hospital Association* **28**, 82–86.

12 Indrieri RJ and Taylor RF (1984) Vestibular dysfunction caused by squamous cell carcinoma involving the middle ear and inner ear in two cats. *Journal of the American Veterinary Medical Association* **184**, 471–473.

13 Luttgen PJ (1994) Deafness in the dog and cat. *Veterinary Clinics of North America* **24**, 981–989.

14 Little CJL (1991) Inflammatory middle ear disease of the dog: the clinical and pathological features of cholesteatoma, a complication of otitis media. *Veterinary Record* **128**, 319–322.

15 Eger C and Lindsay P (1997) Effects of otitis on hearing in dogs characterised by brainstem auditory evoked response testing. *Journal of Small Animal Practice* **38**, 380–386.

16 Braund KG (1994) *Clinical Syndromes in Veterinary Neurology*. 2nd edn. Mosby, St Louis, pp. 81–332.

17 McAnulty JF, Hattel A and Harvey CE (1995) Wound healing and brainstem auditory evoked potentials after experimental total ear canal ablation with lateral tympanic bulla osteotomy in dogs. *Veterinary Research* **24**, 1–8.

18 McAnulty JF, Hattel A and Harvey CE (1995) Wound healing and brainstem auditory evoked potentials after experimental ventral tympanic bulla osteotomy in dogs. *Veterinary Surgery* **24**, 9–14.

19 Marshall AE (1990) Comment on 'Reduction of spiral ganglion neurons in the ageing canine with hearing loss'. *Advances in Small Animal Medicine and Surgery* **2**, 5–7.

20 Sommerlad S, Mackenzie D, Divitni J, Goldstein L and Filippich L (1999) Surgical placement and efficacy of a bone-anchored hearing aid in a dog with conductive deafness. *Australian Veterinary Practitioner* **29**, 70–80.

21 Knowles K, Blauch B, Leipold H, Cash W and Hewett J (1989) Reduction of spiral ganglion in the ageing canine with hearing loss. *Journal of Veterinary Medicine* **36**, 188–199.

22 Luttgen PJ (1990) Diseases of the nervous system in older dogs. Part II: Peripheral nervous system. *Compendium on Continuing Education* **12**, 1077–1081.

23 Petersen-Jones SM (1989) Neuro-ophthalmology. *British Veterinary Journal* **145**, 99–120.

24 Jaggy A, Oliver JE, Ferguson DC, Mahaffey EA and Glaus-T Jnr (1994) Neurological manifestations of hypothyroidism: a retrospective study of 29 dogs. *Journal of Veterinary Internal Medicine* **8**, 328–336.

25 Braund KG, Steiss JE, Amling KA et al. (1987) Insulinoma and subclinical peripheral neuropathy in two dogs. *Journal of Veterinary Internal Medicine* **1**, 86–90.

26 Rendano VT, DeLahunta A and King JM (1980) Extracranial neoplasia with facial nerve paralysis in two cats. *Journal of the American Animal Hospital Association* **16**, 921–925.

27 Braund KG, Luttgen PG, Sorjonen DC and Redding RW (1979) Idiopathic facial nerve paralysis in the dog. *Veterinary Record* **105**, 297–299.

28 Braund KG, Vandevelds M, Walker TL and Redding RW (1978)

Granulomatous meningoencephalomyelitis in six dogs. *Journal of the American Veterinary Medical Association* **172**, 1195–1200.

29 Jones BR and Studdert VP (1975) Horner's syndrome in the dog and cat as an aid to diagnosis. *Australian Veterinary Journal* **51**, 329–332.

30 Innes DC (1973) How temperature changes hair color in the Siamese. *Feline Practice* **3**, 23–29.

31 Laties AM (1972) Specific neurohistology comes of age: a look back and a look forward. *Investigatory Ophthalmology* **11**, 555–584.

32 Morgan RV and Zanotti SW (1989) Horner's syndrome in dogs and cats: 49 cases (1980–1986). *Journal of the American Veterinary Medical Association* **194**, 1096–1099.

33 Theisen SK, Podell M, Schneider T, Wilkie DA and Fenner WR (1996) A retrospective study of cavernous sinus syndrome in four dogs and eight cats. *Journal of Veterinary Internal Medicine* **10**, 65–75.

34 Scagliotti RH (1991) Neuro-ophthalmology. In *Veterinary Ophthalmology*. (ed KN Gelatt) Lea and Febiger, Philadelphia, pp. 707–743.

35 Bistner S, Rubin L, Cox TA and Condon WE (1970) Pharmacologic diagnosis of Horner's syndrome in the dog. *Journal of the American Veterinary Medical Association* **157**, 1220–1224.

36 Kramer SG and Potts M (1969) Iris uptake of catecholamines in experimental Horner's syndrome. *American Journal of Ophthalmology* **67**, 705–713.

37 Gum GG (1991) Physiology of the eye. In *Veterinary Ophthalmology*. (ed KN Gelatt) Lea and Febiger, Philadelphia, pp. 124–161.

38 Broek AHM van den (1987) Horner's syndrome in cats and dogs: a review. *Journal of Small Animal Practice* **28**, 929–940.

39 Kern TJ (1991) The canine orbit. In *Veterinary Ophthalmology*. (ed KN Gelatt) Lea and Febiger, Philadelphia, pp. 239–255.

40 Raw ME (1994) Horner's syndrome in the dog and cat. *Veterinary Annual* **34**, 181–188.

41 Slatter D (1990) *Fundamentals of Veterinary Ophthalmology*. 2nd edn. WB Saunders, Philadelphia, pp. 451–452.

42 Brightman AH, Helper LC and Parker AJ (1977) Congenital Horner's syndrome. *Canine Practice* **4**, 19–20.

43 Pauli ML and Carer JD (1970) Horner's syndrome in a cat: a case report. *Iowa State University Veterinarian* **31**, 55–57.

44 Manning PD (1998) Horner's syndrome secondary to metastatic squamous cell carcinoma of a retropharyngeal lymph node in a cat. *Australian Veterinary Journal* **76**, 322–324.

45 Carpenter JL, King NW and Abrams KL (1987) Bilateral trigeminal nerve paralysis and Horner's syndrome associated with myelomonocytic neoplasia in a dog. *Journal of the American Veterinary Medical Association* **191**, 1594–1596.

46 Murphy CJ, Koblik P, Bellhorn RW, Pino M, Hacker D and Burling T (1989) Squamous cell carcinoma causing blindness and ophthalmoplegia in a cat. *Journal of the American Veterinary Medical Association* **195**, 965–968.

47 Birchard SJ, Peterson ME and Jacobson A (1984) Surgical treatment of feline hyperthyroidism: results of 85 cases. *Journal of the American Hospital Association* **20**, 705–709.

48 Kallet AJ, Richter KP, Feldman EC and Brum DE (1991) Primary hyperparathyroidism in cats: seven cases (1984–1989). *Journal of the American Veterinary Medical Association* **199**, 1767–1771.

49 Steidl T and Zimmerman M (1989) Operationbedings Horner-Syndrom beim Hund. *Kleintierpraxis* **34**, 363–364.

50 Boydell P, Pike R, Crossley D and Torrington A (1997) Horner's syndrome following intrathoracic tube placement.

Journal of Small Animal Practice **38**, 466–467.

51 Kneller SK, Lewis RE and Oliver JE (1972) Horner's syndrome following common carotid artery catheterization in cats. *Journal of Small Animal Practice* **13**, 595–599.

52 Kern TJ, Aromado MC and Erb HN (1989) Horner's syndrome in dogs and cats: 100 cases (1975–1985). *Journal of the American Veterinary Medical Association* **195**, 369–373.

53 Boydell P (1995) Idiopathic Horner's syndrome in the Golden Retriever. *Journal of Small Animal Practice* **36**, 382–384.

54 Sullivan PS and Pardo AD (1993) Challenging cases in internal medicine: what's your diagnosis (*Toxoplasma gondii*). *Veterinary Medicine* **88**, 309–320.

55 Greene CE and Braun KG (1989) Diseases of the brain. In *Textbook of Veterinary Internal Medicine*. (ed S Ettinger) WB Saunders, Philadelphia, pp. 578–623.

56 LeCouteur RA and Child G (1989) Diseases of the spinal cord. In *Textbook of Veterinary Internal Medicine*. (ed S Ettinger) WB Saunders, Philadelphia, pp. 684–701.

57 Greene CE and Higgins RJ (1976) Fibrocartilaginous emboli as the cause of ischemic myelopathy in a dog. *Cornell Veterinarian* **66**, 131–142.

58 Rubin LF (1971) Neuro-ophthalmology. In *Canine Neurology: Diagnosis and Treatment*. 2nd edn. (ed BF Hoerlein) WB Saunders, Philadelphia, pp. 502–516.

NEUROLOGIC SIGNS RELATED TO INNER EAR DISEASE

1 LeCouteur RA (1994) Vestibular disorders of cats and dogs. *Proceedings of the XIX Annual Meeting of the World Small Animal Veterinary Association*, Durban, pp 417– 422.

2 Schunk KL (1990) Diseases of the vestibular system. *Progress in Veterinary Neurology* **1**, 247–254.

3 DeLahunta A (1983) *Veterinary Neuroanatomy and Clinical Neurology*. 2nd edn. WB Saunders, Philadelphia, pp. 238–254.

4 Holliday TA (1990) Clinical signs caused by experimental lesions in the vestibular system. *Proceedings of the 8th Annual Congress of the American College of Veterinary Internal Medicine*, Washington DC, pp. 1025–1028.

5 Stirling J and Clarke M (1981) Congenital peripheral vestibular disorder in two German Shepherd Dogs. *Australian Veterinary Journal* **57**, 200.

6 Forbes S and Cook JR (1991) Congenital peripheral vestibular disease attributed to lymphocytic labyrinthitis in two related litters of Doberman Pinscher pups. *Journal of the American Veterinary Association* **198**, 447–449.

7 Wilkes M and Palmer A (1986) Congenital deafness in Dobermanns. *Veterinary Record* **115** (letter), 218.

8 Bedford PGC (1979) Congenital vestibular disease in the English Cocker Spaniel. *Veterinary Record* **105**, 530–531.

9 Bower JM (1983) Head tilt in Tibetan Terrier puppies. *Veterinary Record* **112**, 46.

10 Barker J and Sansom J (1983) Head tilt in puppies. *Veterinary Record* **112**, 207.

11 Jaggy A, Oliver JE, Ferguson DC, Mahaffey and Glaus T jnr (1994) Neurological manifestations of hypothyroidism: a retrospective study of 29 dogs. *Journal of Veterinary Internal Medicine* **8**, 328–336.

12 Bichsel P, Jacobs G and Oliver JE (1988) Neurologic manifestations associated with hypothyroidism in four dogs. *Journal of the American Veterinary Medical Association* **192**, 1745–1749.

13 Carpenter JL, Andrews LK and Holzworth J (1997) Tumors and tumor-like lesions. In *Diseases of the Cat*. (ed J Holzworth)

WB Saunders, Philadelphia, pp. 565–569.

14 Lane IF and Hall DG (1992) Adenocarcinoma of the middle ear with osteolysis of the tympanic bulla in a cat. *Journal of the American Veterinary Medical Association* **201**, 463.

15 Indrieri RJ and Taylor RF (1984) Vestibular dysfunction caused by squamous cell carcinoma involving the middle ear and inner ear in two cats. *Journal of the American Veterinary Medical Association* **184**, 471–473.

16 Birchard SJ and Bradley RL (1994) Surgery of the respiratory tract and thorax. In *The Cat: Diseases and Clinical Management*. (ed RG Sherding) Churchill Livingstone, New York, pp. 1093–1116.

17 Stanton ME, Wheaton LG, Render JA and Blevins WE (1985) Pharyngeal polyps in two feline siblings. *Journal of the American Veterinary Medical Association* **186**, 1311–1313.

18 Burke EE, Mosie NS, DeLahunta A and Erb HN (1985) Review of idiopathic feline vestibular syndrome. *Journal of the American Veterinary Medical Association* **187**, 941–943.

19 Fenner WR (1994) Diseases of the brain, spinal cord, and peripheral nerves. In *The Cat: Diseases and Clinical Management*. (ed RG Sherding) Churchill Livingstone, New York, pp. 1507–1568.

20 Schunk KL and Averill DR (1983) Peripheral vestibular syndrome in the dog: a review of 83 cases. *Journal of the American Veterinary Medical Association* **182**, 1354–1357.

21 Cole L, Kwochka KW, Kowalski JJ, Hillier A et al. (1998) Microbial flora and antimicrobial susceptibility patterns of isolated pathogens from the horizontal ear canal and middle ear in dogs with otitis media. *Journal of the American Veterinary Medical Association* **212**, 534–538.

22 Mayhew IG (1989) *Large Animal Neurology: A Handbook for Veterinary Clinicians*. Lea and Febiger, Philadelphia, pp. 133–146.

23 Oliver JE, Lorenz MD, and Kornegay JN (1989) *Handbook of Veterinary Neurology*. 3rd edn. WB Saunders, Philadelphia, pp. 208–228.

24 Evans HE (1993) The ear. In *Miller's Anatomy of the Dog*. (ed HE Evans) WB Saunders, Philadelphia, pp. 988–1008.

25 Myers D, Schlosser WD and Wolfson RJ (1970) Otologic diagnosis and treatment of deafness. *Clinical Symposia* **22**, 34–69.

26 Strain G (1991) Congenital deafness in dogs and cats. *Compendium on Continuing Education* **13**, 245–253.

27 Foss I and Flottorp G (1974) A comparative study of the development of hearing and vision in various species commonly used in experiments. *Acta Otolaryngology* **77**, 202–214.

28 Heffner HE (1983) Hearing in large and small dogs: absolute thresholds and size of the tympanic membrane. *Behavioral Neuroscience* **97**, 310–318.

29 Heffner RS and Heffner HE (1985) Hearing range of the domestic cat. *Hearing Research* **19**, 85–88.

30 Strain G, Tedford B and Jackson R (1991) Postnatal development of the brainstem auditory evoked potential in dogs. *American Journal of Veterinary Research* **52**, 410–414.

31 Buchwald JS and Shipley C (1986) Development of auditory evoked potentials in the kitten. In *Advances in Neural and Behavioral Development*. (ed RN Aslin) Ablex Publishing Company, Norwood, pp. 95–118.

32 Shiu J, Munro K and Cox C (1997) Normative auditory brainstem response data for hearing threshold and neuro-otological diagnosis in the dog. *Journal of Small Animal Practice* **38**, 103–107.

33 Luttgen PJ (1994) Deafness in the dog and cat. *Veterinary Clinics of North America* **24**, 981–989.

34 Strain GM (1996) Aetiology, prevalence and diagnosis of deaf-

ness in dogs and cats. *British Veterinary Journal* **152**, 17–36.

35 Rawitz B (1896) Gehororgan and Gehirn eines weissen Hundes mit blauen Augen. *Morphol Arbeit* **6**, 545–554.

36 Darwin C (1898) Variation under domestication. In *Origin of Species by Means of Natural Selection*. W Clowes and Sons, London, pp. 5–30.

37 Hayes H, Wilson GP, Fenner WR, and Wyman M (1981) Canine congenital deafness: epidemiologic study of cases. *Journal of the American Animal Hospital Association* **17**, 473–476.

38 Little CC (1957) *The Inheritance of Coat Color in Dogs*. Howell Book House, New York, pp. 180–188.

39 Brown KS, Bergma DR and Barrow MV (1971) Animal models of pigment and hearing abnormalities in man. In *Birth Defects: Original Article Series*. (ed DR Bergma) Williams and Wilkins, Baltimore, pp. 102–109.

40 Bergsma DR (1971) White fur, blue eye and deafness in the domestic cat. *Journal of Heredity* **62**, 171–185.

41 Strain G, Kearney MT, Gignac IJ et al. (1992) Brainstem auditory evoked potential assessment of congenital deafness in Dalmatians: association with phenotypic markers. *Journal of Veterinary Internal Medicine* **6**, 175–182.

42 Strain G (1992) Deafness in dogs and cats. *Proceedings of the 10th Annual Congress of the American College of Veterinary Internal Medicine*, San Diego, pp. 275–278.

43 Anderson H, Henricson B, Lundquist PG, Wedenberg E and Wersall J (1968) Genetic hearing impairment in the Dalmatian dog. *Acta Otolaryngologica* **(Suppl 23)**, 1–34.

44 Fraser JS (1924) Congenital deafness in a dog. *Proceedings of the Royal Society of Medicine* **17**, 29–31.

45 Lurie MH (1948) The membranous labyrinth in the congenitally deaf Collie and Dalmatian dog. *Laryngoscope* **58**, 279–287.

46 Hudson WR, Durham NC, and Reuben RJ (1962) Hereditary deafness in the Dalmation dog. *Archives of Otolaryngology* **75**, 213–219.

47 Ferrara ML and Halnan CRE (1983) Congenital structural brain defects in the deaf Dalmatian. *Veterinary Record* **112**, 344–346.

48 Igarashi M, Alford BR, Cohn AM, Saito R and Watanabe T (1972) Inner ear abnormalities in dogs. *Annals of Otology, Rhinology and Laryngology* **81**, 249–255

49 Alexander G and Tandler J (1905) Untersuchungen an kongenital tauben Hunden, Katzen und an jungen kongenital tauber Katzen. *Archives Ohrenheilkd* **66**, 161–179.

50 Adams E (1956) Hereditary deafness in a family of Foxhounds. *Journal of the American Veterinary Medical Association* **15**, 302–303.

51 Wilkes MK and Palmer AC (1992) Congenital deafness and vestibular deficit in the Dobermann. *Journal of Small Animal Practice* **33**, 218–224.

52 Anniko M, Fabiansson E and Nilsson O (1977) Deafness in an Old English Sheepdog. *Archives of Otology, Rhinology and Laryngology* **218**, 1–7.

53 Steinberg S, Kelin E, Killens R and Uhde TW (1989) Inherited deafness among nervous Pointer dogs. *Proceedings of the 7th Annual Meeting of the American College of Veterinary Internal Medicine*, San Diego, pp. 953–956

54 Foss I (1981) Development of hearing and vision in deaf white Norwegian Dunkerhounds and normal dogs (black and dappled Norwegian Dunkerhound). *MSc Thesis*, University of Cornell.

55 Schucknecht HF (1955) Presbycusis. *Laryngoscope* **65**, 402–419.

56 Schuknecht HF and Gacek MR (1993) Cochlear pathology in presbycusis. *Annals of Otology, Rhinology and Laryngology* **102**, 1–16.

57 Knowles K, Blauch B, Leipold H, Cash H and Hewett J (1989) Reduction of spiral ganglion in the ageing canine with hearing loss. *Journal of Veterinary Medicine* **36**, 188–199.

58 Shimada A, Ebisu M, Morita T, Takeuchi T and Unemara T (1998) Age-related changes in the cochlea and cochlear nuclei of dogs. *Journal of Veterinary Medical Science* **60**, 41–48.

59 Knowles K, Cash W and Blauch B (1988) Auditory evoked responses of dogs with different hearing abilities. *Canadian Journal of Veterinary Research* **52**, 394–397.

60 Peterson APG (1980) *Handbook of Noise Measurement.* Gen-Rad, Massachusetts.

61 Flottorp, G (1990) Treatment of noise-induced hearing loss. *Scandinavian Audiology* **34**, 123–130.

62 Munro K and Cox C (1997) Investigation of hearing impairment in Cavalier King Charles Spaniels using auditory brainstem response audiometry. *Journal of Small Animal Practice* **38**, 2–5

63 Cook JR, Tyler DE, Coulter DB and Chandler FW (1984) Disseminated protot.hecosis causing acute blindness and deafness in a dog. *Journal of the American Veterinary Medical Association* **184**, 1266–1272.

64 Pickerell JA, Oehme FW and Cash WC (1993) Ototoxicity in dogs and cats. *Seminars in Veterinary Medicine and Surgery* **8**, 42–49.

Chapter Eight

Ototoxicity and Other Side-Effects of Otic Medication

INTRODUCTION

KEY POINTS

- Clinical cases of true ototoxicity following medical management of otitis externa are very rare.
- Almost all the risks associated with otopharmacy can be obviated provided the clinician can document an intact tympanic membrane before applying the otopharmaceutical agent.
- Side-effects from otic administration of chemicals include local inflammation, otitis media, vestibular or cochlear damage, and systemic absorption.
- Almost any chemical will cause inflammation within the middle ear or inner ear if instilled through the tympanum.
- The round window is an important portal for the passage of drugs, toxins, and inflammatory mediators from the middle to the inner ear.
- The non-pharmaceutical component of an otic preparation (penetrance enhancer, detergent) may significantly affect the toxic potential of the product.

Many types of medication are applied to the external ear canal of dogs and cats. In addition to specific medications, such as anti-inflammatory agents, acaricides, antimicrobial agents, and ceruminolytics, there may be substances included to enhance penetration and to act as vehicle components and preservatives.

The anatomy of the external ear canal is such that liquid medications, in excess, will tend to pool in the horizontal canal. High concentrations of medication may thus come into contact with inflamed epithelium and the potential for intra- and percutaneous absorption is readily apparent. In some circumstances this is desirable. For example, the anti-inflammatory effect of a topical glucocorticoid must be exerted on dermal tissues. In contrast, an antimicrobial, antifungal, or acaricidal agent will usually be applied to the external ear canal for their topical effect and absorption is not necessary.

Inflammation within, and overt damage to, the tympanic and round window membranes may permit inflammatory mediators or drugs to enter the middle ear or inner ear, respectively. Furthermore, it is not known to what extent penetration enhancers such as propylene glycol (a common ingredient in otic preparations) may increase the passage of these substances across these membranes.

The unwanted effects of otic medication may be classified into four groups:
- Direct effects on the meatal and tympanic epithelium and underlying dermis.
- Effects within the middle ear.
- Effects on vestibular and cochlear functions (ototoxicity).
- Systemic sequelae of the otic administration of medications.

One of the greatest difficulties facing clinicians is assessing the relevance of experimental studies, particularly if they are performed in another species. Much experimental research into ototoxicity is performed on guinea pigs and chinchillas. It could be argued that these tests are so artificial, and interspecies anatomic and physiologic variation is so great, that the conclusions drawn from experimental animals cannot be applied to dogs with clinical ear disease[1]. Merchant *et al.*[2] demonstrated that chlorhexidine exhibited very little ototoxic effect in dogs, in contrast to experimental studies which reported both vestibular and cochlear toxicity to chlorhexidine in guinea pigs[3, 4]. However, in a recent experimental study using guinea pigs and dogs there was a good correlation between the two species[5], suggesting that extrapolation might be valid in some instances.

MEATAL AND TYMPANIC INFLAMMATION

The effects of various constituents of commercial otic pharmaceutical products on the meatal epithelium and the tympanic membrane were studied in an experimental model[6]. Benzalkonium chloride (a quaternary ammonium preservative) produced profound effects such as acanthosis and surface ulceration. A mixed inflammatory infiltrate in the dermis was also noted. Propylene glycol (a solvent and penetrance enhancer) induced acanthosis and hyperkeratosis but no histo-pathologic evidence of inflammation was noted. Not surprisingly, both products also induced a statistically significant increase in the epidermal mitotic index. Similar effects were exerted on the tympanic epithelium. The only noted effect of topical hydrocortisone was a significant reduction in the epidermal mitotic index. The authors made the point that it was the supposedly 'inactive' components, rather than the pharmacologically active ingredients, of commercial otopharmaceutical products which induced most change. It may be that these iatrogenic inflammatory effects are, in reality, very mild in nature and are probably masked by the more marked changes consequent upon otitis externa. Thus, they may be of little clinical significance. However, until definitive studies are performed this cannot be relied upon.

Otic maceration may result from overenthusiastic or prolonged application of aqueous or propylene glycol-based cleansers. This might particularly be the case when otic preparations are used for the long-term management of ear disease, such as in allergic otitis externa[7]. Suspicion should be raised when examination of the external ear canal reveals moderate inflammation accompanied by an accumulation of white, moist debris composed of sloughed squames, with no inflammatory cells present.

EFFECTS WITHIN THE MIDDLE EAR

Several types of otic medication can induce inflammation within the middle ear, if they reach it via a ruptured tympanum. Several commercial ceruminolytic preparations were recently shown to cause acute inflammation within the middle ear[5]. Propylene glycol is well documented as an irritant of middle ear epithelium[8]. Indeed, almost all antibacterial agents (carbenicillin is a notable exception) and most solvents (with the exception of water and saline) cause inflammation in the middle ear if instilled into it[9].

Chronic inflammation within the middle ear is thought to be associated with cholesteatoma formation[10, 11]. Propylene glycol is the main agent used for experimental induction of cholesteatomas[11] and it is a common ingredient in many commercial otic pharmaceuticals. Whether this, or other, chemotherapeutic agents are involved in the induction of cholesteatomas in dogs is not known. However, many polypharmaceutical otic preparations contain glucocorticoids in addition to putative irritants, and intratympanic administration of prednisolone with propylene glycol has been shown to inhibit propylene glycol-induced inflammation and subsequent cholesteatoma formation[11].

OTOTOXICITY

An ototoxic agent produces cochlear or vestibular damage by injuring structures within the inner ear[1, 12]. The effects may reflect uni- or bilateral toxicity. Clinical signs of vestibular damage may be reflected very early after the insult has been effected and these include nystagmus, strabismus, ataxia, head tilt, and circling. Clinical signs of cochlear damage usually go unnoticed until complete deafness is recognized[1]. The early signs of cochlear damage in man include tinnitus and although this would be difficult to document in dogs and cats, it may be that an inappropriate, or unusually strong, response to an auditory stimulus is a reflection of early cochlear damage[13].

In order for a drug to exert ototoxicity it must reach the inner ear. This may be the result of hematogenous spread following oral or parenteral dosage. However, more commonly it follows topical application of ototoxic agents into the external ear canal and their subsequent passage into the middle ear via a ruptured tympanum. Subsequent diffusion into the middle ear is enhanced by the presence of otitis media, which induces increased permeability through the round window membrane[14, 15, 16]. The round window membrane is an important portal for the passage of inflammatory mediators, toxins, and drugs from the middle ear to the inner ear[16].

The potential for a drug to cause ototoxicity will vary: the vehicle, chemical composition, and concentration of the agent in question; the route, frequency, and duration of administration; the concentrations of other components in the otic preparation used; and, in some cases, concurrent administration of other drugs[13]. In summary:

- Direct instillation of most substances into the inner ear is likely to induce ototoxicity.
- Topical administration into the external ear canal in the presence of a ruptured tympanum and/or otitis media increases the risk of ototoxicity.
- Certain detergents may increase the ototoxic potential of chlorhexidine.
- Certain agents, such as aminoglycosides, are selectively ototoxic, by whatever route they are administered.
- Loop diuretics potentiate aminoglycoside toxicity by increasing their relative concentration in the endolymph.
- Salicylates may potentiate the toxicity of gentamycin.
- Familial sensitivity to aminoglycoside toxicity has been demonstrated in man[17] and may be relevant in veterinary medicine.

CERUMINOLYTICS

Mansfield *et al.*[5] recently demonstrated that instillation of some commercial ceruminolytic preparations into the middle ear of both guinea pigs and dogs resulted in measurable loss of cochlear function, although whether the damage resulted from one or several of the ingredients was not clear.

PROPYLENE GLYCOL

Propylene glycol is a solvent and penetrance enhancer found in many proprietary otic preparations[6]. When instilled into the middle and inner ear in experimental studies it is ototoxic[8, 9]. In one study[5] some commercial ceruminolytic preparations were shown to induce inflammatory reaction within the middle ear. Some of the dogs exhibited signs of vestibular damage and altered brainstem auditory evoked response. Two of the three products which were associated with these changes contained propylene glycol, although whether this was the sole agent responsible for the effects is not clear.

ANTIMICROBIAL AGENTS

Chlorhexidine

Chlorhexidine is ototoxic, affecting both the vestibular and cochlear systems[18]. Vestibular effects may be noted very rapidly, even on awakening from anesthesia[3], whereas the signs of cochlear damage are more subtle and difficult to detect early. Ultimately, the functional disturbances of the vestibular and cochlear systems are accompanied by fibrosis and degeneration of the sensory epithelia[4].

Although there are no licensed chlorhexidine-based otic preparations, the chemical is readily available in clinical practice and is frequently used for irrigation of the external ear canal. Care must be taken to ensure that adequate dilution is achieved. If it is formulated too weakly, it loses its antimicrobial potency, particularly against gram-negative bacteria; if formulated too strongly, it is ototoxic[18]. However, used as a 0.05% solution (2% solution diluted 1 in 40), chlorhexidine has a broad-spectrum antimicrobial action and may even have some residual activity. A recent study[2] investigated the ototoxic potential of 0.2% chlorhexidine acetate instilled into canine ears before and after experimental myringotomy. No significant effects were noted, suggesting that at 0.2% concentration, or less, chlorhexidine is safe as an irrigating solution in dogs, even in the presence of a ruptured tympanum. Chlorhexidine may exert a transient ototoxicity in cats[19].

The ototoxicity of chlorhexidine is markedly enhanced in the presence of some, but not all, nonionic or cationic detergents[20, 21]. Quaternary ammonium compounds (cetrimide for example) appear to potentiate the toxic effects of chlorhexidine[18] and commercial mixtures of the two compounds (Savlon® for example) should not be instilled into the external ear canal.

Povidone-iodine preparations

Aqueous solutions of certain iodine preparations were found to be non-ototoxic in guinea pigs[22] whereas alcohol-based preparations of iodine[22] and povidone-iodine solutions[20] were ototoxic. Both vestibular and cochlear damage was caused.

Antibacterial agents

Aminoglycosides are recognized to be selectively ototoxic, by whatever route, although the various agents exhibit differing effects, particularly at low doses[23]. Thus, neomycin and dihydrostreptomycin affect the cochlea whereas gentamycin and streptomycin exert effects primarily on the vestibular organ[23, 24]. Topical otic administration of gentamycin, even in the presence of a ruptured tympanum, did not produce a noticeable degree of cochlear or vestibular toxicity after 21 days therapy[25].

Aminoglycosides preferentially, but not exclusively, damage the outer hair cells of the cochlea[23]. The exact mechanism by which aminoglycosides exert their toxicity is unclear, but early effects probably relate to their ability to influence the concentrations of ions, particularly calcium, and free radicals in the endolymph. This will subsequently impact on both electrical activity and neuron function. Other effects relate to aminoglycoside-induced inflammatory cascades mediated via membrane phospholipids such as phosphoinositides[23]. To a certain extent the ototoxic effects are dose and duration related but, ultimately, irreversible fibrodegeneration of the organ of Corti and stria vascularis occurs. Thus, in the case of neomycin sulfate intoxication, BAER waveform loss is reported to occur between 22 and 50 days after initiation of the treatment and it is permanent[26].

Other antibacterial substances must be administered directly into the middle ear for effects to be noted[9].

OTHER PHARMACEUTICALS

Furosemide, salicylates, and cisplatin have all been reported to cause ototoxicity in man and experimental animals but only cisplatin has been reported to cause cochlear damage in dogs[1, 13], and then only in situations where it is administered long term.

ALLERGIC CONTACT DERMATITIS AND IRRITANT CONTACT DERMATITIS

Allergic contact dermatitis and irritant contact dermatitis can be very difficult to differentiate and, from a practical point of view, it is not necessary to do so: removal of the triggering agent results in resolution of the problem.

The external ear canal may be predisposed to locally-induced topical drug reactions. Firstly, the anatomy favors pooling of medication, rather than rapid run off, resulting in prolonged exposure. Secondly, the lipid nature of cerumen may result in high concentrations of certain drugs remaining closely apposed to the epidermis, favoring increased local absorption. Thirdly, some products contain solvents and other agents designed to aid penetration (propylene glycol, for example), and these may increase the risk of sensitization. Finally, topical sensitizers such as neomycin, may be incorporated into topical otic products.

Allergic and irritant contact dermatitis present as an erythematous, occasionally erosive or ulcerative, dermatitis. The principal differential diagnosis is gram-negative otitis[7]. Examination of cytologic specimens will reveal a neutrophilic inflammatory reaction in both conditions, but there will be very few micro-organisms in the case of contact dermatitis and multitudes of them in the case of the gram-negative infection.

The most common contact allergen in the canine ear is neomycin[7]. In man both neomycin and gentamycin are commonly implicated in allergic otitis externa[27]. This suggests that trying to avoid neomycin sensitivity by substituting gentamycin might not be helpful.

Problems may occur if the allergen is propylene glycol. This is so widely used that it is difficult to avoid.

SYSTEMIC EFFECTS OF OTIC MEDICATION

Topically applied drugs pass easily into and through the epithelial lining of the external ear canal. This may be enhanced in the presence of propylene glycol and other agents. The facility of systemic absorption following topical otic administration, even into normal ear canals, is demonstrated by the ability of locally applied glucocorticoid to suppress the pituitary adrenococortical axis[28].

Systemic absorption following topical otic administration may not be limited to glucocorticoids.

Measurable serum concentrations of gentamycin occurred in humans and dogs following otic administration[29, 30]. Whether the route of absorption was via the epithelium of the external or middle ear, or even if it was via the auditory tube, is not known, although the latter route is unlikely in view of the poor absorption of aminoglycosides via the gut. Given that most topical otic preparations are administered when the otic epithelium is inflamed, it is most probable that absorption was via this route.

STRATEGIES TO MINIMIZE OTOTOXICITY

In general, ototoxic effects are dose related, *vis a vis* the middle and inner ear. The first principle, therefore, is to avoid using ototoxic chemicals and, if they must be used, reduce the dose and frequency of administration to an absolute minimum. Careful observation and regular follow-up examinations of the patient may allow detection of vestibular signs early enough to allow the clinician to suspend therapy. In some circumstances prompt action may prevent permanent damage[13]. Unfortunately, it is difficult to detect early

cochlear damage[1]. Indeed, it may be virtually impossible to detect unilateral cochlear damage in the clinical setting without recourse to sophisticated investigatory tools, such as BAER, for example.

> Always suspect a ruptured tympanum unless you can demonstrate otherwise.

The use of aminoglycosides such as neomycin and gentamycin, which are concentrated in the endolymph, should be avoided in the presence of otitis media since inflammation of the round window allows increased penetration of drugs into the inner ear. Concomitant use of loop diuretics should be avoided[12].

With regard to the flushing of the external ear canal, it is best to assume that the tympanum is not intact and to use only saline or 0.2% chlorhexidine solution as flushing agents. It is important to remember that certain detergents may potentiate chlorhexidine toxicity and concomitant use should be avoided.

If the tympanum is proven to be intact, cerumenolytics, foamers, and chemical depilatories may be used provided that the ear canal is thoroughly washed, flushed, and dried at the end of the cleaning procedure.

REFERENCES

1 Merchant SR (1994) Ototoxicity. *Veterinary Clinics of North America* **24**, 971–980.

2 Merchant SR, Neer TM, Tedford BL, Tewdt AC, Cheramie OM and Strain GM (1995) Ototoxicity of a chlorhexidine otic preparation in dogs. *Progress in Veterinary Neurology* **4**, 72–75.

3 Aursnes J (1981) Vestibular damage from chlorhexidine in guinea pigs. *Acta Otolaryngology* **92**, 89–100.

4 Aursnes J (1981) Cochlear damage from chlorhexidine in guinea pigs. *Acta Otolaryngology* **92**, 259–271.

5 Mansfield PD, Steiss JE, Boosinger TR and Marshall AE. (1997) The effects of four commercial ceruminolytics on the middle ear. *Journal of the American Animal Hospital Association* **33**, 479–486.

6 Monkhouse WS, Moran P and Freedman A (1988) The histological effects on the guinea pig external ear of several constituents of commonly used aural preparations. *Clinical Otolaryngology* **13**, 121–131.

7 Rosychuck RAW (1994) Management of otitis externa. *Veterinary Clinics of North America* **24**, 921–951.

8 Morozono T (1988) Ototopical agents: ototoxicity in animal studies. *Annals of Otorhinolaryngology* **97** (**supplement 131**), 28–30.

9 Parker FL and James GWL (1978) The effect of various topical antibiotic and antibacterial agents on the middle and inner ear of guinea pigs. *Journal of Pharmacology and Pharmaceutics* **30**, 236–239.

10 Little CJL, Lane JG, Gibbs C and Pearson GR (1991) Inflammatory middle ear disease in the dog: the clinical and pathological features of cholesteatoma, a complication of otitis media. *Veterinary Record* **128**, 319–322.

11 Ozkul A, Gedikogula G and Turan E (1998) Effect of intratympanic steroid application on the development of experimental cholesteatoma. *Laryngoscope* **108**, 543–547.

12 Mansfield PD (1990) Ototoxicity in dogs and cats. *Compendium on Continuing Education* **12**, 331–337.

13 Pickrell JA, Oehme FW and Cash WC (1993) Ototoxicity in dogs and cats. *Seminars in Veterinary Medicine and Surgery (Small Animal)* **8**, 42–48.

14 Goycoolea MM, Paparella MM, Goldberg B et al. (1980) Permeability of the round window membrane in otitis media. *Archives of Otolaryngology* **106**, 430–433.

15 Goycoolea MV and Lundman L (1997) Round window membrane. Structure function and permeability: a review. *Microscopy Research and Technique* **36**, 201–211.

16 Morizono T (1990) Toxicity of ototopical drugs: animal modelling. *Annals of Otolaryngology, Rhinology and Laryngology* **99**, 42–45.

17 Hu DN, Qui WQ, Wu BT et al. (1991) Genetic aspects of antibiotic induced deafness: mitochondrial inheritance. *Journal of Medical Genetics* **28**, 79–83.

18 Gallé HG and Venker van Haagen AJ (1986) Ototoxicity of the antiseptic combination chlorhexidine/cetrimide (Savlon®): effects on equilibrium and hearing. *Veterinary Quarterly* **8**, 56–60.

19 Igashi Y and Oka Y (1988) Vestibular ototoxicity following intratympanic application of chlorhexidine gluconate in the cat. *Archives of Otorhinolaryngology* **245**, 210–217.

20 Morizono T and Sikora MA (1982) The ototoxicity of topically applied povidone-iodine products. *Archives of Otolaryngology* **108**, 210–213.

21 Morizono T and Sikora MA (1982) Reply to correspondence. *Archives of Otolaryngology* **108**, 808.

22 Aursnes J (1982) Ototoxic effect of iodine disinfectants. *Acta Otolaryngolica* **93**, 219–226.

23 Priuska EM and Schacht J (1997) Mechanism and prevention of aminoglycoside toxicity: outer hair cells as targets and tools. *Ear, Nose and Throat Journal* **76**, 164–172.

24 Tran Ba Huy P and Deffrennes D (1988) Aminoglycoside ototoxicity: influences of dosage regimen of drug uptake and correlation between membrane binding and some clinical features. *Acta Otolaryngologica* **105**, 511–515.

25 Strain GM, Merchant SR, Neer TM and Tedford BL (1995) Ototoxicity of a gentamycin sulfate otic preparation in dogs. *American Journal of Veterinary Research* **56**, 532–538.

26 Morgan JL, Coulter DB, Marshall AE and Gortsch DD (1980) Effects of neomycin on the wave form of brainstem auditory evoked potentials in dogs. *American Journal of Veterinary Research* **41**, 1077–1081.

27 Önder M, Önder T, Özünlü A et al. (1994) An investigation of contact dermatitis in patients with chronic otitis externa. *Contact Dermatitis* **31**, 116–117.

28 Moriello KA, Fehrer-Sawyer SL, Meyer DJ and Feder B (1988) Adrenocortical suppression associated with topical otic administration of glucocorticoids in dogs. *Journal of the American Veterinary Medical Association* **193**, 329–331.

29 Green KM, Lappin DW, Curley JW and de Carpentier JP (1997) Systemic absorption of gentamycin ear drops. *Journal of Otolaryngology* **111**, 960–962.

30 Weinstein MJ, Oden EM, Zeman WV and Wagman GH (1965) Antibiotic absorption after otic administration in dogs. *Antimicrobial Agents and Chemotherapy* **5**, 239–244.

Chapter Nine

Cleaning the External Ear Canal

INTRODUCTION

KEY POINTS

- The integrity of the tympanum must be established before anything other than water or saline is put into the external ear canal.
- Many of the commonly used ceruminolytics exhibit ototoxic effects in the middle ear.
- Aural lavage and subsequent drying are the key steps in cleaning the external ear canal.
- Chemical depilation and ceruminolytics may be an aid to cleaning the ear canal.

> If the tympanum is ruptured, the clinician must use the least ototoxic regime available. This means water or saline only, gentle pressure using a syringe and catheter system (see below), careful aspiration of all fluid, gentle manual removal of all debris, and treatment for otitis media (see Chapter 5: Otitis media, otitis externa) in addition to treatment of the otitis externa.

Inflamed ear canals contain increased amounts of moisture, aberrant cerumen, increased numbers of microorganisms, and increased concentrations of microbial toxins. Foreign bodies, neoplasms, or ectoparasites may be present. There may be inflammatory cells in the lumen, an inflammatory reaction within the epithelium, and erosions, or even ulceration, of the epithelium. The animal may well be showing signs of pain. The tympanum may be ruptured.

Aural lavage is beneficial for several reasons (after Little[1] and McKeever[2]):

- It removes exudate, debris, macerated epithelial components, microorganisms, toxins, and some foreign bodies.
- It improves visualization of the proximal external ear canal and allows otoscopic examination of the deeper regions.
- It may permit visualization of the tympanum.
- It facilitates subsequent therapy.
- It may provide relief from pain.

The procedure for cleaning the external ear is straightforward and involves a number of distinct steps:

- Establish the integrity of the tympanum. If this cannot be assessed, use only saline as a lavage agent.
- Pretreat with a ceruminolytic or an oil-based lubricant.
- Flush and remove all debris from the external ear canal.
- Remove as much free fluid as possible with suction or very gentle swabbing.
- Apply a drying agent to ensure complete removal of moisture.
- Consider visual examination in the light of the cytologic results and provide specific treatment.

ASSESSING THE INTEGRITY OF THE TYMPANUM

This step is critical since many cleaning techniques advocate chemicals and some degree of water pressure to flush the external ear canal. Any damage to the tympanum puts the middle and inner ear at risk. A recent study[3] demonstrated that glycerine-based ceruminolytics, including carbamide peroxide/dioctyl sulfosuccinate and triethanolamine polypeptide oleate-condensate preparations, had pathologic effects when instilled directly into the middle ear.

Visual assessment of the tympanum is difficult in normal circumstances and often impossible when otitis externa is present (see Chapter 2: Otoscopic appearance of the external ear canal and tympanum). However, Griffin[4] described a technique which allows indirect assessment of the tympanum. An otoscope is used to visualize the distal horizontal canal. A small, soft rubber feeding tube is passed through the otoscope toward the tympanum. If it continues to pass unhindered, the tympanum is ruptured or there is false middle ear syndrome. If its progress is blocked and the tip remains in view, the tympanum is intact. Assessing the tympanum with a Spreull needle is not advised since such a needle has the potential to rupture the tympanum.

PRODUCTS ADVOCATED FOR CLEANING EARS

CERUMINOLYTICS

Many authors[2, 4–7] advocate an initial application of ceruminolytic agents prior to lavage in cases of otitis externa. The justification for this is that the action of the ceruminolytic, and some of the additives which may potentiate their effect, softens the ceruminous debris and cerumenocellular aggregates, permitting easy removal with subsequent aural lavage. Clinicians should be aware of the difference between a true ceruminolytic and a lubricant:

- A ceruminolytic disrupts the integrity of cerumen by inducing lysis of the squames[8].
- A lubricant merely softens and loosens the cerumen.

A recent study[3] demonstrated that some commercial ceruminolytics were ototoxic (vestibular effects) and caused inflammatory changes within the middle ear. It was not clear which component(s) of the various products was/were responsible for the changes.

Ceruminolysis is optimal in hypo-osmolar, alkaline solutions[8]. Proteins on the surface of squames dissolve into this alkaline solution, binding with free hydroxyl ions. Loss of surface proteins reduces the integrity of the cell membrane and water enters the cell, resulting in swelling and fragmentation[8]. Disruption of the squames results in disintegration of the cerumen, allowing it to be flushed from the external ear canal.

No *in vivo* or *in vitro* studies have been performed on canine or feline cerumen. However, studies on human cerumen demonstrated that aqueous alkaline solutions of sodium hydroxide (0.1 molar), sodium bicarbonate (0.5% and 1.25%), and sodium dodecyl sulfate (0.05% and 0.1%) were superior to organic agents such as glycerine, triethanolamine polypeptide oleate-condensate, and olive oil[8]. Proprietary oil-based ceruminolytics were found to be no better than glycerine or olive oil. None of the oil-based products had any true ceruminolytic effect; all merely lubricated and softened the bolus of cerumen[8, 9]. However, softening and lubricating may be just as useful as true ceruminolysis since a blind, controlled study[10] failed to show significant differences between sterile water, sodium bicarbonate solution, and a lipid-based proprietary 'ceruminolytic'.

Water-based proprietary ceruminolytic preparations usually possess surfactant and emulsifying properties which allow aqueous substances to penetrate and underrun oily masses. These are preferred to oil-based products for two reasons:

- Firstly, they are less messy[6] and are more easily removed from the ear canal, permitting quicker cleaning and drying.
- Secondly, oil-based preparations are occlusive and may, if not thoroughly removed, potentiate bacterial infections[7].

Dioctyl sodium sulfosuccinate and calcium sulfosuccinate are effective emulsifiers[11] but they must not be used in dogs or cats if there is a ruptured tympanum[3, 4]. Carbamate peroxide is a less potent agent than the sulfocuccinates[4] but is still capable of damaging the middle ear[3]. The foaming effect of released urea and oxygen may help to loosen adhered debris. This product is probably most useful in cases of purulent otitis externa[4].

Oil-based proprietary lubricants may have a very mild clinical 'ceruminolytic' effect[4]. Indeed, they are probably best confined to cases characterized by a mild ceruminous otitis, where they may have a lubricant, diluting effect, permitting subsequent flushing out. Squalene, triethanolamine polypeptide oleate condensate, and hexamethyltetracosane are more potent than propylene glycol and mineral oil, but are not as powerful as the aqueous products detailed above which have a powerful surfactant activity[4]. These oil-based products soften the cerumen permitting easier removal from the external ear canal. Squalene appears to be well tolerated in the middle ear[3] and was not associated with otic toxicity in Mansfield's study[3].

CHEMICAL DEPILATORIES

Chemical depilatory compounds have occasionally been advocated as aids in cleaning the external ear canal of dogs[12]. Given that in some dogs the external ear canal may be so hirsute that cleaning and adequate visualization is difficult, depilatory compounds would appear to be useful. Furthermore, chemical depilatory products, because of their alkalinity, might well be of value in helping to break down some of the aggregates of hair and cerumen which occur in some ears.

Most modern chemical depilatories contain thioglycolic acid or glycolate salts, presented as a cream or foam spray[13]. The depilation is accomplished by chemical disruption of disulfide bonds. The chemical effect requires a concentration of at least 2.5% and most contain thioglycolates in the range of 2.5–4%[13]. One drawback of these preparations is that thioglycolates require a very high pH (ideally about

12.5) if the chemical depilation is to occur within a few minutes[13] and as such they might be expected to have an irritant potential to dogs and cats[12]. However, one study[12] looked at the postapplication histopathologic features of the external ear canal of dogs, and no significant evidence of inflammation was reported. Furthermore, experimental studies comparing chemical depilation with shaving found no evidence of either increased bacterial colonization or delayed wound healing[14, 15].

The depilatory compound is applied via a syringe in sufficient quantity to coat the external ear canal and it is allowed to remain for 5–10 minutes before being flushed out. It has been suggested (Fadok, communication on VetDerm Listserv) that an initial test dose should be applied to the concave surface of the pinna as a few individuals may show extreme sensitivity. It is recommended that chemical depilatory compounds do not enter the middle ear.

CLEANING PROCESS

There are three methods, not mutually exclusive, to accomplish removal of cerumen from the external ear canal[16]: mechanical removal; suction; and lavage.

MECHANICAL REMOVAL
This is the safest method for removing cerumen since it does not involve any risk to the tympanum or middle ear. Good visualization is imperative and if possible, both eyes should be used as this increases depth perception[16]. A wire loop, or blunt curette, is gently pulled along the lining of the canal, loosening and rolling cerumen out of the canal as it moves. After pretreatment with lubricants or ceruminolytics, there should be no tightly adherent pieces of cerumen, but if any are remaining, perhaps bound to hair shafts, they should not be subject to undue force as this may result in erosions to the epidermis.

SUCTION
Suction is particularly useful when cerumen is semiliquid or purulent. It is indicated for draining the middle ear[4] and is useful when the tympanum has been ruptured since there is no lavage fluid which might

enter the middle ear cavity. However, there is a risk of the suction tip becoming blocked[16] and in animals the tip is often too large to enter the middle ear[4]. Furthermore, the lack of infusion fluid can make effective cleaning difficult. The length of time involved in cleaning the equipment is also a disadvantage[4].

IRRIGATION
Irrigation is necessary to remove ceruminolytics or chemical depilatory compounds and it is very effective in cleaning the external ear canal[16]. Pressure irrigation is potentially hazardous as a damaged tympanum may be ruptured by powerful jets of fluid[4, 16]. Curved heads on the end of the jets may help to prevent direct pressure on the tympanum[4]. The main disadvantage of these irrigating pumps is the lack of suction, the mess they create, and the time taken to dry the dog and clean up the equipment[5].

Griffin[4] described using a soft rubber feeding tube attached to a syringe, which may be used alternatively to flush and aspirate fluid under direct observation through the otoscope. This method is also ideal for flushing the middle ear cavity.

IRRIGATING SOLUTIONS

Irrigating solutions are used to flush out debris and any cleaning agents, such as ceruminolytics or chemical depilatories. Generally they are administered

in a gentle stream, the overflow being monitored to assess when flushed debris ceases to be present. Extreme care is needed if the tympanum is ruptured.

> Cleaning the external ear canal using cotton buds is not advised. Impaction of cerumen onto the tympanum may occur, as may trauma to the epidermal lining of the canal.

> Chlorhexidine, povidone-iodine, and acetic acid should be used with care in the external ear canal, particularly if the integrity of the tympanum is not known.

A solution of propylene glycol and malic, benzoic, and salicylic acids, 2% or 5% acetic acid alone, or 1:3 povidone-iodine (1%) solution have been recommended if the tympanum is not intact[2, 4, 5].

WATER OR STERILE SALINE

These are the agents of choice when the integrity of the tympanum has not been established[1, 6]. Given that the antimicrobial agents listed below have potential ototoxic effects, particularly in the presence of a ruptured tympanum, the justification for their use is debatable; their main indication is a broad-spectrum antimicrobial activity. However, in most cases the cleaning and irrigation procedure is a preliminary step whose function is to clean the ear canal in preparation for specific topical medication.

CHLORHEXIDINE

A 0.05% solution (2% solution diluted 1:40) of chlorhexidine has a broad-spectrum antimicrobial action, may have some residual activity, and is not toxic in the presence of a ruptured tympanum in dogs, although it may exert a transient ototoxicity in cats[17, 18]. An even more dilute preparation (0.0075%: 15 ml 2% solution in 4.5 liters of water) has been recommended by one author[7, 11]. *Pseudomonas aeruginosa* may be resistant to chlorhexidine at this lower concentration[1].

Although concentrations of chlorhexidine diacetate over 0.013% were shown to be cytotoxic to fibroblasts *in vitro*[19], a concentration of 0.05% was not detrimental to wound healing *in vivo*[20]. However, a 0.5% solution of chlorhexidine has been shown significantly to impair granulation tissue production and wound healing[21].

On the basis of the above research a 0.05% concentration of chlorhexidine would appear to be a safe product with which to irrigate the canine external ear canal, although it might not be an ideal choice for postoperative irrigation following aural surgery. Note that *P. aeruginosa* may be resistant to chlorhexidine at a concentration of 0.05% or lower[1]. Consequently, more potent antimicrobial agents should be used if gram-negative bacterial infection is suspected.

POVIDONE-IODINE

The bactericidal activity of povidone-iodine is related to the concentration of non-complexed iodine in solution[22]. Concentrations of povidone-iodine greater than 0.5% are toxic to fibroblastic cultures[19], somewhat below the 1% minimum concentration required for reliable antistaphylococcal activity[19], although comfortably above the 0.001% dilution reported to be staphylococcicidal in another study[23]. However, povidone-iodine, particularly when combined with a detergent, is potentially ototoxic[24] and it is not recommended for use as a flushing agent[6].

ACETIC ACID

Dilute solutions of acetic acid (5% diluted 1 in 2 or 1 in 3) have been reported to be safe for use as a middle ear flushing agent[6] and several commercial preparations of 2.5% or 5% solutions are available. A 2% solution of acetic acid kills pseudomonids and a 5% solution kills staphylococci[4], although the higher concentration may be irritating.

DRYING AGENTS

Once the ear canal has been cleaned it must be dried, as residual moisture may potentiate bacterial infection. Lavage fluid may be removed by suction, or even gentle use of swabs, but a final application of an alcohol-based product is recommended[1, 2, 5].

Most products contain isopropyl alcohol, often combined with a weak acid such as boric acid, benzoic acid, salicylic acid, or acetic acid[1, 4]. High concentrations of these weak acids may be mildly irritant, particularly in inflamed ear canals.

HOME CLEANING

Animals with chronic otitis externa will benefit from regular ear cleaning and in many cases owners can perform this at home, although patient compliance is mandatory. The most usual candidates are dogs with ceruminous otitis externa, secondary to defects in keratinization or allergy[4]. In these cases flushing debris and preventing secondary microbial proliferation is necessary.

A commercially available ear cleanser containing 2.5% lactic acid, 0.1 % salicylic acid with sodium docusate, propylene glycol, and parachlorometaxylenol has been shown to be particularly effective as a rapidly effective, *in vitro* killer of bacteria and yeast commonly found in canine otitis externa[25]. Furthermore, a controlled *in vivo* study demonstrated effective killing of microorganisms in the external ear canal of Basset Hounds[25].

REFERENCES

1 Little CJ (1996) Medical treatment of otitis externa in the dog and cat. *In Practice* **18**, 66–71.

2 McKeever PJ (1996) Otitis externa. *Compendium on Continuing Education* **18**, 759–772.

3 Mansfield PD, Steiss JE, Boosinger TR and Marshall AE (1997) The effect of four commercially available ceruminolytic agents on the middle ear. *Journal of the American Animal Hospital Association* **33**, 479–486.

4 Griffin CE (1993) Otitis externa and otitis media. In *Current Veterinary Dermatology*. (eds CE Griffin, KW Kwochka and JM MacDonald) Mosby, St Louis, pp. 245–262.

5 McKeever PJ and Richardson HW (1988) Otitis externa. Part 3: Ear cleaning and medical treatment. *Companion Animal Practice* **2**, 24–30.

6 Rosychuck RAW (1994) Management of otitis externa. In *Veterinary Clinics of North America*. (eds RAW Rosychuck and SR Merchant) **24**, 921–952.

7 Chester DK (1988) Medical management of otitis externa. In *Veterinary Clinics of North America*. (ed JG August) **18**, 799–812.

8 Robinson AC, Hawke M, Mackay A, Ekem JK and Stratis M (1989) The mechanism of ceruminolysis. *Journal of Otolaryngology* **18**, 268–273.

9 Robinson AC and Hawke M (1989) The efficacy of ceruminolytics: everything old is new again. *Journal of Otolaryngology* **18**, 263–267.

10 Bruyette DS and Lorenz MD (1993) Otitis externa and otitis media: diagnostic and medical aspects. *Seminars in Veterinary Medicine and Surgery (Small Animal)* **8**, 3–9.

11 Wilcke JR (1988) Otopharmacology. In *Veterinary Clinics of North America*. (ed JG August) **18**, 783–798.

12 Hammond DL, Conroy JD and Woody BJ (1990) The histological effects of a chemical depilatory on the auditory canal of dogs. *Journal of the American Animal Hospital Association* **26**, 551–554.

13 Wilkinson JB and Moore RJ (1982) Depilatories. In *Harry's Cosmeticology*. 7th edn. (eds HB Wilkinson and RJ Moore) Longman Scientific, Harlow, pp. 142–152.

14 Jaffray B, King PM, Macleod DA and Wiseman R (1990) Bacterial colonisation of the skin after chemical depilation. *Journal of the Royal College of Surgeons (Edinburgh)* **35**, 243–244.

15 De Koos T and McComas B (1983) Shaving versus skin depilatory cream for preoperative skin preparation: a prospective study of wound infection rates. *American Journal of Surgery* **145**, 377–378.

16 Wilson PL and Roeser RJ (1997) Cerumen management: professional issues and techniques. *Journal of the American Academy of Audiology* **8**, 421–430.

17 Merchant SR, Neer TM, Tedford BL, Tewdt AC, Cheramie OM and Strain GM (1995) Ototoxicity of a chlorhexidine otic preparation in dogs. *Progress in Veterinary Neurology* **4**, 72–75.

18 Igashi Y and Oka Y (1988) Vestibular ototoxicity following intratympanic application of chlorhexidine gluconate in the cat. *Archives of Otorhinolaryngology* **245**, 210–217.

19 Sanchez IR, Nusbaum KE, Swaim SF, Hale AS, Henderson RA and McGuire JA (1988) Chlorhexidine diacetate and povidine-iodine cytotoxocity to canine embryonic fibroblasts and *Staphylococcus aureus*. *Veterinary Surgery* **17**, 182–185.

20 Sanchez IR, Swaim SF, Nusbaum KE, , Hale AS, Henderson RA and McGuire JA (1988) Effects of chlorhexidine diacetate and povidine-iodine on wound healing in dogs. *Veterinary Surgery* **17**, 291–295.

21 Lee AH, Swaim SF, McGuire JA and Hughes KS (1988) Effects of chlorhexidine diacetate, povidine iodine and polyhydroxydine on wound healing in dogs. *Journal of the American Animal Hospital Association* **24**, 77–84.

22 Rackur H (1985) New aspects of mechanism of action of povidine-iodine. *Journal of Hospital Infection* **6**, 13–23.

23 Lineaweaver W, McMorris S, Soucy D and Howard R (1985) Cellular and bacterial toxicities of topical antimicrobials. *Plastic and Reconstructive Surgery* **75**, 394–396.

24 Morizono T and Sikora MA (1982) The ototoxicity of topically applied povidone-iodine preparations. *Archives of Otolaryngology* **108**, 210–213.

25 Lloyd DH, Bond R and Lamport I (1998) Antimicrobial activity *in vitro* and *in vivo* of a canine ear cleanser. *Veterinary Record* **143**, 111–112.

Chapter Ten

Aural Hematoma, and Other Pinnal Surgery

INTRODUCTION

KEY POINTS
- Aural hematoma must be properly drained but surgical fixation is not always necessary.
- Pinnal lesions tend to bleed profusely and are easily traumatized, particularly in dogs with pendulous pinnae.
- Wound healing at the pinnal margins may be slow; even small lacerations need aggressive treatment.
- Pinnal lacerations require prompt attention if a good cosmetic result is to be obtained.
- Pedicle flaps may be indicated if large pinnal defects are present.

The pinna is composed of a flared cartilaginous extension of the annular cartilage covered with skin[1, 2]. The relatively hairless skin of the concave side is more tightly adherent than the haired skin of the convex side[1]. The pinna is supplied by branches of the external carotid artery and the great auricular artery which branches and courses up the convex aspect of the pinna (342). The concave aspect is supplied by branches

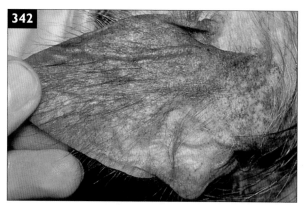

342   Prominent, longitudinal veins are visible on the convex aspect of the pinna of this dog.

which pass through foramina in the middle third of the pinna[2] or which wrap around the pinnal margins. This pattern of vascular supply explains the tendency for pinnal lacerations to bleed profusely and is the reason for placing mattress sutures parallel to the long axis of the pinna when dealing with aural hematoma.

AURAL HEMATOMA

The underlying cause of aural hematoma is unknown[3]. Various factors have been proposed to account for the pathogenesis of the lesion itself and for the underlying cause which incites the process: most of these have been shown subsequently to be inadequate in some degree.

UNDERLYING CAUSES
Association with *Otodectes cynotis*
Stephenson[4] noted the association with otitis externa and observed that otodectic mange was present in most cases. Fifty nine percent of dogs and 76% of cats with aural hematoma were affected with *O. cynotis* in one study[5]. It has been suggested that antigens released from ear mites, in the process of feeding, might be involved in an immune-mediated action which culminates in aural hematoma[5, 6]. However, otodectic mites are not present in all the ears in which aural hematoma occurs, suggesting that if there is a relationship, it is not direct.

Association with otitis externa
Seventy two percent of dogs and 81% of cats were affected with some macroscopic evidence of otitis externa in one study[5], lending support to the hypothesis that otitis externa, and the head shaking which accompanies it, are involved in the pathogenesis of aural hematoma[4]. However, Joyce[7] found evidence of otitis externa in only 36% of her series, again suggesting only a tenuous connection.

Association with trauma
Trauma to the pinna is most frequently cited as the cause of aural hematoma[8, 9]. Traumatic injury to the pinna can occur from directly inflicted trauma from the ipsilateral rear foot or from violent head shaking. Given that trauma from a dog's foot, for example, would most likely affect the convex aspect of the pinna, it seems unlikely that direct trauma is the cause[5]. Furthermore, Kuwahara[5] was unable to produce aural hematoma by either applying direct force to the pinna or by injecting sterile saline or autogenous blood between the skin and the cartilage.

Trauma might occur secondary to head shaking and underlying otitis externa. Ectoparasite infestations, allergy, and otic foreign bodies have been proposed as common causes[8]. However, the author had never seen aural hematoma in cases of scabies, possibly the most pruritic dermatosis in dogs, notwithstanding the severe pinnal self-trauma which occurs. Also, otitis externa is not often associated with aural hematoma[7].

Association with autoimmunity

Kuwahara[5, 6] proposed that aural hematoma had an immune-mediated, possibly autoimmune, cause. This hypothesis was based on positive direct and indirect immunofluorescence on pinnal excised tissue, antinuclear antibody titers, and a response to glucocorticoids[5]. This hypothesis has subsequently been challenged by Joyce and Day[3] who found no evidence of antinuclear antibody activity and minimal evidence of tissue immunofluorescence.

Association with underlying hypersensitivity

Many cases of aural hematoma appear to be associated with underlying hypersensitivity[3] and in atopy, the most common canine hypersensitivity, lesions are often present on the concave aspect of the pinnae. Certainly, otitis externa is a common manifestation of atopy, as is pruritus of the head and face. Furthermore, Joyce and Day[3] reported that in two thirds of their case series there was a significant dermal infiltrate of eosinophils and mast cells.

PATHOGENESIS OF THE LESION

Quite why aural hematoma occurs on the concave aspect of the pinna is not known. That there is some damage to the pinnal cartilage is unquestionable, but whether this results from trauma is not known. A dog with acute otitis externa will attempt to scratch the ear but in that case the trauma is more likely to be on the convex aspect of the pinna, at least in dogs with pendulous pinnae, or in the external ear canal itself, and

neither of these sites suffer from hematoma. The site of the fluid accumulation is within the cartilage[5, 10, 11] and this led investigators to search for mechanisms of cartilage damage. Violent head shaking resulting in stress or standing-wave-induced fractures was proposed[11] but no experimental evidence has been put forward to support this theory. Similarly, Kuwahara[5] was unable to reproduce aural hematoma by inflicting cartilage damage with hemostats.

It has recently been proposed[3] that the initiating event may be an immunologic process which results in damage to the pinnal cartilage. Joyce and Day[3] reported that in 93% of their series there was cartilage degeneration with fibrovascular granulation tissue-filling defects within the cartilage. This finding suggests that at least some of the cartilage damage occurs weeks before the aural hematoma develops, which is at odds with the clinical signs which are acutely uncomfortable to the dog and usually prompt rapid presentation to the veterinary surgeon.

The fluid within the lesion is more akin to seroma fluid than that found in true hematomas[5] and this also suggests a more chronic nature to the etiology than clinical findings would suggest.

CLINICAL FEATURES

Aural hematoma is a relatively common condition in small animal practice and it has a pathognomonic appearance (**343, 344**). The initial lesion usually develops at the base of the concave aspect of the pinna, subsequently enlarging towards the apex[5]. The lesion is a cause of acute discomfort to the dog and rapid presentation is the norm. This is supported by a study[6] in which over 80% cases were in the acute stages of the disease. Aural hematomas are warm, tense, and painful.

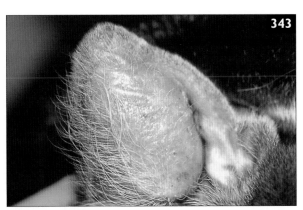 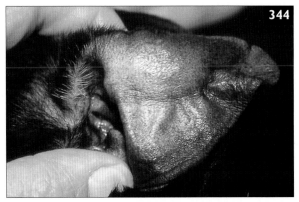

343, 344   Aural hematoma in a cat (**343**) and a dog (**344**). Such lesions are tense, rounded, occasionally bluish purple in color, and fluid filled.

In cases where drainage or surgical intervention is not performed, chronic scarring fibrosis develops which distorts the pinna, the so-called 'cauliflower ear' (**345**).

MANAGEMENT

The lesion must be drained. In addition, recurrence, both immediate and long term, must be prevented. There are three techniques described in the literature which achieve the first aim, but only a carefully taken history and complete physical examination will allow identification of the underlying cause, if indeed there is one. General anesthesia may be necessary to treat the lesion. None of the three techniques described achieve a rapid resolution and all are relatively expensive in financial terms for what the owner might consider simply a large 'blood blister'. Good communication with the owner is important.

Aural hematomas that are acute respond to drainage and pressure dressings better than those which have been present for more than seven days. These latter cases require drainage and sutures to obliterate dead space[12]. Although surgery is more painful, more expensive, and requires general anesthesia, it does resolve the condition more rapidly than passive drainage[12].

Surgical incision, drainage, and suture

Incisional drainage and suturing is probably the most consistently successful technique for dealing with aural hematomas[9]. Early and complete drainage ensures good apposition with minimal fibrin deposits to curette out. The principle disadvantage of this method is the necessity for general anesthesia. The technique (after Henderson and Horne[8], Cechner[9], and Swaim and Henderson[12]) is as follows:

- The pinna is prepared surgically and the hematoma incised with a single, straight cut along its long axis (**346**). Additional excision is not necessary[9].

> Client management and an attempt to prevent recurrence are important.

- The cavity is drained, fibrin is curetted out, and the cavity flushed with sterile saline.
- Full-thickness sutures are placed in rows parallel with the incision (**347, 348**). The longitudinal placing of these sutures is mandatory as it minimizes the risk of iatrogenic damage to the blood vessels of the pinna. The major vessels may be visualized on the concave aspect of the pinna but incorrect placement and blockage of even a small vessel can lead to necrosis of an area of the pinna. The free ends of the sutures, on the convex aspect of the pinna, are cut short (**349**).
- The principle role of these sutures is to obliterate dead space, rather than to appose tissue, and consequently the number of rows placed will depend on the size of the cavity. Generally, one to three rows are required, each some 5–10 mm (0.2–0.4 in) from the next.
- Pressure wrapping is necessary (see Chapter 12: Perioperative analgesia and management). An absorbent pad is placed on the crown, the pinna is folded back over the head, and the ear is bandaged. The free pinna may poke through a window (**350**). In some animals an Elizabethan collar may be necessary.
- Postoperative pain relief is necessary for the first 24–48 hours (see Chapter 12: Perioperative analgesia and management).
- Sutures are removed after a minimum of two weeks; more usually three weeks is allowed.

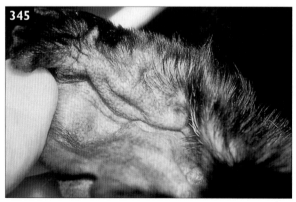

345 Gnarled and distorted pinna, a consequence of leaving an aural hematoma to resolve without treatment.

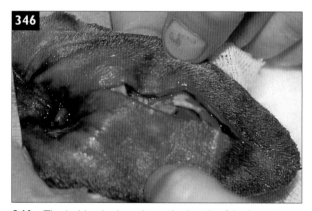

346 The incision is along the entire length of the hematoma.

Postsurgical problems

The following may occur:

- Some animals may shake their heads so violently that hemorrhage occurs. Sedation may be necessary in these cases, although good control of pain usually prevents self-trauma.
- Localized necrosis as a result of poor suture placement will necessitate symptomatic management.
- Recurrence, and permanent scarring of the pinna (**351, 352**), may follow poor drainage, incorrect suture placement, or, more usually, too few sutures. Recurrence should prompt a search for an underlying pruritus if the surgical technique was good.

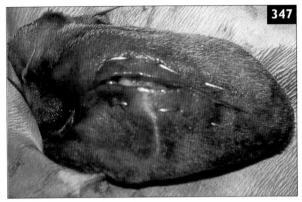

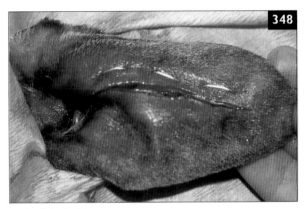

347, 348   The sutures are placed longitudinally along the entire length of the incisions.

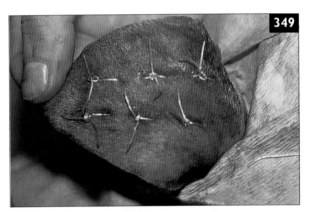

349   The free ends of the sutures are cut short.

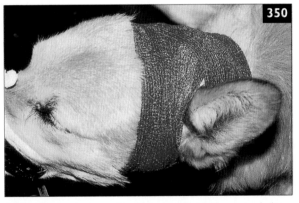

350   The ear is dressed and bandaged with the normal pinna allowed to stand free.

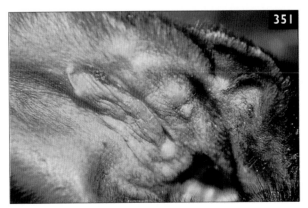

351   Localized scarring and distortion of the pinna secondary to poor surgical technique.

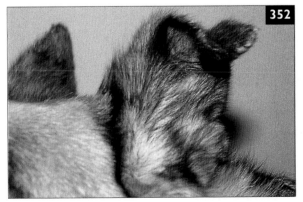

352   Distortion of the pinna following inadequate surgical management of an aural hematoma.

Surgical incision, drainage, and taping

This technique is reported to have an advantage over that described above in that no sutures are required and there is therefore less risk of pinnal distortion[13]. The major disadvantages of this technique are the necessity for general anesthesia and the unnatural position of the pinna, which may upset some owners. The technique (after Bojrab and Constantinescu[13]) is as follows:

- The hematoma is drained as described above but no sutures are placed.
- Dressings are applied as described above and the wound cleaned daily.
- Dressings are changed as necessary and the taped pinna is freed after three weeks.

Drainage with an indwelling Penrose drain or teat tube

This procedure may be carried out under heavy sedation or ultrashort anesthesia. The hematoma is incised distally and drained via a stab incision or biopsy punch[7, 14]. A Penrose drain is inserted through the incision to exit proximally via another similar incision (**353**). Both ends of the drain are left exposed and stay sutures are placed. No dressings are applied, although the owner is advised to clean the drain holes gently on

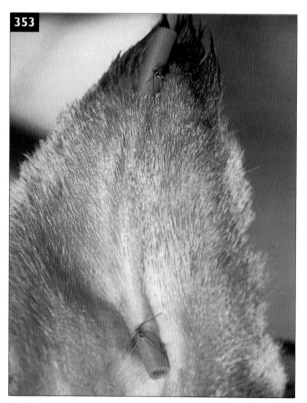

353 A Penrose drain has been inserted through this aural hematoma.

a daily basis. The dog is checked weekly and the drain removed when the lesion is quiescent. A similar approach was reported using a teat tube rather than a Penrose drain[15]. In one study[7], Penrose drain insertion was supplemented by oral prednisolone (1 mg/kg q12h for two weeks followed by a further two weeks at 1 mg/kg q24h). Twenty four of 27 hematomas were successfully treated with this technique.

Drainage and glucocorticoid instillation

The huge advantage of this technique is that general anesthesia is not required. Furthermore, a more rapid resolution of the condition occurs[6]. The principle disadvantage is that repeated visits to the clinic are necessary as regular drainage is required. This tends to negate any cost benefit that may be gained by obviating a general anesthetic and it may prove logistically tedious to the client. In addition, the instillation of gluco-corticoids into the wound may delay healing and the technique has been criticized on this basis[8]. The technique (after Kuwahara[6]) is as follows:

- The hematoma is cleaned and sprayed with spirit.
- An 18G needle and syringe was described initially to drain the hematoma fluid. However, the authors found that a butterfly connection (with a length of soft tubing interposed between needle and syringe) allowed for some movement by the dog and was a much less painful procedure (**354, 355**).
- Dexamethasone (0.2% solution) diluted 5–10 times in sterile saline is instilled into the hematoma cavity, although not in sufficient quantity to cause distension of the skin overlying the cavity.
- The puncture is sealed with a piece of adhesive tape to prevent leakage.
- The procedure is repeated daily until no fluid is aspirated, typically on the third to fifth day[6].

Closed-suction drainage

Closed-suction drainage depends on fluid following a negative pressure gradient. A technique has been described which exploits this principle in the management of aural hematoma[16]. Although a good response to treatment has been reported, this technique appears to hold no advantage over the other, more straightforward, methods described above. A 19G butterfly adapter with swaged-on tubing is used in this technique[16]. The length of the hematoma is measured on the tubing and it is repeatedly fenestrated so that the fenestrated length of tube lies completely within the hematoma. The hematoma is drained via a 19G needle and if there are clots of fibrin within, it is incised, drained, and sutured as described above. If the aspirated fluid contains no clots, the closed-suction

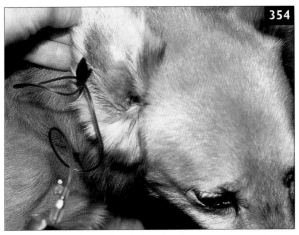

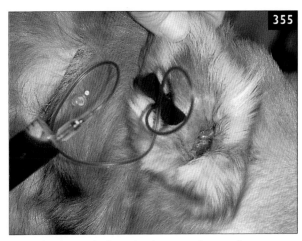

354, 355   A loose butterfly connection is preferred to a simple needle and syringe as it allows the dog some degree of movement.

technique is progressed. The technique (after Swaim and Bradley[16]) is as follows:

- A small incision is made to enlarge the needle puncture just so that the fenestrated tube can pass into the hematoma. The tube is pushed to the apex of the hematoma cavity so that all the fenestrations are within the cavity. The distal end of the tube is fixed with a simple interrupted percutaneous non-absorbable suture. A purse-string suture is passed around the proximal end to ensure a tight seal.
- The needle at the end of the tubing is passed through the stopper of a 3 ml or 5 ml evacuated blood collection tube. Proper placement of the fenestrated tube is confirmed by noting that the hematoma 'collapses' onto the tube as

pressure become negative. The first evacuated tube is immediately replaced with another.
- The pinna is reflected back over the head, as described above, and the evacuated tube packed between surgical sponge on the dog's head and secured with adhesive tape.
- Periodically the vacuum tube is 'unpacked' and replaced to ensure a steady draw of fluid. Initially, this is necessary two or three times daily, falling to once daily as fluid production within the hematoma decreases.
- After seven days the bandages are removed, the stay sutures removed, and the tube withdrawn.
- The bandages are replaced to ensure that the pinna is held firm for another ten days to allow complete healing.

TRAUMATIC INJURY TO THE PINNA

Traumatic injuries to the pinnae are common. Dogs and cats frequently suffer pinnal laceration and even pinnal defects during fights, and wound infection invariably occurs. The general principles of treatment are cleaning, debridement, tissue apposition, protection, and prevention of secondary infection[8]. Lacerations may be full thickness or partial, in which case pinnal cartilage may or may not be involved. Small lacerations may be treated conservatively by clipping and cleaning

PINNAL LACERATION
Hydroactive dressings
Adhesive, hydroactive dressings may be useful in the management of small lacerations. They are ideal in

circumstances where general anesthesia is not indicated (or cannot be funded) but the end result is not quite as good as can be achieved with careful surgical apposition and suturing. The dressing is cut to shape and applied to the cleaned and dried wound such that there is at least 1 cm (0.4 in) margin of overlap. The dressing must be held gently in place for a few minutes until it has adhered. Once firmly attached, no further dressing is needed. Hydroactive dressings are light and generally very well tolerated. They suppress bacterial infection and encourage epithelialization. A discharge is often noted under these dressings as they break down; this should not be confused with infection. The remains of the hydroactive dressing may be gently peeled off after two weeks.

Surgical repair

Early surgical intervention is recommended[8]. The pinna must be surgically prepared and carefully debrided. The first sutures are placed at the pinnal margin to ensure good alignment. If a full-thickness laceration has occurred, it must be closed with sutures on both the concave and convex aspects, either with rows of simple interrupted sutures on both aspects or with simple interrupted sutures on one face and vertical mattress sutures on the other[8].

PINNAL DEFECTS

Large pinnal defects may be repaired with pedicle flaps[8]:

- The edges of the defect are debrided and straightened, excising as little tissue as possible. Topical antibacterial ointment is applied and the dressings changed, as necessary, for seven days, when a clean proud epithelial line is visible.
- A donor site is chosen to close the convex aspect of the defect first. It is selected on the basis of hair color, texture, density, and direction of growth, usually in the cervicobuccal region, avoiding the ventral midline of the neck.
- Both the recipient and donor site are aseptically prepared.

- The outline of the pinnal defect is marked on the donor site, allowing 5 mm (0.2 in) excess in all directions. The edges of the pinnal lesion are debrided.
- The pedicle is incised on the two edges which are to be sutured into the pinna and the graft is incorporated with simple interrupted sutures.
- The wound is dressed and bandaged. Regular redressing is performed for two weeks.

Three options are now available for management of the defect on the convex side of the pinna:

- The base of the pedicle is severed and the concave side left to granulate. This is usually cosmetically acceptable in dogs with pendulous ears.
- The base of the pedicle is severed and a new pedicle prepared for the defect on the concave aspect.
- The base of the original pedicle is used as a base for a new pedicle matching the defect on the concave aspect. Since the flap has revascularized it is not necessary to create a new pedicle, simply 'flip' the flap over and suture it into position. This technique is quick but runs the risk of avascular necrosis following collapse of vessels in the folded flap.

REFERENCES

1 Fraser G, Gregor WW, Mackenzie CP, Spreull JSA and Withers AR (1970) Canine ear disease. *Journal of Small Animal Practice* **10**, 725–754.
2 Getty R, Foust HL, Presley ET and Miller ER (1956) Macroscopic anatomy of the ear of the dog. *American Journal of Veterinary Research* **17**, 364–375.
3 Joyce JA, and Day MJ (1997) Immunopathogenesis of canine aural hematoma. *Journal of Small Animal Practice* **38**, 152–158.
4 Stephenson HC (1941) Some diseases of the ear of dogs. *Journal of the American Veterinary Medical Association* **98**, 138–142.
5 Kuwahara J (1986) Canine and feline aural hematomas: clinical, experimental, and clinicopathological observations. *American Journal of Veterinary Research* **47**, 2300–2308.
6 Kuwahara J (1986) Canine and feline aural hematomas: results of treatment with corticosteroids. *Journal of the American Animal Hospital Association* **22**, 641–647.
7 Joyce JA (1994) Treatment of canine aural haematoma using an indwelling drain and corticosteroids. *Journal of Small Animal Practice* **35**, 341–344.
8 Henderson RA and Horne RD (1993) The pinna. In *Textbook of Small Animal Surgery*. 2nd edn. (ed D Slatter) WB Saunders, Philadelphia, pp. 1545–1559.
9 Cechner PE (1998) Suture technique for repair of aural

hematoma. In *Current Techniques in Small Animal Surgery*. 4th edn. (ed MJ Bojrab) Williams and Wilkins, Baltimore, pp. 95–97.
10 Larsen S (1968) Intrachondrial rupture and hematoma formation in the external ear of dogs. *Pathologica Veterinaria* **5**, 442–450.
11 Dubielzig RR, Wilson JW and Serieg AA (1984) Pathogenesis of canine aural hematomas. *Journal of the American Veterinary Medical Association* **185**, 873–875.
12 Swaim SF and Henderson RA (1990) Wounds of the head. In *Small Animal Wound Management*. (eds SF Swaim and RA Henderson) Williams and Wilkins, Baltimore, pp. 191–233.
13 Bojrab MJ and Constantinescu GM (1998) Sutureless technique for repair of aural hematoma. In *Current Techniques in Small Animal Surgery*. 4th edn. (ed MJ Bojrab) Williams and Wilkins, Baltimore, pp. 97–98.
14 Kagan KG (1983) Treatment of canine aural hematoma with an indwelling drain. *Journal of the American Veterinary Medical Association* **182**, 972–974.
15 Wilson JW (1983) Treatment of auricular hematoma using a teat tube. *Journal of the American Veterinary Medical Association* **182**, 1081–1083.
16 Swaim SF and Bradley DM (1996) Evaluation of closed-suction drainage for treating auricular hematomas. *Journal of the American Animal Hospital Association* **32**, 36–43.

Chapter Eleven

Surgical Resection, Aural Ablation, and Bulla Osteotomy

INTRODUCTION

KEY POINTS

- Surgical resection and ablation of the ear canal is useful in the management of chronic ear disease, provided a critical assessment of the individual case is made on each occasion.
- Do not underestimate the medical aspects of chronic ear disease. In particular, recognize the contribution that dermatologic conditions can make to poor surgical outcome.
- Lateral wall resection is most probably over-performed and the technique has very few, if any, indications in the Cocker Spaniel.
- Vertical canal ablation is associated with the fewest postoperative complications.
- Total ablation and bulla osteotomy is best performed by an experienced surgeon.

The various surgical resections of the external ear canal are generally indicated as a means of resolving chronic otitis externa or as aids in the management of otitis media. The decision on how much of the external ear canal to resect is crucial, since the outcome of the surgical procedure will be assessed by the alleviation of the chronic otitis. For example, failure fully to assess the patient and make a definitive diagnosis of the cause of the otitis externa is the main reason why lateral wall resection fails. Thus, if the underlying cause is atopy or dietary intolerance, the otitis will continue to affect the remaining medial wall of the external ear canal, even after a technically perfect lateral wall resection.

Surgical management of ear disease cannot be divorced from the medical necessity of fully investigating all the components of the otic structure and recognizing that the epithelial lining of the external ear canal is an extension of the skin of the head and neck. Chronic otitis externa, at least in the dog, is usually a manifestation of a more generalized dermatologic process such as a defect in keratinization, hypersensitivity, endocrinopathy, or an immune-mediated disease. Furthermore, many cases are associated with otitis media. These diseases and associated problems must all be fully investigated before surgery is contemplated. Clinicians are urged to read the relevant chapters and sections of this book for further information.

PRESURGICAL INVESTIGATIONS

Presurgical assessment of the entire structure of the ear is essential[1, 2, 3]. In many cases some of the procedures advocated below will have been performed by way of routine management and work up of a case of otitis media or externa. A fuller description of these procedures can be found elsewhere in this book.

Palpation of the external ear canal may reveal thickening and ossification of the cartilaginous components. Local thickening, particularly in the parotid area, or the presence of a sinus adjacent to the external ear canal may reflect para-aural abscess[4, 5]. Changes to the vertical part of the external ear canal are often accompanied by chronic changes to the concave aspect of the pinna, which may be thickened and lichenified.

Otoscopy (see Chapter 2: Otoscopic appearance of the external ear canal and tympanum) is essential and a clear view is mandatory if meaningful conclusions are to be drawn. Visual examination via an otoscope can provide information on the state of the epithelial lining of the otic canal, the degree of stenosis of the lumen and, sometimes, an indication that neoplasia is present. The status of the tympanic membrane cannot always be assessed fully by otoscopy, even in a normal external ear canal[6].

Neurologic examination (see Chapter 2: Neurologic examination of the ear) of the facial, oculosympathetic, and vestibular (CN VIII) nerves provides a baseline for assessing the significance of any postoperative neurologic signs. Similarly, assessing a dog's auditory ability preoperatively may give a useful measure against which to compare postoperative deafness.

Bacteriological culture and sensitivity testing will often have been performed before surgery is considered. However, repeated use of various topical antibacterial agents may well influence the bacterial population and its antibacterial susceptibility. Preoperative sampling to provide an up-to-date antibacterial susceptibility is advisable if postoperative infection is to be managed effectively. However, if otitis media is present, intraoperative sampling is essential since it has been shown that in the presence of otitis media there is little correlation between the flora of the horizontal ear canal and that of the middle ear[7].

Radiographic assessment (see Chapter 2: Radiographic features of the normal and abnormal ear) of the external ear may reveal ossification of the auricular cartilage and absence of the luminal air shadow, both findings suggestive of chronic, inflammatory, proliferative otitis externa[8, 9]. Positive contrast ear canalography may be useful in establishing the status of the tympanum if tympanometry is not available or is impracticable, for instance if the external ear canal is stenosed[8, 10]. Radiographic examination of the middle ear is essential in the work up of otitis media[9, 10, 11], although CT (see Chapter 2: Imaging of the middle and inner ears) may be more sensitive for evaluation of otitis media than radiography[12].

Biopsy (see Chapter 2: Other investigatory procedures) of the epithelial lining of the external ear canal is rarely performed but, conceivably, it may help to influence whether surgery takes place. For example, if the histopathologic pattern is inflam-

> Owners should be cautioned that all aural resections, but particularly those involving ablation of the entire vertical canal, may adversely affect ear carriage in dogs with erect pinnae.

matory, with little evidence of fibrosis and glandular hyperplasia, aggressive glucocorticoid therapy may reduce luminal stenosis, thus obviating the need for surgery. Biopsy of neoplastic lesions may provide information which influences the type of surgical resection required, and it is therefore a useful presurgical investigation, particularly if the lesion is accessible. Cytologic examination of otic cerumen may help provide information on the tumor type but it cannot grade malignancy; this requires histopathologic examination of biopsy samples.

RESECTION AND ABLATION OF THE EXTERNAL EAR CANAL

INDICATIONS
Lateral wall resection
Resection of the lateral wall of the external ear canal is accompanied by a small, but measurable, reduction in the humidity within the lumen of the canal[13]. Whether this is clinically relevant is debatable. However, the provision of good drainage at the most ventral part of the external ear canal probably results in an improved otic microenvironment by reducing humidity and surface maceration. Zepp's modification[14] of an earlier technique[15] was the first report to describe the crucial step of making a drainplate (baffle) which provides the mechanism for markedly increased drainage of the ventral parts of the external ear canal.

Clinicians should note that lateral wall resection is probably contraindicated in the Cocker Spaniel for two reasons. Firstly, the otic disease is almost always too far advanced and secondly, the breed is very likely to have ear disease severe enough to warrant total ear canal ablation[2]. This is supported by a retrospective study which demonstrated that Cocker Spaniels, as a breed, correlate highly with surgical failure[16].

Lateral wall resection is indicated in the following circumstances[3, 17, 18]:

- Persistent, or recurrent, otitis externa with mild, potentially reversible, hyperplasia of the epithelium and adnexae.

- Neoplasia of the lateral wall of the vertical ear canal.
- In the management of otitis media to facilitate flushing and drainage of the bulla, although in most cases a total ear canal ablation and bulla osteotomy is probably the treatment of choice.

Vertical canal ablation
The purpose of vertical canal ablation is to remove the portion of the external ear canal which contains the most potential for chronic hyperplastic change. In reality, most surgery is performed in patients with irreversible changes already in place, i.e. it is salvage surgery rather than pre-emptive surgery. Furthermore, most cases of chronic otitis externa exhibit varying degrees of luminal stenosis within the horizontal portion of the external ear canal, in addition to changes within the vertical portion, and in theory this should also be removed. However, the horizontal canal is short and ablation of the vertical canal (provided a good

> It is important to stress that lateral wall resection will fail if there are chronic, irreversible, hyperplastic changes to the luminal epithelium[17, 18] or if there is ongoing otic inflammation. If in doubt, ablate the entire vertical canal.

drainplate is fashioned) establishes good drainage, resulting in an improvement of the microenvironment within the remaining portions of the canal.

Vertical canal ablation is indicated in the following circumstances[17, 18, 19]:

- Chronic, or recurrent, otitis externa associated with irreversible, hyperplastic changes in the luminal epithelium.
- Neoplasia of the vertical ear canal.

Total ear canal ablation (and lateral bulla osteotomy)

Total ear canal ablation is always performed with a lateral bulla osteotomy. The removal of the entire external ear canal can only be accomplished if the external canal is resected to the level of the tympanum, which marks the boundary between the external and the middle ear. This necessitates resection of bone.

Total ear canal ablation and lateral bulla osteotomy is rarely indicated in cats[2, 20]. Although bulla osteotomy alone (usually ventral) may be indicated for the management of polyps, for example, the otitis externa usually resolves and chronic changes are rarely severe enough to warrant vertical canal ablation.

Total ear canal ablation and lateral bulla osteotomy are indicated in the following circumstances[2, 3, 18, 21]:

- Chronic, or recurrent, otitis externa associated with irreversible, hyperplastic changes in the luminal epithelium.
- Failure of more conservative surgery to alleviate otitis externa or media.
- Neoplasia of the external ear canal.
- Otitis media.

Total ear canal ablation and lateral bulla osteotomy renders the ear dysfunctional as a hearing organ. Bilateral surgery may result in deafness[21].

Total ear canal ablation and lateral bulla osteotomy is a technically difficult procedure with potential for long-term postoperative neurologic deficiencies. This procedure should not be attempted by inexperienced surgeons. Referral is indicated.

RESECTION

Because of the difficulty of adequately preparing the entire surgical field, systemic antibiotics should be used in the intraoperative period and for ten days postoperatively. Antibiotic selection should be based on culture and sensitivity of the ear canal obtained prior to intravenous medication. If empirical drug selection is necessary, first generation cephalosporins[3] most often provide an adequate antibacterial spectrum, although the effect of previous therapy must be borne in mind.

Lateral wall resection

The crucial steps in this procedure are:

- Careful delineation of the tissue to be resected; do not let the incisures wander rostromedially.
- Construction of the drainplate (baffle).

A basic surgery kit supplemented with rongeurs, Gelpi retractors, periosteal elevators, Steinmann pins (**356**), drains, and small-gauge absorbable and non-absorbable suture materials is necessary. The external ear canal is flushed with 0.05% chlorhexidine solution. Both sides of the pinna are prepared aseptically, as well as the area of head surrounding the external acoustic meatus. It is helpful if the patient is positioned in lateral recumbency with the head supported over a sandbag; this helps to keep the tissues around the surgical field taut[17]. The pinna is hung with atraumatic forceps and a full draping of the field is performed[3, 18, 19].

The junction of the vertical and horizontal canal is determined by palpation or by inserting a curved hemostat, facing laterally, into the vertical canal to the level of the horizontal ear canal.

The incisions start at the incisures of the tragus (**357**) and continue parallel to the vertical canal (**358**), terminating below the level of the horizontal canal.

The flap is reflected, using blunt, superficial dissection (**359**), and removed.

Careful, blunt dissection is used to expose the cartilage of the canal (**360**). **NB:** The parotid salivary gland will be found at the base of the vertical canal, and care must be taken not to disrupt this structure. It is not necessary to dissect deeper than the vertical cartilage and the dissection should not be performed ventral to the horizontal canal, as damage to the facial nerve (CN VII) may occur.

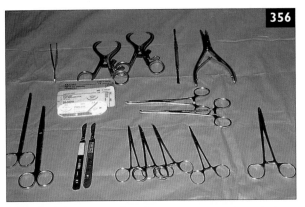

356   Basic instruments for otic surgery are supplemented with rongeurs, Gelpi retractors, and periosteal elevators.

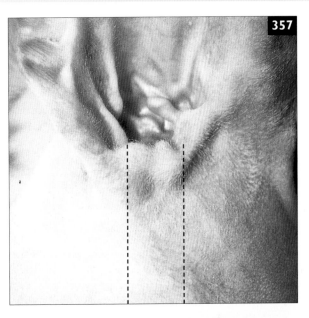

357   Illustration depicting the amount of skin to be removed during lateral wall resection.

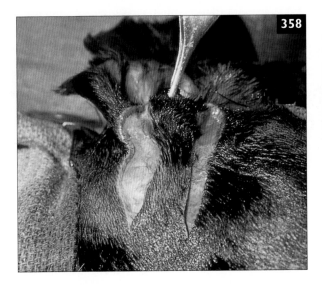

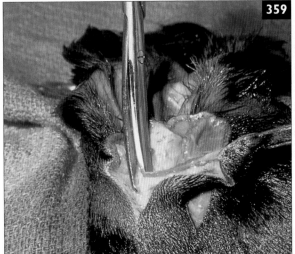

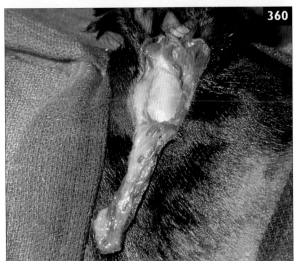

358   Lateral wall resection. The incisions are parallel to the vertical canal.

359   The skin flap is reflected using careful, superficial, blunt dissection.

360   The dissection is carried deeper to expose the cartilaginous wall of the external ear canal.

Using a tissue forceps at the lateral aspect of the external acoustic meatus for traction, the vertical canal is incised from the tragal incisures to the junction of the vertical and horizontal canals, to permit resection of the lateral one third to one half of the vertical canal (**361**). The local anatomy tends to force the incision rostro-medially. It is critical that this does not occur. Lane[7] advocated preliminary scoring (on the outer surface of the exposed ear canal prior to beginning the incisions) from the ligament between the conchal and annular cartilages dorsally to the tragal incisures, i.e. in the opposite direction to which the actual incisions will subsequently be performed. This scoring provides a guide for incision and prevents the line of incision wandering rostromedially. This is crucial for surgery success as any tendency for the incision to deviate from the lateral aspect of the vertical canal results in a narrowed exposure and an inadequate drainplate[3, 17, 19, 23, 24].

The incised section of vertical wall is reflected (**362**). A section of the lateral cartilage is left attached at the base, 2–3 cm (0.8–1.2 in) above the level of the junction between the conchal and annular cartilages (**363**). This will allow creation of a drainplate[17, 24]. The creation of a functional drainplate is essential for the success of this technique.

The drainplate is created by reflecting the residual flap of the lateral wall of the vertical canal ventrally (**364**), using the ligament between the conchal and annular cartilages as a hinge[24]. Simple interrupted subcuticular monofilament absorbable sutures (3/0) should be used to suture the flap in place. It is easiest to suture the four corners first to ensure proper positioning. Apposition of the remaining exposed cartilage to the skin is then performed in the same manner (**365**). Absorbable, or non-absorbable, skin sutures are used if necessary.

Postoperative care

Postoperative self-trauma may be a problem and adequate analgesia must be ensured; taping the pinnae over the head may help to minimize disruption of the suture line[5, 18] and in some cases an Elizabethan collar may be necessary until the incision has healed (see Chapter 12: Perioperative analgesia and management). Postoperative use of anti-inflammatory doses of prednisolone (0.5–1.0 mg/kg p/o q24h) may be of use in helping to minimize soft tissue swelling[5], although care should be taken not to use prednisolone in conjunction with non-steroidal anti-inflammatory drugs (NSAIDs). Gentle application of a warm moist towel helps to minimize swelling and facilitate cleaning of the surgical site.

If non-absorbable sutures are used, they should be left in place for 14 days[18], although regular postoperative checks are important. Caution owners that wound healing and complete recovery may take some time. It may take 10–14 days for obvious improvement to take place and several weeks for re-epithelialization of any defects around the drainplate to be completed[5]. Mild postoperative surgical dehiscence is left to heal by second intention[18]. Complete dehiscence necessitates surgical revision; postoperative infection should be suspected in these cases and bacterial culture and sensitivity testing performed.

It may prove necessary to sedate the animal to facilitate suture removal. To avoid this the use of long-life absorbent materials such as PDS should be considered. Regular clipping of long hair in the area helps ensure cleanliness.

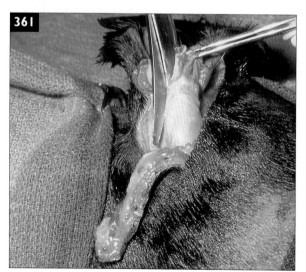

361   Starting at the tragus, the vertical ear canal is incised to the level of the horizontal ear canal.

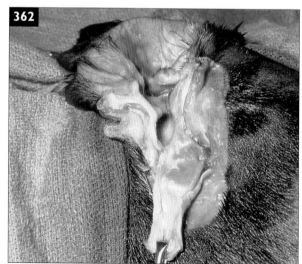

362   The reflected skin flap has been removed. The excised section of lateral wall is reflected ventrally.

Postsurgical problems

Reviews of lateral wall resections cite a 34–47% failure rate[15, 25]. There are three common reasons for failure of this procedure, two medical and one surgical[23]:

- Failure to appreciate that this procedure should not be relied upon as the sole treatment for otitis externa. Concurrent medical therapy of underlying

disorders and concomitant infections is imperative if resolution of otitis externa is to be achieved. Inflammatory changes will continue in the medial wall irrespective of the surgical technique (**366**).
- Unrecognized otitis media.
- Failure to provide adequate drainage for the remnants of the horizontal canal by way of a functional drainplate.

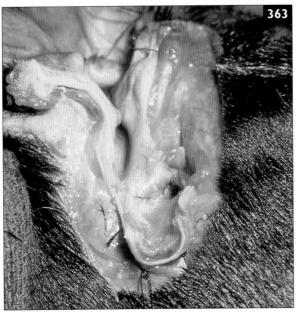

363 The major part of the reflected cartilage is removed, ensuring that a 2–3 cm (0.8–1.2 in) flap is left with which to make the drainplate.

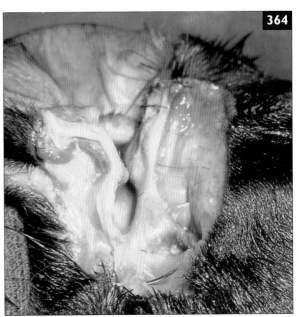

364 The reflected drainplate is sutured to surrounding skin, starting at the corners.

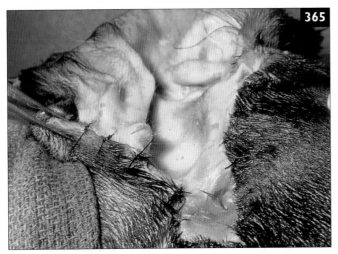

365 The exposed walls of the vertical canal are then sutured to surrounding skin, to close the operation.

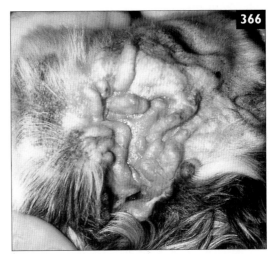

366 This English Setter has atopy. The lateral wall resection was technically sound, but it failed in its objective because otitis continued.

Options in the face of postsurgical problems

If the results of surgery are disappointing, it is important to understand why, rather than to persist with ineffectual topical medications in the face of ongoing pathologic change and aural discomfort, or even frank pain. Surgical options include:

- Corrective surgery. In reality this is limited to providing a functional drainplate and this should only be performed in cases where there is no ongoing inflammation in the medial wall.
- Converting the lateral wall resection to a vertical canal ablation. This option should only be considered if there is no evidence of otitis media and if the horizontal canal is normal and provided with a fully patent opening and a functional drainplate.
- Performing a total ablation and bulla osteotomy.

VERTICAL EAR CANAL ABLATION

The crucial steps in this procedure are:

- Construction of an effective drainplate.
- Careful closure of all dead space.

Preparation of the field is identical to that for a lateral ear resection.

An initial 'T'-shaped incision is made. The lower point of the incision, the base of the 'T', is just below the level of the horizontal portion of the external ear canal[3, 17, 23, 24, 26]. The bar of the 'T' follows a circumferential path across the medial wall of the conchal cartilage (**367**), immediately dorsal to the large antihelicine tubercle[17]. In dogs with erect pinnae a dorsally curved incision may be performed; this results in a crescent-shaped base for the pinna and helps to maintain a normal carriage postoperatively[27].

Incision through the auricular cartilage is made, taking care not to penetrate the lateral aspect of the pinna. The 'trumpet' of conchal cartilage is grasped with tissue forceps and a combination of blunt and sharp dissection is used to isolate the vertical canal, which can be pulled free from the underlying tissues (**368**). It is essential to keep the dissection as close to the cartilage as possible as this minimizes iatrogenic damage to blood vessels and nerves.

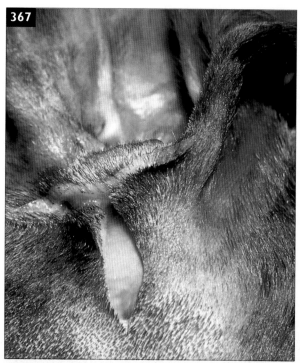

367   Vertical canal ablation. A 'T'-shaped incision is made over the vertical ear canal.

The excised canal is sectioned above the level of the horizontal canal to allow creation of a drainplate (**369**). The ligamentous connection between the annular and conchal cartilages is used as a hinge to allow reflection of the cartilage, as in the lateral wall resection described above. At the new acoustic meatus, exact closure of skin to canal epithelium with 4/0 absorbable monofilament subcuticular sutures is attempted so as to minimize stricture at the site (**370**). Skin sutures are placed if necessary.

The suture line is closed above the drainplate (**371**), incorporating subcutaneous tissues deep to the excised conchal cartilages with the sutures to eliminate dead space[17]. Failure to close dead space may result in postoperative dehiscence.

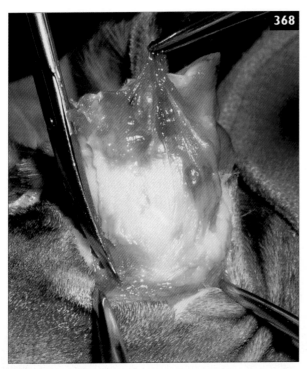

368 Circumferential dissection of the soft tissues is performed keeping as close to the cartilaginous ear canal as possible.

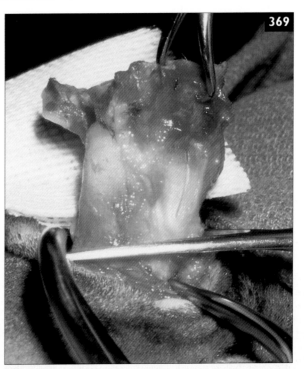

369 The base of the freed vertical ear canal is resected at a level below the diseased tissue, at the level of the horizontal ear canal.

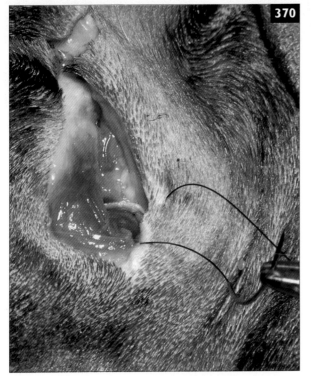

370 A permanent stroma is constructed by ensuring that the cartilaginous portion of the horizontal ear canal remains patent when sutured to the skin.

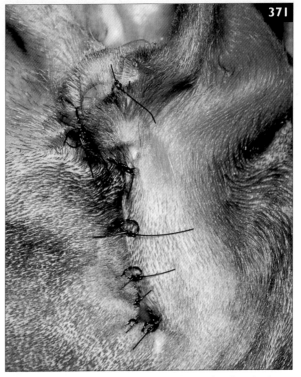

371 The rest of the incision is closed, ensuring that dead space is eliminated.

Pull-through modification[28]

This modification of vertical canal ablation results in less incised tissue to suture than with standard techniques, less trauma to subcutaneous tissues, less risk of damage to associated structures such as the salivary glands, less postoperative discomfort, fewer sutures, more rapid healing, and less dead space. Although the original authors did not describe the creation of a drainplate, it is generally considered appropriate to do so.

The circumferential incision is identical to that described above except that a subsequent vertical incision is not made (**372**). Instead, the conchal cartilage is gradually worked free by digital and blunt dissection until the entire 'trumpet' of the vertical canal is freed from its soft tissue attachments and exposed via the dorsal incision (**373, 374**).

The skin is palpated at the level of the horizontal canal (**375**) and a circular incision, roughly one and a half times the diameter of the horizontal canal, is made (**376**).

The entire, exposed conchal cartilage 'trumpet', which was previously exposed by blunt dissection, is pulled through this ventral incision (**377**) and cut 1.5 cm (0.6 in) above the level of the horizontal canal (**378**).

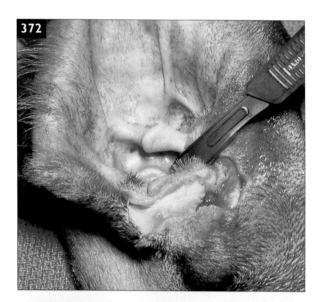

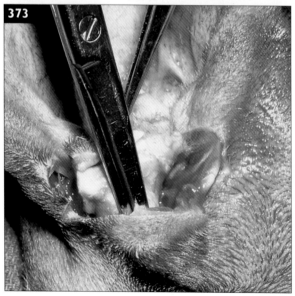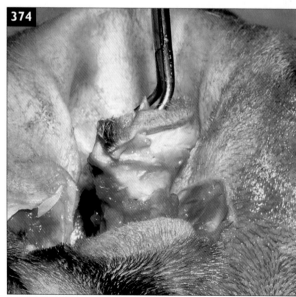

372 Tigari modification. A circumferential incision is made at the entrance to the vertical ear canal.

373, 374 Using traction and blunt dissection, the vertical ear canal is gradually freed from its surroundings.

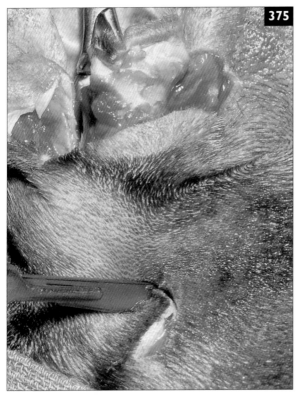

375 The level of the horizontal ear canal is palpated.

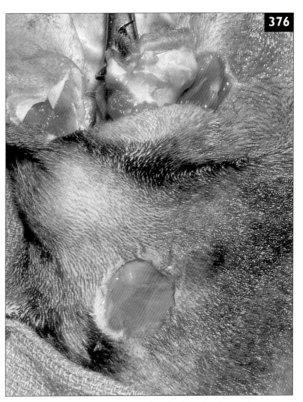

376 The skin is incised at the level of the horizontal ear canal.

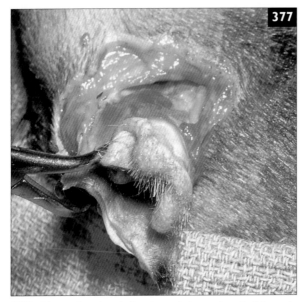

377 The entire, already freed, conchal cone is pulled through the incision.

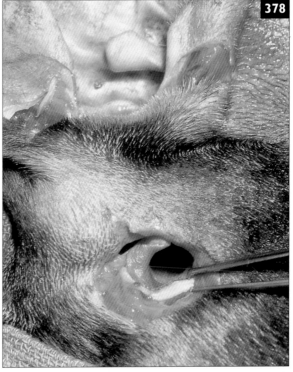

378 The exposed vertical ear canal is excised at the level of the horizontal ear canal.

A drainplate is constructed as described above (**379**) and the distal incision closed (**380**).

Postoperative care

Postoperative analgesia is mandatory (see Chapter 12: Perioperative analgesia and management). Postoperative antibacterial therapy should be continued for at least ten days, or until the sutures are removed. Surgical aftercare is similar to that provided for lateral ear resection, although the wound is less likely to dehisce[18].

Postsurgical problems

Postsurgical complications with this technique are much less common than those seen after lateral wall resection[17, 18, 26]. Furthermore, improper patient selection occurs less frequently than with lateral wall resection[17]. In one study[26], dehiscence of the suture line occurred in 12% of cases, with stenosis of the external acoustic meatus occurring in 7% of cases. Damage to the facial nerve is possible, particularly if deep sectioning of the external acoustic meatus is attempted. Stenosis of the external acoustic meatus (**381**) is usually a consequence of inadequate construction of the drainplate, resulting in a failure to support the canal and impairment of natural drainage[16].

Options in the face of postsurgical problems

- Postoperative, acute, inflammatory stenosis of the external acoustic meatus may be suppressed if the lumen is packed with glucocorticoid-impregnated gauze for a few days[17].
- Dehiscence is best treated aggressively with systemic antibacterial agents and drainage[26]. Consideration should be given to obtaining a culture and sensitivity report if dehiscence occurs in dogs receiving postoperative antibacterial therapy. Surgical closure is indicated as soon as infection is under control[6].
- Stenosis of, or impaired drainage from, the external acoustic meatus warrants investigation since it implies one of two problems, neither mutually antagonistic: inadequate drainplate construction or ongoing otitis media.

Dealing with ossification of the external ear canal

Mineralization of the cartilaginous components of the external ear canal may occur as a consequence of chronic inflammation[5]. The initial changes appear to occur in the horizontal canal[5], although with time, and in particular in Cocker Spaniels, the vertical canal may also become ossified. Although the ossified vertical canal may be removed relatively easily by ablation, the surgical resection of ossified horizontal canals is more difficult[5].

A surgical technique has been described[5, 29] for dissecting out the ossified portions of the horizontal and vertical canals, although if the condition has progressed to this stage, total ablation and bulla osteotomy may be indicated. However, since total ablation and bulla osteotomy sometimes results in loss of hearing, owners may want to avoid such a radical step, particularly if the contralateral ear has already been ablated. Although the pain associated with chronic otitis externa was largely controlled in the dogs subjected to this procedure[29], most required occasional treatment to clean the ear canals.

The technique for dissecting out the ossifications is as follows (after Hobson[5] and Elkins *et al.*[29]):

- If the vertical canal is still present (and is to be ablated, as described above), it is exposed and the dissection is continued ventrally to expose the ventral wall of the ossified horizontal canal, taking great care to avoid the facial nerve.
- In the presence of an ossified vertical canal, ronguers are used to remove ossified cartilage from the lateral surface of that portion of the vertical canal destined to form the drainplate. In effect, the drainplate is constructed from the epithelial components of the vertical canal rather than from the cartilaginous portion.
- An incision is made on the distal aspect of the junction of the annular and auricular cartilages. This allows an osteotome (or a small rounded periosteal elevator) gradually to elevate the soft tissue lining of the horizontal canal. The ossified cartilage can then be gradually removed with ronguers while leaving the soft tissue lining of the ear canal intact.
- Once the ossified material has been removed a drainplate is created from the remnants of the lateral wall of the vertical canal, taking care to ensure that the horizontal canal is patent.

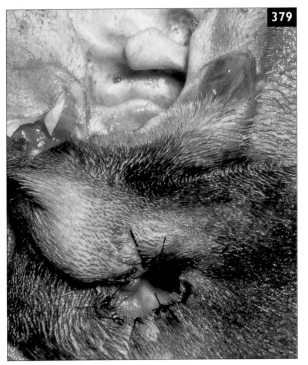

379   The stoma at the horizontal ear canal is closed, taking care to ensure that the drainplate keeps the opening patent.

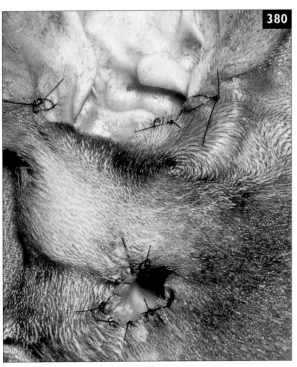

380   The initial circumferential incision is closed in a routine manner.

381   Stenosis of the horizontal ear canal following inadequate construction of the drainplate. The problem was exacerbated by a failure to identify underlying atopy, which resulted in ongoing disease in the remnants of the vertical ear canal and concave aspect of the pinna.

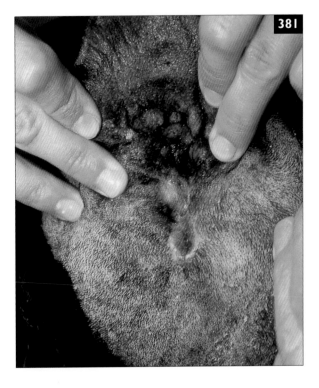

TOTAL EAR CANAL ABLATION AND LATERAL BULLA OSTEOTOMY

The crucial steps in this procedure are:

- Avoid damage to the round window and the facial nerve.
- Ensure that all secretory epithelium is removed from the bulla and from the site of the horizontal ear canal.
- Treat tissues gently; ensure good hemostasis and close all dead space.

It is now generally accepted that it is prudent to perform a lateral bulla osteotomy (LBO) with every total ear canal ablation[2, 3, 19, 30, 31, 32]. Given the difficulty of definitively documenting otitis media by radiography[8], or even by CT[33], it is almost impossible to justify not performing a bulla osteotomy. Any residual discharge or secretion which might result from continuing otitis media, or indeed any portions of epithelial tissue inadvertently left behind, will accumulate and may well result in para-aural abscessation[3, 31]. Most authorities recommend LBO in association with ablation of the external ear canal, since to perform ventral bulla osteotomy would require repositioning of the animal during surgery, an unnecessary complication since the ventral approach has no advantage over the lateral[34].

Presurgical evaluation of the facial, oculosympathetic, and vestibular (CN VIII) nerves is useful[2, 33, 35] as it provides a baseline for assessing the significance of any postoperative neurologic signs. Bilateral total ear canal ablation (TECA) performed simultaneously has been reported to cause pharyngeal swelling[2], a complication of hypoglossal nerve damage. This complication may necessitate a tracheostomy to alleviate upper airway obstruction. For this reason some surgeons stage the procedure by allowing at least 2–3 weeks to lapse before performing a second TECA on a patient. However, other surgeons take the view that the advantages of a single episode of anesthesia and a single period of postoperative pain outweigh the small risk of pharyngeal problems.

Total ablation and bulla osteotomy should render the ear deaf but, somewhat surprisingly, this does not always occur[2, 22, 36]. It is wise to try and assess the dog's auditory ability preoperatively and to demonstrate this to the owners[2] in an attempt to forestall unwarranted accusations of surgical ineptitude.

Systemic antibacterial therapy is indicated both pre- and postoperatively, beginning 7–14 days preoperatively[35]. The patient is anesthetized and the surgical area prepared as described above. The pinna is hung with atraumatic forceps and a full draping of the field is performed. A small rolled towel placed under the neck of the dog, to elevate the head to the level of the chest wall, facilitates exposure[2].

A circumferential incision is made around the acoustic meatus, severing the auricular cartilage but not penetrating the lateral skin surface of the pinna. The incision is continued to the level of the junction of the horizontal and vertical ear canals (**382**). It may be necessary to resect large areas of infected, hyperplastic tissue in some cases, with consequent implications for postoperative pinnal carriage.

Blunt dissection is used to expose the lateral surface of the vertical canal (**383**). The vertical canal is freed from the surrounding tissue using a combination of blunt and sharp dissection (**384, 385**). A dry gauze sponge can be helpful for bluntly rubbing the connective tissue from the vertical canal. Care should be taken to avoid hemorrhage from the rostral auricular artery and vein and from the auriculopalpebral (branch of the facial) and auriculotemporal (branch of the trigeminal) nerves in the cranial aspect of the dissection[35]. Damage to blood vessels in this area may lead to avascular necrosis of the pinna[2]. Hemorrhage may be controlled with electrocautery in the area around the vertical canal but not the horizontal canal; the risk to the facial nerve is too great[5].

Blunt dissection, keeping as close to the perichondrium as possible, is continued around the angle that forms the transition between the vertical and horizontal canals, which represents the transition from auricular cartilage to annular cartilage (**386**). Care should be taken to identify the facial nerve as it exits from the stylomastoid foramen and curves rostroventrally around the horizontal canal. It should be carefully retracted ventrally. The advantage of performing this dissection after freeing the vertical canal is that there is maximal tissue laxity, which allows the fullest retraction[21]. In some cases the facial nerve may be intimately associated with perichondrial connective tissue or even buried within the reactive tissue surrounding ossified cartilage[1, 31]. This will require careful dissection if significant postoperative morbidity is to be avoided. Gelpi retractors may be useful at this point. If the facial nerve proves hard to find, Smeak[21] advocated searching the caudal and more superficial aspect of the horizontal ear canal for small branches of the internal auricular nerve which penetrate the cartilage; these may be followed back to the facial nerve trunk. Gentle traction and tissue manipulation in this area is mandatory.

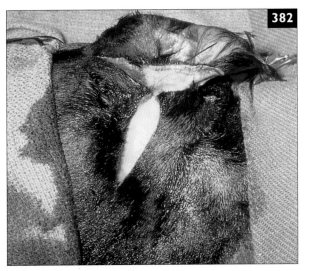

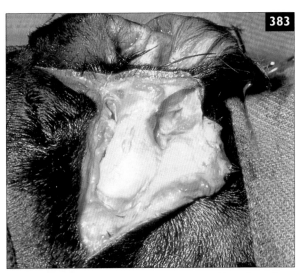

382 Total ear canal ablation and bulla osteotomy. The initial incisions are made.

383 The vertical ear canal is exposed, using blunt dissection.

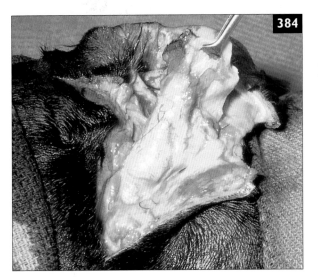

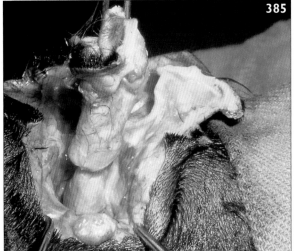

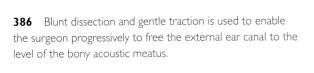

384, 385 The external ear canal is gradually freed.

386 Blunt dissection and gentle traction is used to enable the surgeon progressively to free the external ear canal to the level of the bony acoustic meatus.

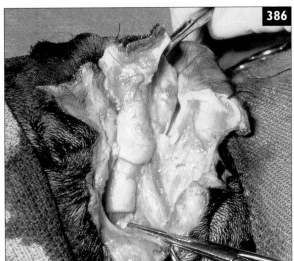

Blunt dissection is continued along the horizontal canal to the level of the skull. The entire horizontal canal is exposed to the level of the bony acoustic meatus, and then sharply transected, with scissors, at this level (**387**). If chronic disease has caused ossification of the horizontal canal, a small osteotome may be necessary to transect the ear canal. A clamp across the base of the horizontal canal before transection minimizes contamination from debris within the canal.

A bone curette is used to scrape all epithelial tissue from the osseous external acoustic meatus[32, 35, 37]. It is critical that all secretory tissue is removed as failure to achieve this will result in postoperative para-aural abscessation. The bony external acoustic meatus is removed (**388**) using a sharp, small rongeur (such as a Lempert rongeur) or an air drill. This will allow increased visualization of the tympanic cavity. When enlarging the external auditory meatus it is best to stay rostral and ventral to avoid the oval and round windows (on the opposite wall of the bulla to the tympanum) and the facial nerve[37].

The ventrolateral portion of the tympanic bulla is removed (**389**) with rongeurs or an air-driven bur. It may prove necessary to extend the osteotomy rostrally and caudally in order adequately to visualize the caudal aspects of the tympanic cavity. It is imperative that the shelf of bone ventromedial to the external acoustic meatus is removed if adequate exposure is to be achieved for optimum curettage[37].

The surgeon should avoid advancing onto the ventral aspect of the bulla. Some ventral retraction of the soft tissues will have been performed to allow dissection of the annular cartilage, but both the facial nerve and the external carotid artery are in this area and extreme caution is warranted. If hemorrhage is encountered, definitive hemostasis is important; use hemostatic clips[37].

Suction is usually necessary at this point to maintain adequate visibility of the surgical field. The tympanic cavity is curetted or abraded, using a dry gauze sponge wrapped on the end of a hemostat to remove any inspissated contents, secretory epithelium, and remnants of the tympanic membrane and the malleus, if not removed earlier. Care should be taken not to evulse the stapes off the oval window; peripheral vestibular problems may result. Paradoxically, removal of chronically inflamed epithelia is often more easily

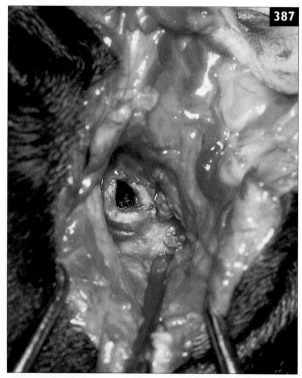

387 The external ear canal is excised to expose the tympanic aperture.

accomplished than removal of minimally inflamed tissue. Extreme care should be taken not to disrupt the epitympanic recess, the round window (mid-dorsal aspect), or the oval window (craniodorsal). Samples from the middle ear should be submitted for bacterial culture and sensitivity.

NB: This part of the procedure is critical, for if infected secretory tissue is left within the bulla, postoperative abscessation and fistulation can be expected.

The tympanic cavity is thoroughly flushed with warmed saline solution (**390**). A drain (latex, active, or ingress/egress) (**391**) may be placed, entering via the tympanic orifice and exiting the tympanic cavity through the osteotomy and passing through the skin via a stab incision. This is beneficial if clearing of the bulla is not complete or if a large amount of discharge is expected[2]. Drainage may not be necessary with strict adherence to good surgical techniques[38].

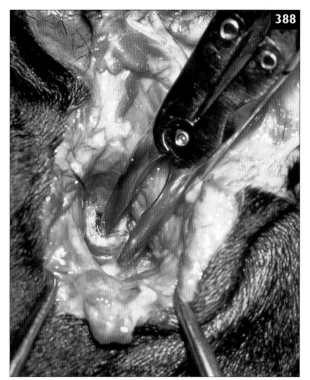

388 Using rongeurs, the bony external acoustic meatus is removed to expose further the tympanic cavity.

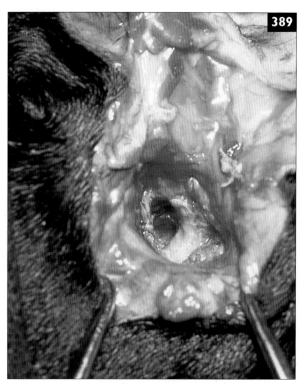

389 The ventrolateral wall of the tympanic bulla has now been breached.

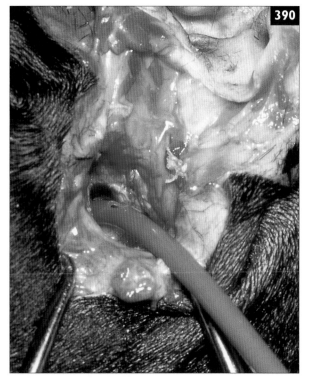

390 After the tympanic cavity has been curetted it is flushed to ensure removal of all debris.

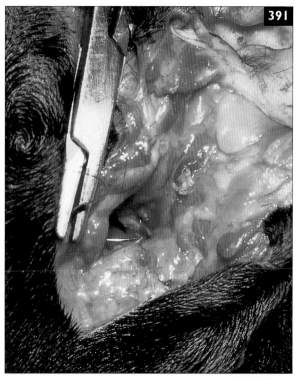

391 A drain tube is placed (through a separate stab incision) and closure begun.

Closure is performed using monofilament absorbable sutures in the subcutaneous tissue (**392–394**). Great care must be taken to close all potential dead space as this will help to minimize postoperative cellulitis. Routine skin closure is performed in the shape of a 'T', with care taken to effect a cosmetic ear carriage when closing the area of the former tragus and antitragus.

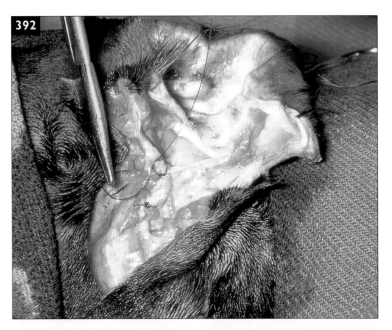

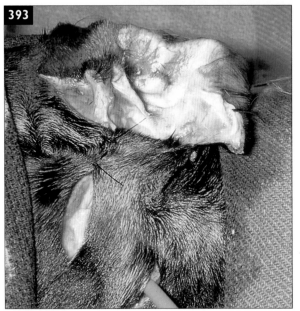

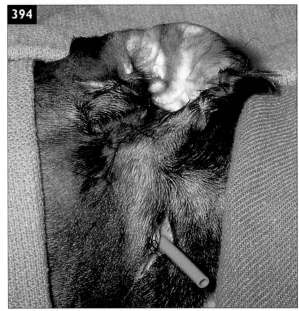

392–394 Routine closure, ensuring elimination of dead space, ends the surgery.

Postsurgical care

Postoperative analgesia is mandatory (see Chapter 12: Perioperative analgesia and management). Postoperative systemic antibacterial therapy is usually warranted and must be continued for 10–21 days[2, 35]. The choice of antibacterial agent may need to be reviewed in the light of bacterial culture and sensitivity testing of tissue obtained at surgery. Postoperative glucocorticoids have been recommended[5]. Used in anti-inflammatory doses (0.5–1.0 mg/kg divided q12h) prednisolone may help to decrease postoperative swelling. Glucocorticoids should not be used for more than three days and care must be taken to ensure that they are not used concurrently with NSAIDs as there is an increased risk of gastric ulceration.

Generally, it is not necessary to irrigate postoperatively; the drains are placed (**395, 396**) to allow local exudate to clear the surgical site rather than to facilitate flushing[35]. If a drain is inserted, soft, padded dressings should be used to cover the surgical site and the drain egress until the drain is removed, typically after 2–5 days. Care should be taken that these dressings do not constrict the pharynx[21]. Sutures are removed after 10–14 days.

Careful neurologic observations should be made. In the immediate postoperative period, hypoglossal damage may be apparent and although it does not usually require specific treatment, animals should be closely observed for the 24 hours immediately post surgery[2]. Respiratory function, in particular, should be monitored postoperatively as significant pharyngeal swelling may occur following bilateral surgery[21]. Ocular lubricants may be indicated until normal blink reflex is regained.

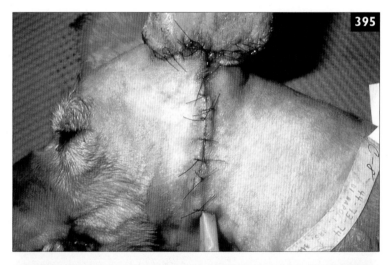

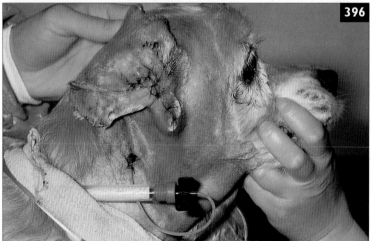

395, 396 Passive and active drains, put in place after surgery, ensure that any exudate is removed.

Postsurgical problems

Postsurgical problems are a reflection of two main factors: the surgical complexity of the procedure and the degree of bacterial contamination of the surgical site[2, 21, 35].

Discharge from the surgical site is common[2, 31, 32, 33, 37]. Discharge and postoperative swelling may be treated with hot compresses for five minutes, three times daily. Drainage may be facilitated by removing the most ventral sutures. Fistula formation (para-aural sinus) (**397**) may occur 3–12 months post surgery in cases in which incomplete removal of infected and secretory tissue was achieved. Para-aural sinuses may create more clinical problems than the original otitis[21] (see Chapter 6: Para-aural abscess).

Pinnal necrosis (which is usually limited to the caudal aspect of the pinna) is a consequence of compromised blood supply. Management is based on local cleansing, debridement if necessary, and awaiting re-epithelialization.

Postoperative nerve damage is relatively common, and in about 10% of cases some degree of permanent neuropathy can be expected[2, 32, 35, 38]. Hypoglossal nerve damage (drooling, dysphagia) is usually short term. Facial nerve damage is the most common postoperative neuropathy[2, 32, 35, 38]. Mild, transient paresis of the auriculopalpebral nerve is also common[21]. Ninety percent of these cases resolve within a few weeks of surgery and they can be managed by application of artificial tears, for example[35, 37]. However, absence of blink reflex, lip paralysis, or pinnal paralysis may be long term and the prognosis is poor if no evidence of improvement is apparent four weeks post surgery[21]. The practical consequences of long-term facial nerve damage are minimal provided tear production is normal and exophthalmia is not present[21].

Postoperative Horner's syndrome and damage to the facial nerve (ptosis, midriasis, nystagmus, head tilt, flaccid facial paralysis) is usually confined to the cat and will resolve within a few weeks, as long as the otitis media has resolved[2].

Options in the face of postsurgical problems

Short-term complications such as incisional abscess, dehiscence, or swelling can be seen with TECA-LBO. Most are short lived and resolve with conservative treatment, although extensive complications may require surgical revision.

If damage to the epitympanic recess, oval window, or round window occurs, abnormalities such as nystagmus, head tilt, and general vestibular abnormalities can occur. This complication is often temporary, and resolves within 7–10 days with only supportive care. If a patient displayed a head tilt prior to surgery, it will often persist in the acute post-operative period, with some patients remaining persistently abnormal.

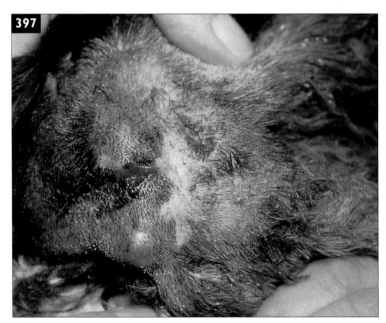

397 Para-aural sinus following incomplete removal of all secretory tissues at surgery.

Long-term complications usually involve abscessation of the middle ear and/or fistulation of tissues ventral to the middle ear (see Chapter 6: Para-aural abscess). Most commonly this is due to incomplete excision of the membranous lining of the bulla[3, 38]. Medical therapy of persistent or recurrent infection is rarely curative. Surgical re-exploration of the bulla to remove remaining epithelial tissue, combined with debridement of infected tissue and appropriate drainage, is used to control infection and this is effective in up to 85% of dogs with recurrent postoperative otitis[39, 40].

Deafness and loss of hearing ability after total ablation and bulla osteotomy is a common concern of owners. Studies vary, but patients with severe proliferative canal disease tend to retain the same level of hearing they had prior to surgery, hence the value of preoperative assessment[22]. This also is true in most cases when comparing preoperative and postoperative brainstem auditory evoked responses[6, 40].

BULLA OSTEOTOMY

INDICATIONS
The principle indication for bulla osteotomy is the treatment of refractory otitis media[34, 35, 37]. The procedure is most commonly performed in the dog in association with total ablation of the external ear canal, in which case a lateral bulla osteotomy is performed. The alternative approach to the bulla is a ventral approach, most often performed in the cat in the management of inflammatory polyps arising from the middle ear. Other, much less common, indications are the excision of neoplastic masses and the removal of cholesteatomas[21].

SURGICAL TECHNIQUE
Lateral bulla osteotomy as a separate procedure
Lateral bulla osteotomy is more easily performed after total ear canal ablation has been carried out, principally because of increased visualization[41].

The surgical technique is as follows (after Krahwinkel et al.[40], Barrett and Rathfon[42], and Booth[43]):
- A skin incision is made over the external ear canal and extended ventrally beyond the level of the horizontal ear canal. The subcutaneous tissues are gently dissected to reveal the apposition of the parotid salivary gland and the horizontal ear canal.
- Gentle, ventral retraction of the parotid gland should reveal the facial nerve, which is carefully retracted caudoventrally to reveal the lateral aspect of the tympanic bulla.
- The bulla is further exposed using a periosteal elevator and broached with a Steinmann pin in a hand chuck. Care is needed here because the density of the bulla varies and is unpredictable; too much pressure and the pin may impact on the opposite side of the tympanic cavity. The pin enters on the caudolateral aspect of the bulla and is directed from a caudoventral direction so that if it impacts on the medial wall it avoids the mediodorsal wall.
- The osteotomy site is enlarged with rongeurs, observing the precautions outlined above.
- Samples for microbiological culture and sensitivity testing are taken and the tympanic cavity is flushed with warm isotonic saline until the run-out is clear of debris.
- If purulence is evident in the tympanic cavity, a drain tube is sometimes placed. This is sutured to adjacent soft tissues with 4/0 catgut and exited adjacent to the initial skin incision. Twice daily flushing with an appropriate antibacterial agent is performed until the drain is removed after seven days. Flushing may not always be effective unless an ingress (dorsal via the tympanic opening)/egress (ventral) drain is used[31]. Passive ventral drainage may suffice in many cases.

Ventral bulla osteotomy
Ventral bulla osteotomy provides less opportunity for iatrogenic nerve damage, better visualization of the tympanic cavity, and more consistent ventral drainage than the lateral approach[44, 45]. The reason that this approach is not used more frequently in dogs is that in most cases middle ear infection is associated with chronic external ear disease and both areas are then addressed in a unified field. Furthermore, in one study[34] there was little difference in postoperative complications compared with the lateral approach.

Ventral bulla osteotomy is the most frequently used approach in the cat, a reflection of otitis media occurring in the absence of chronic otitis externa in this species. Note that the bulla of the cat differs from that of the dog (see page 255).

The surgical technique is as follows (after Fossum[3], Harari[19], Smeak and de Hoff[31], Booth[44], Seim[45], Denny[46], and McNutt and McCoy[47]):

- A sagittal incision is made immediately medial to the mandibular salivary gland, at a level midway between the angle of the mandible and the wings of the atlas (**398**). The thin myelohyoid muscle is split.
- The digastricus muscle is separated from the hyoglossal and styloglossal muscles by blunt dissection.
- The hypoglossal nerve and branches of the internal carotid artery are identified on the lateral aspect of the hyoglossal muscle and carefully retracted medially.
- Further retraction of the digastricus muscle (laterally) and of the hyoglossal muscle (medially) reveals the rounded bulge of the bulla between the jugular processes of the skull (caudal to the bulla) and the angular process of the mandible (rostral).
- The thin muscular covering of the bulla is incised and reflected with a periosteal elevator (**398**).
- The bulla is broached with a Steinmann pin in a hand chuck (**399**). Care is needed here because sudden penetration may result in the pin impacting on the dorsal aspect of the tympanic cavity and damaging the oval or round windows.
- The pin is removed and the osteotomy site enlarged with rongeurs (**400, 401**).
- Samples for microbiological culture and sensitivity testing are taken and the tympanic cavity is flushed with warm isotonic saline until the run-out is clear of debris.
- A drain tube is placed if necessary (see above) in the tympanic cavity, sutured to adjacent soft tissues with 4/0 catgut, and exited adjacent to the initial skin incision. Twice daily flushing with an appropriate antibacterial agent is performed until drain removal after seven days.

Postsurgical problems

Possible complications to bulla osteotomy are principally neurologic[42]. As with those encountered after total ear canal ablation and bulla osteotomy (described above), these relate principally to the hypoglossal nerve (drooling, dysphagia) and branches of the sympathetic and parasympathetic nerve supply (ipsilateral Horner's syndrome and keratoconjunctivitis sicca, respectively).

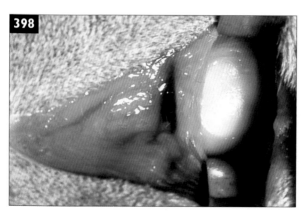

398   The bulla has been exposed.

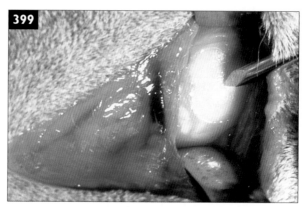

399   A Steinmann pin has been used to broach the bulla.

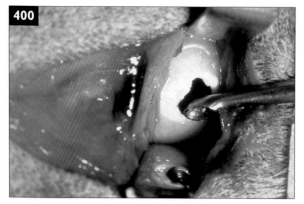

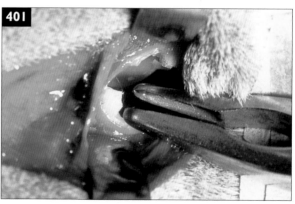

400, 401   The osteotomy is progressively enlarged with rongeurs.

SPECIAL PROBLEMS RELATING TO SURGERY OF THE MIDDLE EAR IN CATS

Middle ear disease in cats usually relates to otitis media or inflammatory polyps, although neoplasia may occur rarely[20, 47].

The tympanic bullae of cats are easily palpable on the ventral aspect of the feline skull and they are easily accessible with a straightforward dissection (**402**), as outlined above. However, the ventral chamber of the tympanic cavity is characterized by an incomplete bony septum[44]. It is this septum which is visible upon opening the ventral wall of the tympanic bulla and it divides the ventral cavity into two. The larger ventromedial chamber is entered via the bulla osteotomy and the smaller dorsolateral chamber, in effect the tympanic cavity proper, lies beyond the septum.

The two chambers communicate via the space between the septum and the caudomedial wall of the tympanic cavity[44]. The round window of the cochlea, the promontory, and the postganglionic fibers of the cervical sympathetic trunk are in this region of the medial wall and are thus vulnerable to damage, particularly if the septum is removed. Horner's syndrome will result if the sympathetic fibers are damaged. It may be necessary to open the septum if access to inflammatory polyps in the dorsolateral chamber is required or to facilitate drainage and, if so, care should be taken to avoid the region adjacent to the promontory[20]. Postoperative Horner's syndrome occurred in 57% of cases in one series[48]. Although the majority of cases resolved within eight days of surgery, the signs persisted, albeit mildly, after four weeks in

21% of cases. Some facial paresis and inner ear disease (head tilt, ataxia) may also be noted postoperatively in a proportion of cases, again usually temporary[20].

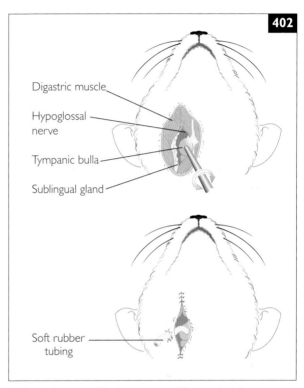

402 Feline ventral bulla osteotomy. The surgical site. (Illustration reproduced from *NVMS Small Animal Surgery*, 1996, courtesy of Williams and Wilkins, Media, PA, USA.)

REFERENCES

1 Layton CE (1993) The role of lateral wall resection in managing chronic otitis externa. *Seminars in Veterinary Medicine and Surgery* **8**, 24–29.
2 Smeak DD and Kerpsack SJ (1993) Total ear canal ablation and lateral bulla osteotomy for management of end-stage otitis. *Seminars in Veterinary Medicine and Surgery* **8**, 30–41.
3 Fossum TW (1997) Surgery of the ear. In *Small Animal Surgery*. (ed TW Fossum) Mosby, St Louis, pp. 153–178
4 Lane JG and Watkins PE (1986) Para-aural sinus in the dog and cat. *Journal of Small Animal Practice* **27**, 521–531.
5 Hobson HP (1988) Surgical management of advanced ear disease. *Veterinary Clinics of North America* **18**, 821–844.
6 Little CJ and Lane JG (1989) An evaluation of tympanometry, otoscopy and palpation for assessment of the canine tympanic membrane. *Veterinary Record* **124**, 5–8.
7 Cole LK, Kwochka KW, Kowalski JJ and Hillier A (1998) Microbial flora and antimicrobial susceptibility patterns of isolated pathogens from the horizontal ear canal and middle ear in dogs with otitis media. *Journal of the American Veterinary Medical Association* **212**, 534–538.
8 Remedios AM, Fowler JD and Pharr JW (1991) A comparison of radiographic versus surgical diagnosis of otitis media. *Journal of the American Animal Hospital Association* **27**, 183–188.
9 Trower ND, Gregory SP, Renfrew H and Lamb CR (1998) Evaluation of the canine tympanic membrane by positive contrast ear canalography. *Veterinary Record* **142**, 78–81.
10 Penrod JP and Coulter DB (1980) The diagnostic use of impedance audiometry in the dog. *Journal of the American Animal Hospital Association* **16**, 941–948

11 Neer TM (1982) Otitis media. *Compendium on Continuing Education* **4**, 410–417.

12 Love NE and Kramer RW (1995) Radiographic and computed tomographic evaluation of otitis media in the dog. *Veterinary Radiography and Ultrasound* **36**, 375–379.

13 Grono LR (1970) Studies of the microclimate of the external auditory canal in the dog. III: Relative humidity within the external auditory meatus. *Research in Veterinary Science* **11**, 316–319.

14 Zepp CP (1949) Surgical technique to establish drainage of the external ear canal and corrections of hematoma of the dog and cat. *Journal of the American Veterinary Medical Association* **115**, 91–92.

15 Tufvesson G (1955) Operation for otitis externa in dogs according to Zepp's method. *American Journal of Veterinary Research* **16**, 565–570.

16 Sylvestre AM (1998) Potential factors affecting the outcome of dogs with a resection of the lateral wall of the vertical ear canal. *Canadian Veterinary Journal* **39**, 157–160.

17 Lane JG (1979) Canine aural surgery. *In Practice* **1**, 5–11.

18 Krahwinkle DJ (1993) External ear canal. In *Textbook of Small Animal Surgery*. 2nd edn. (ed D Slatter D) WB Saunders, Philadelphia, pp. 1561–1567.

19 Harari J (1996) Ear. In *Small Animal Surgery*. (ed J Harari) Williams and Wilkins, Baltimore, pp. 193–199.

20 Trevor PB and Martin RA (1993) Tympanic bulla osteotomy for treatment of middle ear disease in cats: 19 cases (1984–1991). *Journal of the American Veterinary Medical Association* **202**, 123–128.

21 Smeak DD (1998) Total ear canal ablation and lateral bulla osteotomy. In *Current Techniques in Small Animal Surgery*. 4th edn. (ed MJ Bojrab) Williams and Wilkins, Baltimore, pp. 102–109.

22 Krahwinkel DJ, Pardo AD, Sims MH and Bubb WJ (1989) Effect of ear ablation on auditory function as determined by brainstem auditory evoked response and subjective evaluation. *Veterinary Surgery* **18**, 60.

23 Lane JG and Little CJL (1986) Surgery of the canine external auditory meatus: a review of failures. *Journal of Small Animal Practice* **27**, 247–254.

24 Bradley RL (1988) Surgical management of otitis externa. *Veterinary Clinics of North America* **15**, 813–844.

25 Gregory CR and Vasseur PB (1983) Clinical results of lateral ear resection in dogs. *Journal of the American Veterinary Medical Association* **182**, 1087–1090.

26 McCarthy RJ and Caywood DD (1992) Vertical ear canal resection for end-stage otitis externa in dogs. *Journal of the American Animal Hospital Association* **28**, 546–552.

27 Pohlman DDL (1981) A modified surgical approach to chronic otitis externa. *Veterinary Medicine Small Animal Clinician* **76**, 334–335.

28 Tirgari M and Pinniger RS (1986) Pull-through technique for vertical canal ablation for treatment of otitis externa in dogs and cats. *Journal of Small Animal Practice* **27**, 123–131.

29 Elkins AD, Hedlund CS and Hobson HP (1981) Surgical management of ossified ear canals in the canine. *Veterinary Surgery* **10**, 163–168.

30 White RAS (1995) Total ear canal ablation in the dog and cat. *Waltham Focus* **5**, 23–28.

31 Smeak DD and de Hoff WD (1986) Total ear canal ablation: clinical results in the dog and cat. *Veterinary Surgery* **15**, 161–170.

32 Mason LK, Harvey CE and Orsher RJ (1988) Total ear canal ablation combined with lateral bulla osteotomy for end-stage otitis in dogs: results in 30 dogs. *Veterinary Surgery* **17**, 263–268.

33 Love NE, Kramer RW, Spodnick GJ and Thrall DE (1995) Radiographic and computed tomographic evaluation of otitis media in the dog. *Veterinary Radiology and Ultrasound* **36**, 375–379.

34 Sharp NJH (1990) Chronic otitis externa and otitis media treated by total ear canal ablation and ventral bulla osteotomy in 13 dogs. *Veterinary Surgery* **19**, 162–166.

35 Matthiesen DT and Scavelli T (1990) Total ear canal ablation and lateral bulla osteotomy in 38 dogs. *Journal of the American Animal Hospital Association* **26**, 257–267.

36 Payne JT, Shell LG, Flora RM, Martin RA and Shires PK (1989) Hearing loss in dogs subjected to total ear canal ablation. *Veterinary Surgery* **18**, 70.

37 Beckman SL, Henry WB and Cechner P (1990) Total ear canal ablation combining bulla osteotomy and curretage in dogs with chronic otitis externa and media. *Journal of the American Veterinary Medical Association* **196**, 84–90.

38 Devitt CM, Seim HB, Willer R, McPherron M and Neely M (1997) Passive drainage versus primary closure after total ear canal ablation/lateral bulla osteotomy in dogs: 59 dogs (1985–1995). *Veterinary Surgery* **26**, 210–216.

39 Holt D and Brockman DJ (1996) Lateral exploration of fistulas developing after total canal ablations: 10 cases (1989–1993). *Journal of the American Animal Hospital Association* **32**, 527–530.

40 Krahwinkel DJ, Pardo AD, Sims MH and Bubb WJ (1993) Effect of total ablation of the external acoustic meatus and bulla osteotomy on auditory function in dogs. *Journal of the American Veterinary Medical Association* **202**, 949–952.

41 Smeak DD, Crocker BS and Birchard SJ (1996) Treatment of recurrent otitis media that developed after total ear canal ablation and lateral bulla osteotomy in dogs: nine cases (1986–1994). *Journal of the American Veterinary Medical Association* **209**, 937–942.

42 Barrett RE and Rathfon BL (1975) Lateral approach to bulla osteotomy. *Journal of the American Animal Hospital Association* **11**, 203–205.

43 Boothe HW (1988) Surgical management of otitis media and otitis interna. *Veterinary Clinics of North America* **18**, 901–911.

44 Boothe HW (1998) Ventral bulla osteotomy: dog and cat. In *Current Techniques in Small Animal Surgery*. 4th edn. (ed MJ Bojrab) Williams and Wilkins, Baltimore, pp. 109–112.

45 Seim HB III (1993) Middle ear. In *Textbook of Small Animal Surgery*. 2nd edn. (ed D Slatter) WB Saunders, Philadelphia, pp. 1568–1576.

46 Denny HR (1973) The results of surgical treatment of otitis media and interna in the dog. *Journal of Small Animal Practice* **14**, 585–600.

47 McNutt GW and McCoy JH (1980) Bulla osteotomy in the dog. *Journal of the American Veterinary Medical Association* **77**, 617–628.

48 Ader PL and Boothe HW (1979) Ventral bulla osteotomy in the cat. *Journal of the American Animal Hospital Association* **15**, 757–762.

Chapter Twelve

Perioperative Analgesia and Management

INTRODUCTION

KEY POINTS
- Animals will be in considerable pain following ear surgery and they may have difficulty drinking and eating.
- Pain causes physiologic changes in the animal. It also distresses clinicians, nurses, and owners.
- Patient selection, surgical skill, optimal pain relief, good nursing, and appropriate antibacterial therapy all contribute to a rapid recovery.

Surgical intervention results in direct stimulation of nerve endings and the liberation of inflammatory mediators from damaged tissue. There are measurable physiologic changes following surgery[1, 2], mediated by the neuronal, physiologic, and endocrine changes which result in:
- Increased skeletal muscle tone.
- Inhibition of smooth muscle.
- Increased sympathetic tone.

These changes may predispose to metabolic acidosis, constipation and urinary retention, increased heart rate, increased blood pressure, increased metabolic rate, increased release of catecholamines,

Clinicians should consider pre- and postoperative analgesia, nutrition, and nursing to be as important as good surgical technique when contemplating aural surgery.

and a shift to a catabolic state. The animal may resent both movement and handling if pain results[3]. Appetite is reduced, inefficient metabolic pathways kick in, and a delayed return to good health ensues.

The consequence of these events is a vicious circle of pain, apprehension, and weight loss on the part of the animal and apprehension, concern, and even guilt on the part of the owner.

There are a number of aims for effective and successful postoperative nursing care:
- Minimize pain.
- Prevent postoperative infections and surgical complications arising from trauma to the wound.
- Minimize postoperative anorexia and dehydration.
- Ensure a rapid return to the owner.

PERI- AND POSTOPERATIVE ANALGESIA

Pre-emptive analgesia blocks afferent noxious stimuli from sensitizing the central nervous system during surgery and helps to prevent postoperative pain[2, 3, 4, 5, 6]. Furthermore, effective pre-emptive analgesia reduces the amount of postoperative analgesic required to control pain[3]. Pre-emptive analgesia even negates the benefit of supplementary local anesthetic application (splash block) around the surgical site[7].

With these facts in mind, an effective analgesic protocol for dogs undergoing drainage and suture of an aural hematoma, lateral wall resection, vertical canal ablation, and/or bulla osteotomy would be:
- Carprofen (4 mg/kg s/c) 90–120 minutes preoperatively.
- Buprenorphine (0.01–0.02 mg/kg i/m) 45 minutes preoperatively.
  OR butorphanol (0.3–0.6 mg/kg i/m) 20 minutes preoperatively
  OR morphine (0.3–0.6 mg/kg i/m) 20 minutes preoperatively.

OR pethidine (3–5 mg/kg i/m) 10 minutes preoperatively.
OR methadone (0.1–0.5 mg/kg i/m) 20 minutes preoperatively.
NB: Butorphanol should be repeated every 60 minutes during surgery.
All of these morphine-type agents may be repeated postoperatively, if necessary.
- Acepromazine (0.0625–0.125 mg/kg i/m or s/c) 20 minutes preoperatively.
- Carprofen (2 mg/kg s/c) postoperatively at 12 hours.
- Carprofen (2 mg/kg p/o q12h) for 4–7 days.

For feline patients undergoing major otic surgery the same protocol can be used, but generally only two doses of morphine are required (0.3–0.5 mg/kg), one dose preoperatively and then one dose either as required postoperatively or four hours later.

PERIOPERATIVE SYSTEMIC ANTIBACTERIAL THERAPY

Most otic cases which go forward to surgery will be classified as contaminated or dirty[8]. However, classifying a procedure as contaminated or dirty is not an excuse to forgo normal aseptic surgical procedures, i.e. minimizing tissue trauma and eliminating dead space. Nonetheless, some degree of wound contamination is likely and this, plus a degree of self-trauma, may result in postoperative problems. Reported studies of postoperative infection rates in dogs following otic surgery cite an incidence of between 0% and 41%[9-17] depending, among other things, on the type of surgery (*Table 17*). Postoperative infection in cats subjected to aural surgery appears much less of a problem[18-20].

Rational use of prophylactic antibacterial therapy dictates that the antibacterial agent is present in appropriate concentrations in the tissues before surgery begins, and that the antibacterial agent is effective against known and potential pathogens.

The most likely pathogens are *Staphylococcus intermedius*, *Escherichia coli*, *Proteus mirabilis*, and *Pseudomonas aeruginosa*. These bacteria are most likely to have been exposed to a variety of topical and systemic antibacterial agents and they will most probably express resistance to some of them. However, given that most otic surgery is elective there is plenty of opportunity for an up-to-date bacteriological culture and sensitivity. An appropriate agent should be chosen and the correct dose administered at least 24 hours before surgery. Deep, shielded samples should be taken during surgery in order to update the bacteriological susceptibility information; if indicated, a different agent can be used for postoperative treatment. The antibacterial treatment is continued until the wound is healing well, typically 3–4 weeks post surgery[21, 22, 23].

Table 17: Reported rates of postoperative wound dehiscence and postoperative infection in dogs.

Reference	Technique	Number of ears	% postoperative dehiscence	% infection
8	LWR	27	18.5	25.9
9	VCA	68	19	1
10	VCA	18	0	0
11	TECA/LBO	39	7.6	41
12	TECA/LBO	14	0	14.3
13	TECA/LBO	72	0	6.0
14	TECA/LBO	39	21	38
15	TECA/LBO	46	8.6	23.9
16	TECA/LBO	100	11	0

LWR = lateral wall resection

VCA = vertical canal ablation

TECA/LBO = total external canal ablation and lateral bulla osteotomy

POSTOPERATIVE DRESSINGS AND WOUND MANAGEMENT

Postoperative wound dehiscence occurs in between 1% and 21% of cases subjected to aural surgery involving the external ear canal (*Table 17*). Patient selection and surgical technique will influence this figure; however, wound dehiscence is most likely to reflect postoperative infection and/or self-trauma. Therefore, nursing as much as surgical skill plays a part in the degree of complications which may be experienced.

Animals which have been subjected to bulla osteotomy should be monitored for respiratory embarrassment, particularly after bilateral surgery when pharyngeal swelling may occur[23]. Postoperative respiratory distress reflects pharyngeal edema and will require anti-inflammatory medication and, possibly, more aggressive intervention.

Dogs which have had major ear surgery should have their ears dressed after surgery to prevent inadvertent removal of drains or sutures and trauma to the wound[22]. A 2.4–4.8 cm (0.9–1.9 in) piece of 0.8 cm (0.3 in) wide adhesive tape is placed on the concave surface, such that half the width can be reflected over onto the convex aspect[24]. The fold is continued along the length of the tape, even where it becomes free of the pinna. These extra lengths are passed over the head to anchor the pinna[24]. The pinna is reflected back over the head, with gauze sponges between the pinna and the head to prevent development of moist dermatitis[22]. A non-adhesive dressing is placed over the incision and the head is bandaged to include the pinna. The free pinna may poke through a 'window' (**403–407**). This double layer allows the top dressings to be removed to facilitate wound cleaning, without having to rebandage completely on every occasion[23].

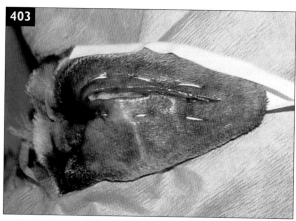

403 A piece of adhesive tape some 48 cm (19 in) long is affixed to the pinnal margin so that half adheres to the concave side and the other half is reflected to adhere to the convex aspect. The free portion of the tape is folded onto itself.

Bandages should be checked twice daily to ensure that they do not become soiled or damp[24]. Dressings should be gently freed from wounds on a daily basis to allow lavage with 1:40 chlorhexidine[2, 23]. If postoperative swelling is marked, a hot pack should be applied to the area several times daily.

If a passive or ingress/egress drain is placed, daily flushing is necessary until the discharge is minimal[14, 22]. It may prove difficult to flush a passive drain effectively, but an ingress/egress drain may be flushed through with sterile saline, dilute chlorhexidine (1:40), dilute povidone iodine (1:10), or modified EDTA-tris[21, 23] (*Table 18*).

Table 18: Formula for EDTA-tris.

- 1 liter distilled water
- 1.2 g EDTA
- 6.05 g tris
- 1 ml glacial acetic acid
- adjust pH to 8

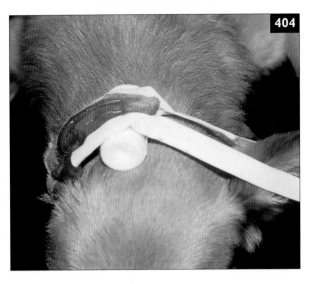

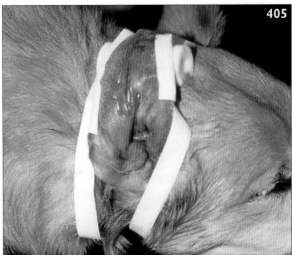

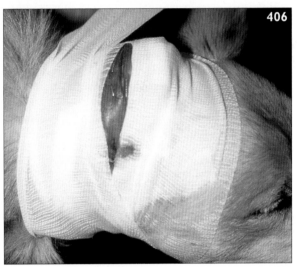

404   The pinna is reflected back over the head. A roll of bandage or gauze is placed between the pinna and the head.

405   The free ends of the tape are passed around the head, to secure the pinna.

406   The head is bandaged in such a way that the free pinna is allowed to 'poke through'. The wound remains visible and this allows dressing changes to be carried out without having to redress the ear completely.

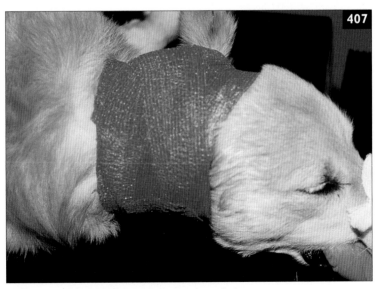

407   A final layer of protective dressing is applied.

POSTOPERATIVE NUTRITIONAL MANAGEMENT

After major surgery, such as total ablation or bulla osteotomy, the metabolic changes that take place can be summarized as follows:

- A relatively short hypometabolic ('shock') phase, which lasts a few hours to a day or so.
- A hypermetabolic, catabolic phase which can be subdivided into:
  - A catabolic phase. The hypermetabolism is maximal at around 110% of normal following elective surgery, usually about a week postoperatively[1]. Postoperative inflammation and wound repair is a glucose-dependent, glycolytic process which is relatively inefficient in energy terms. Thus, even modest surgery may result in a considerable glucose drain[1]. There may also be considerable protein catabolism and, if anorexia is prolonged, there may be postoperative weight loss as skeletal muscle and fat is broken down to provide for increased requirements at the site of surgery.
  - An anabolic convalescent phase characterized by a return of metabolism, weight, and lifestyle to normal.

The initial hypometabolic phase is not generally regarded as being amenable to nutritional management, but its duration may be minimized with attention to intravenous fluid therapy, analgesia, and provision of warmth. Preventing postoperative loss of body heat is important and this becomes more critical with small dogs and cats as they have minimal buffering capacity due to a low body mass. Intravenous fluids should be administered until normal drinking begins.

The subsequent catabolic phase is best met with an energy rich, high protein, highly digestible diet. Concentrated diets (such as Waltham Veterinary Diet: Whiskas or Pedigree Concentrated Instant Diet) are ideal since they provide an essential nutrient source with minimal volume. An animal which has undergone aural surgery might find eating painful, and thus the minimal volume of concentrated diets is helpful. Furthermore, the small volume and high digestibility of these diets reduces the risk of vomiting and diarrhea.

Careful nursing and effective analgesia are usually sufficient to return an animal to good health within a few days of surgery. Chemical stimulation of appetite should not be needed in most cases, although some cats may prove difficult to tempt back to eating. Intravenous diazepam (1–2 mg total dose) may be sufficient to initiate voluntary intake in cats, and this is then sustained[1].

REFERENCES

1 Butterwick RF and Torrance A (1995) Nutrition and malnutrition in the hospitalised small animal. *Waltham Focus* **5**, 15–21.

2 Lascelles BDX, Cripps PJ, Jones A and Waterman-Pearson AE (1997) Postoperative central hypersensitivity and pain: the pre-emptive value of pethidine for ovariohysterectomy. *Pain* **73**, 461–471.

3 Brock N (1995) Treating moderate and severe pain in small animals. *Canadian Veterinary Journal* **36**, 658–660.

4 Lascelles BDX, Cripps PJ, Jones A and Waterman-Pearson AE (1998) Efficacy and kinetics of carprofen, given pre-or postoperatively, for the prevention of pain in dogs undergoing ovariohysterectomy. *Veterinary Surgery* **27**, 568–582.

5 Welsh EM, Nolan AM and Reid J (1997) Beneficial effects of administering carprofen before surgery on dogs. *Veterinary Record* **141**, 251–253.

6 Lascelles BDX, Butterworth SJ and Waterman AE (1994) Postoperative analgesic and sedative effects of carprofen and pethidine in dogs. *Veterinary Record* **134**, 187–191.

7 Buback JL, Boothe HW, Carroll GL and Green RW (1996) Comparison of three methods for relief of pain after ear canal ablation in dogs. *Veterinary Surgery* **25**, 380–385.

8 Fossum TW (1997) Surgical infection and antibiotic selection. In *Small Animal Surgery*. (ed TW Fossum) Mosby, St Louis, pp. 57–63.

9 Gregory CR and Vasseur PB (1983) Clinical results of lateral ear resection in dogs. *Journal of the American Veterinary Medical Association* **182**, 1087–1090.

10 McCarthy RJ and Caywood DD (1992) Vertical ear canal resection for end-stage otitis externa in dogs. *Journal of the American Animal Hospital Association* **28**, 546–552.

11 Tirgari M and Pinniger RS (1986) Pull-through technique for vertical canal ablation for treatment of otitis externa in dogs and cats. *Journal of Small Animal Practice* **27**, 123–131.

12 Smeak DD and de Hoff WD (1986) Total ear canal ablation: clinical results in the dog and cat. *Veterinary Surgery* **15**, 161–170.

13 Sharp NJH (1990) Chronic otitis externa and otitis media treated by total ear canal ablation and ventral bulla osteotomy in thirteen dogs. *Veterinary Surgery* **19**, 162–166.

14 Beckman SL, Henry WB and Cechner P (1990) Total ear canal ablation combining bulla osteotomy and curretage in dogs with chronic otitis externa and media. *Journal of the American Veterinary Medical Association* **196**, 84–90.

15 Mason LK, Harvey CE and Orsher RJ (1988) Total ear canal ablation combined with lateral bulla osteotomy for end-stage otitis in dogs: results in 30 dogs. *Veterinary Surgery* **17**, 263–268.

16 Matthiesen DT and Scavelli T (1990) Total ear canal ablation and lateral bulla osteotomy in 38 dogs. *Journal of the American Animal Hospital Association* **26**, 257–267.

17 White RAS and Pomeroy CJ (1990) Total ear canal ablation and lateral bulla osteotomy (TECA/LBO) in the dog: indications, complications, and long-term results in 100 procedures. *Veterinary Surgery* **19**, 81.

18 Ader PL and Boothe HW (1979) Ventral bulla osteotomy in the cat. *Journal of the American Animal Hospital Association* **15**, 757–762.

19 Trevor PB and Martin RA (1993) Tympanic bulla osteotomy for treatment of middle-ear disease in cats: 19 cases (1984–1991). *Journal of the American Veterinary Medical Association* **202**, 123–128.

20 Pope ER (1995) Feline inflammatory polyps. *Seminars in Veterinary Medicine and Surgery* **10**, 87–93.

21 Fossum TW (1997) Surgery of the ear. In *Small Animal Surgery*. (ed TW Fossum) Mosby, St Louis, pp. 153–178.

22 Henderson JT and Radasch RM (1995) Total ear canal ablation with lateral bulla osteotomy for the management of end-stage otitis in dogs. *Compendium on Continuing Education* **17**, 157–164.

23 Smeak DD and Kerpsack SJ (1993) Total ear canal ablation and lateral bulla osteotomy for management of end-stage otitis. *Seminars in Veterinary Medicine and Surgery* **8**, 30–41.

24 Swaim SF and Henderson RA (1990) Wounds of the head. In *Small Animal Wound Management*. (eds SF Swaim and RA Henderson) Williams and Wilkins, Baltimore, pp. 191–233.

Index